Infections and Rheumatic Diseases

Guest Editor

LUIS R. ESPINOZA, MD

RHEUMATIC DISEASE CLINICS OF NORTH AMERICA

www.rheumatic.theclinics.com

February 2009 • Volume 35 • Number 1

SAUNDERS an imprint of ELSEVIER, Inc.

W.B. SAUNDERS COMPANY

A Division of Elsevier Inc.

1600 John F. Kennedy Blvd., Suite 1800 ● Philadelphia, PA 19103-2899

http://www.theclinics.com

RHEUMATIC DISEASE CLINICS OF NORTH AMERICA Volume 35, Number 1
February 2009 ISSN 0889-857X, ISBN 13: 978-1-4377-1271-1, ISBN 10: 1-4377-1271-1

Editor: Rachel Glover

Rheumatic Disease Clinics of North America (ISSN 0889-857X) is published quarterly by Elsevier Inc., 360 Park Avenue South, New York, NY 10010-1710. Months of issue are February, May, August, and November. Business and editorial offices: 1600 John F. Kennedy Boulevard, Suite 1800, Philadelphia, PA 19103-2899. Customer Service offices: 11830 Westline Industrial Drive, St. Louis, MO 63146. Periodicals postage paid at New York, NY and additional mailing offices. Subscription prices are USD 244.00 per year for US individuals, USD 414.00 per year for US institutions, USD 122.00 per year for US students and residents, USD 288.00 per year for Canadian individuals, USD 512.00 per year for Canadian institutions, USD 342.00 per year for international individuals, USD 512.00 per year for international institutions, and USD 171.00 per year for Canadian and foreign students/residents. To receive student/resident rate, orders must be accompanied by name of affiliated institution, date of term, and the *signature* of program/residency coordinator on institution letterhead. Orders will be billed at individual rate until proof of status received. Foreign air speed delivery is included in all *Clinics* subscription prices. All prices are subject to change without notice. **POSTMASTER:** Send address changes to *Rheumatic Disease Clinics of North America*, Elsevier Journals Customer Service, 11830 Westline Industrial Drive, St. Louis, MO 63146. **Customer Service: 1-800-654-2452 (US and Canada). From outside of the US and Canada: 314-453-7041. Fax: 314-453-5170. For print support, e-mail: JournalsCustomerService-usa@elsevier. com. For online support, e-mail: JournalsOnlineSupport-usa@elsevier.com.**

Reprints. For copies of 100 or more of articles in this publication, please contact the Commercial Reprints Department, Elsevier Inc., 360 Park Avenue South, New York, New York, 10010-1710; Tel.: (+1) 212-633-3813, Fax: (+1) 212-462-1935, and E-mail: reprints@elsevier.com.

Rheumatic Disease Clinics of North America is covered in *MEDLINE/PubMed (Index Medicus), Current Contents/Clinical Medicine, Science Citation Index, ISI/BIOMED,* and *EMBASE/Excerpta Medica.*

Printed and bound in the United States of America
Transferred to Digital Print 2011

Contributors

GUEST EDITOR

LUIS R. ESPINOZA, MD
Professor and Chief, Section of Rheumatology, Department of Internal Medicine, Louisiana State University Health Sciences Center, New Orleans, Louisiana

AUTHORS

EDUARDO ACEVEDO-VÁSQUEZ, MD, DR
Professor of Medicine, Universidad Nacional Mayor de San Marcos; and Department of Rheumatology, Guillermo Almenara Hospital, Lima, Peru

NOAH ALBERTS-GRILL, BA
PhD Student, Lowance Center for Human Immunology and Rheumatology, Emory University School of Medicine, Atlanta, Georgia

ALEJANDRO BALSA, MD, PhD
Associate Professor, Department of Rheumatology, Universitario La Paz, Madrid, Spain

DAN BUSKILA, MD
Professor, Division of Internal Medicine, Department of Medicine H, Soroka Medical Center, Faculty of Health Sciences, Ben Gurion University, Beer Sheva, Israel

PATRICE CACOUB, MD
Professor, Service de Médicine Interne, AP, HP Pitié-Salpetriè Hospital Group; and Université Pierre and Marie Curie, Paris, France

JOHN D. CARTER, MD
Associate Professor of Medicine, Department of Internal Medicine, Division of Rheumatology, University of South Florida, Tampa, Florida

INES COLMEGNA, MD
Post-Doctoral Research Fellow, Lowance Center for Human Immunology and Rheumatology, Emory University School of Medicine, Atlanta, Georgia

RAQUEL CUCHACOVICH, MD
Assistant Professor, Section of Rheumatology, Department of Internal Medicine, Louisiana State University Health Sciences Center, New Orleans, Louisiana

LUIS R. ESPINOZA, MD
Professor and Chief, Section of Rheumatology, Department of Internal Medicine, Louisiana State University Health Sciences Center, New Orleans, Louisiana

ROCÍO GAMBOA-CÁRDENAS, MD
Department of Rheumatology, Guillermo Almenara Hospital, Lima, Peru

IGNACIO GARCÍA-DE LA TORRE, MD
Head, Department of Rheumatology and Immunology, Hospital General de Occidente, Secretaría de Salud; and Professor of Immunology and Rheumatology, Centro Universitario de Ciencias de la Salud, Universidad de Guadalajara, Guadalajara, Jalisco, México

ABRAHAM GEDALIA, MD
Professor of Pediatrics and Head, Division of Pediatric Rheumatology, Department of Pediatrics, Louisiana State University Health Sciences Center, New Orleans, Louisiana

HERVÉ C. GÉRARD, PhD
Senior Research Scientist, Department of Immunology and Microbiology, Wayne State University School of Medicine, Detroit, Michigan

ALAN P. HUDSON, PhD
Professor, Department of Microbiology and Immunology, Wayne State University School of Medicine, Detroit, Michigan

EMILIO MARTIN-MOLA, MD, PhD
Associate Professor, Department of Rheumatology, Universitario La Paz, Madrid, Spain

ARNULFO NAVA-ZAVALA, MD, MSc
Department of Rheumatology and Immunology, Hospital General de Occidente, Secretaría de Salud; and Associated Researcher, Unidad de Investigacion en Epidemiología Clinica, UMAE, HE, CMO, IMSS, Guadalajara, Jalisco, México

NEEJ PATEL, BS
Research Student, Section of Rheumatology, Louisiana State University Health Sciences Center, New Orleans, Louisiana; Undergraduate Student, College of Arts and Sciences, University of Pennsylvania, Philadelphia, Pennsylvania

NIRUPA PATEL, MD
Clinical Assistant Professor of Medicine, Section of Rheumatology, Louisiana State University Health Sciences Center, New Orleans, Louisiana

DARÍO PONCE DE LEÓN, MD
Department of Internal Medicine, Guilllermo Almenara Hospital, Lima, Peru

FRANCISCO P. QUISMORIO, Jr., MD
Professor, Division of Rheumatology, Department of Internal Medicine, Keck School of Medicine, University of Southern California, Los Angeles, California

BENJAMIN TERRIER, MD
Service de Médicine Interne, AP, HP Pitié-Salpetriè Hospital Group; and Université Pierre and Marie Curie, Paris, France

KARINA D. TORRALBA, MD
Assistant Professor, Division of Rheumatology, Department of Internal Medicine, Keck School of Medicine, University of Southern California, Los Angeles, California

JUDITH A. WHITTUM-HUDSON, PhD
Professor, Department of Immunology and Microbiology, Wayne State University School of Medicine, Detroit, Michigan

Contents

> Severe and chronic inflammatory arthritis sometimes follows urogenital infection with Chlamydia trachomatis or gastrointestinal infection with enteric bacterial pathogens. A similar clinical entity can be elicited by the respiratory pathogen Chlamydophila (Chlamydia) pneumoniae. Arthritogenesis does not universally require viable enteric bacteria in the joint. In arthritis induced by either of the chlamydial species, organisms are viable and metabolically active in the synovium. They exist in a "persistent" state of infection. Conventional antibiotic treatment of patients with Chlamydia-induced arthritis is largely ineffective. The authors outline the current understanding of the molecular genetic and biologic aspects underlying bacterially-induced joint pathogenesis, available information regarding host-pathogen interaction at that site, and several directions for future study to inform development of more effective therapies.

> Reactive arthritis (ReA) is an inflammatory arthritis that arises after certain gastrointestinal or genitourinary infections, representing a classic interplay between host and environment. It belongs to the group of arthritidies known as the spondyloarthropathies. The classic syndrome is a triad of symptoms, including the urethra, conjunctiva, and synovium; however, the majority of patients do not present with this triad. Diagnostic criteria for ReA exist, but data suggest new criteria are needed. Epidemiologic and prospective studies have been difficult to perform because of over-reliance on the complete classic triad of symptoms and the different terms and eponyms used. Studies assessing various treatment strategies are ongoing.

> Soft tissue infections are common and potentially fatal conditions. Infections are a major cause of morbidity and mortality in patients who have rheumatic disease. Patients who have rheumatic diseases may be at increased risk for soft tissue infections because of various factors, including inherent immunologic defects, genetics, and use of immunomodulatory therapy, including biologic agents. Timely diagnosis and management with the institution of antibiotics with or without surgical intervention is imperative for effective resolution of infection. This article provides a review

of recent literature on the presentation and clinical course of infectious tenosynovitis, septic bursitis, pyomyositis, and necrotizing fasciitis, especially in relation to patients who have rheumatic disease.

Acute bacterial arthritis usually is caused by gonococcal or nongonococcal infection of the joints. Nongonococcal and gonococcal arthritis are the most potentially dangerous and destructive forms of acute arthritis. These bacterial infections of the joints are usually curable with treatment, but morbidity and mortality are still significant in patients who have underlying rheumatoid arthritis, patients who have prosthetic joints, elderly patients, and patients who have severe and multiple comorbidities. This article reviews the risk factors, pathogenesis, clinical manifestations, diagnosis, and treatment of nongonococcal and gonococcal arthritis.

Systemic lupus erythematosus (SLE) is an inflammatory and multisystemic autoimmune disorder characterized by an uncontrolled autoreactivity of B and T lymphocytes leading to the production of autoantibodies against self-directed antigens and tissue destruction. Environmental factors, such as infections, which are an important cause of morbidity and mortality, are potential triggers of the disease. This article discusses bacterial, viral, and opportunistic microorganism infections in SLE, and the role of immunosuppressive therapy and immunodeficiencies in the disease.

B19 infection–associated joint symptoms occur most frequently in adults, usually presenting as a self-limited, acute symmetric polyarthritis affecting the small joints of the hands, wrists, and knees. A small percentage of patients persist with chronic polyarthritis that mimics rheumatoid arthritis raising the question of whether B19 virus may have a role as a concomitant or precipitating factor in the pathogenesis of autoimmune conditions. Comprehensive and updated reviews address different aspects of human parvovirus infection. This article focuses on the evidence supporting the arthritogenic potential of the B19 virus and the proposed mechanisms that underlie it.

Hepatitis C virus (HCV) is an important causative agent of liver diseases. However, HCV infection is also associated with numerous hematologic, renal, dermatologic, rheumatic, and autoimmune disorders. These include arthralgia, arthritis, vasculitis, sicca syndrome, myalgia, and fibromyalgia. The purpose of this article is to review the prevalence and spectrum of rheumatic disorders and autoimmune phenomena in HCV-infected patients. It evaluates and current treatment options including nonsteroidal anti-inflammatory drugs, low-dose corticosteroids, hydroxychloroquine, methotrexate, penicillamine, combined antiviral therapy, cyclosporin A, anti–TNF-a agents, and rituximab. It concludes that larger, controlled studies are needed to establish further the treatment indications, efficacy, and safety of these agents.

This article focuses on autoimmune manifestations related to the hepatitis B virus (HBV). Although the HBV vaccination has resulted in the decline of the virus, approximately 400 million individuals are infected worldwide. Up to twenty percent of the afflicted may develop extrahepatic manifestations ranging from the severe polyarteritis nodosa to the many, varied, and less severe clinical and biologic forms. Currently, control of the viral infection is mainly based on the use of antiviral drugs (with the current availability of potent agents). Discussion of two hypotheses of the pathophysiology of the virus is followed by descriptions of the general, renal, rheumatologic, neurologic, skin, ophthalmologic, and hematologic manifestations.

In this article, the authors discuss the occurrence and prevalence of rheumatic syndromes before and after highly active antiretroviral therapy became the usual mode of treatment. The immunologic, environmental, and genetic factors behind the combination of HIV infection and rheumatic manifestation contribute to the complexity of these diseases. Miscellaneous case reports are discussed in relation to HIV infection. The authors conclude that geriatric care of HIV patients is on the horizon as more people have access to newer, more effective therapy and mortality is on the decline. Younger HIV patients will be committed to a lifetime of therapy to address bone disease and other chronic problems. In the future, newer agents may steer the clinical scenario in unforeseen directions.

New drug classes, biologics, have been developed over the past 10 years based on human or chimeric antibodies against cytokines or receptors with pivotal roles in the inflammatory pathways of immune-mediated inflammatory disease. Anti–tumor necrosis factor agents carry the largest infection risk of all the biologics, predisposing patients to mycobacterial infections. Patients receiving biologics are at higher risk for developing tuberculosis. New cases of tuberculosis or reactivation of latent tuberculosis infections may occur during the course of treatment, so a high level of vigilance is highly recommended.

Infection is a frequent complication in rheumatoid arthritis (RA) and other autoimmune diseases. Since 2000, the spectrum of therapeutic possibilities (ie, biologic agents) for treating RA has expanded rapidly and many safety reports of patients treated with these drugs have been published. In most studies, biologics are associated with an increased incidence of infections with the use of tumor necrosis factor antagonists. Reported risks for developing infection differ among studies. This article provides an overview of which studies the authors consider the most relevant.

RELATED INTEREST
Infectious Disease Clinics of North America
Volume 21, Issue 4 (December 2007)
Fever of Unknown Origin
Burke A. Cunha, MD, *Guest Editor*

THE CLINICS ARE NOW AVAILABLE ONLINE!

Access your subscription at:
www.theclinics.com

Preface

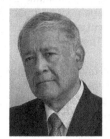

Luis R. Espinoza, MD
Guest Editor

Infection remains an important cause of morbidity and mortality in the general population and also affects the natural course, disease manifestations, progression, and clinical response to current therapeutic management of many musculoskeletal disorders. The latter issue merits particular attention, especially concerning the use of newer biologic agents in inflammatory joint disorders. Their significant clinical efficacy is associated with an increasing array of infectious complications by both routine and opportunistic pathogens. This issue of *Rheumatic Disease Clinics of North America* is devoted to exploring the interesting relationship between infections and the musculoskeletal system.

The opening article by Gérard and colleagues reviews the role of the molecular biology of infectious agents in chronic arthritis. Particular attention is given to the potential role of *Chlamydia trachomatis* as an etiologic agent of reactive arthritis. The next article by Carter and Hudson reviews important clinical aspects of reactive arthritis and discusses in detail the therapeutic management of this interesting clinical disorder, particularly the use of antibiotics.

Torralba and Quismorio subsequently provide an extensive and comprehensive overview of soft-tissue infections, with emphasis on common and uncommon infections, predisposing risk factors, and specific therapeutic management recommendations. García-De La Torre and Nava-Zavala then present a review of gonococcal and non-gonococcal arthritis with emphasis on predisposing risk factors, and the use of newer antibiotic agents in the management of septic arthritis.

The next article by Cuchacovich and Gedalia reviews the pathophysiology and clinical spectrum of infections in systemic lupus erythematosus—both in children and in adults. Infection remains an important cause of morbidity and mortality in lupus, and the authors provide an extensive and in-depth discussion of the underlying predisposing immunologic defects and other risk factors, as well as the common microorganisms involved.

The next four articles of this issue deal with the role of viral disorders in the etiology, disease manifestations, and clinical complications in patients who have musculoskeletal disorders. Therapeutic management is also discussed.

Rheum Dis Clin N Am 35 (2009) xi–xii
doi:10.1016/j.rdc.2009.05.001
0889-857X/09/$ – see front matter © 2009 Elsevier Inc. All rights reserved.

First, Colmegna and Alberts-Grill attempt to characterize the potential role of Parvovirus B19 in the etiology of chronic arthritis. A comprehensive review of the appropriate literature is included. Buskila then reviews the rheumatic manifestations associated with hepatitis C infection, as well as its therapeutic management. Cacoub and Terrier, based on their extensive experience, subsequently present an overview of the autoimmune clinical manifestations associated with hepatitis B. They also discuss the current therapeutic management recommendations.

The important role of HIV infection in the development of arthritis and autoimmune disorders is discussed next. Patel and colleagues present an up-to-date review of inflammatory musculoskeletal and autoimmune disorders triggered by infection with the human immunodeficiency virus seen prior to the advent of highly active antiretroviral therapy (HAART) and following its use. The changing clinical spectrum and development of newer clinical syndromes, such as the immune reconstitution syndrome, following the use of HAART in developing countries is reviewed.

The last two articles of this issue are devoted to the diagnosis and management of infectious complications directly related to the use of biologic agents in patients who have articular inflammatory disorders, especially rheumatoid arthritis. Acevedo-Vásquez and colleagues present an overview of latent infection and tuberculosis disease in patients who have rheumatoid arthritis, based on their original observations. Emphasis is placed on early recognition, current diagnostic procedures, and therapeutic management of this important infectious complication. The last article by Martin-Mola provides an in-depth discussion of the infectious complications associated with the use of biologic agents, especially tumor necrosis factor-alpha inhibitors. This is of great clinical relevance and importance in view of the increasing use of these agents in the management of patients who have rheumatoid arthritis and other arthritides.

This issue of *Rheumatic Disease Clinics of North America* attempts to discuss the major advances in the field and represents the concerted effort of experienced investigators. I am most grateful to Rachel Glover, editor at Elsevier, for her confidence and support in the preparation of this issue.

Luis R. Espinoza, MD
Section of Rheumatology
Department of Internal Medicine
Louisiana State University Health Sciences Center
2020 Gravier Street
New Orleans, LA 70112-2822 USA

E-mail address:
luisrolan@msn.com (L.R. Espinoza)

Molecular Biology of Infectious Agents in Chronic Arthritis

Hervé C. Gérard, PhD[a], Judith A. Whittum-Hudson, PhD[a],
John D. Carter, MD[b], Alan P. Hudson, PhD[a],*

KEYWORDS

- Reactive arthritis • Bacterial infection • Pathogenesis
- *Chlamydia* • Persistent infection

The first report in the modern literature to describe inflammatory arthritis following an episode of bacterially induced dysentery was published in 1916, although physicians had noticed the phenomenon in the early 19th century, the 18th century, and even before[1,2] (see article by Carter and Hudson in this issue for further discussion of this topic). Since that 1916 report, several bacterial species known to be responsible for gastrointestinal diseases have been associated firmly with development of Reiter syndrome, now known more generally as reactive arthritis.[3] Studies over the last three decades have demonstrated that urogenital infection with the obligate intracellular eubacterial pathogen *Chlamydia trachomatis*, and more recently with the related respiratory pathogen *Chlamydophila (Chlamydia) pneumoniae*, can elicit an inflammatory joint disease with characteristics similar to the arthritis caused by infection with the various gastrointestinal pathogens.[4–7] Detailed understanding of the mechanisms of pathogenesis used by all the relevant bacterial pathogens to elicit the inflammation that characterizes the arthritis has increased significantly over the last two decades; however, many aspects of disease genesis and maintenance remain to be elucidated. For example, the incidence of new cases of acute bacterially-induced reactive arthritis is in the range of a few percent of those infected with any of the bacterial species at issue, and only about half of those individuals who develop the acute disease will progress to chronicity.[2–5] The overall number of people who develop an infection

This work was supported by grants AR-42541 (APH), AR-47186 (HCG), AR-48331 (JAW-H), and AR-53646 (JDC) from the US National Institutes of Health. APH has also been supported in part by grants from the Department of Veterans Affairs Medical Research Service.

[a] Department of Immunology and Microbiology, Wayne State University School of Medicine, 540 East Canfield Avenue, Detroit, MI 48201, USA

[b] Department of Internal Medicine, Division of Rheumatology, University of South Florida College of Medicine, 12901 Bruce B. Downs Blvd., Tampa, FL 33612, USA

* Corresponding author.

E-mail address: ahudson@med.wayne.edu (A.P. Hudson).

with *Salmonella* or other relevant gastrointestinal pathogens is large, of course, as is the incidence and prevalence of genital infections with *C trachomatis*. Infection with *C pneumoniae* is virtually ubiquitous in all geographic regions examined to date.[8] However, it is not understood why only a small proportion of patients who develop a gastrointestinal or chlamydial infection develop the arthritis initially, and why only a portion of those individuals go on to chronic disease. Whereas it is the case that the clinical characteristics of inflammatory arthritis elicited by any of the gastrointestinal pathogens or by the two chlamydial species are similar, many studies indicate that the biochemical and molecular biologic or molecular genetic attributes of chlamydiae in the synovium differ profoundly from those of the gut pathogens in the same context. Thus, it is not at all clear what underlies the generation of a consistent suite of clinical attributes by bacterial pathogens that interact with the host in different manners. In this article, the authors review what is known or strongly suspected concerning the molecular biology of the organisms that elicit reactive arthritis, with emphasis on *C trachomatis* and *C pneumoniae*, and discuss the means by which those detailed characteristics engender inflammatory joint disease. Based on that understanding, directions for further research that should point the way toward new and effective therapies to treat this form of arthritis are suggested.

EPIDEMIOLOGY AND DISEASE CHARACTERISTICS

Detailed discussion of the clinical characteristics of reactive arthritis induced by gastrointestinal pathogens and by chlamydiae, and discussion of management and therapy of patients with the disease, will be found in another article in this issue. It will be useful, though, to include a brief summary of those and other disease aspects to provide a context for what follows. Current criteria specified by the American College of Rheumatology (ACR) for diagnosis of reactive arthritis require documented prior urogenital infection with *C trachomatis* or gastrointestinal infection with any of several enteric bacterial species, including those from the genera *Yersinia*, *Salmonella*, *Campylobacter*, *Shigella*, and others.[3,9–11] Infection with *C pneumoniae* is not indicated as a causative agent in the official ACR diagnostic criteria (see below). The acute clinical picture of the articular syndrome (ie, the inflammatory response characteristic of the disease) is similar regardless of specific infecting organism. Largely because of its generally high prevalence in the population, *C trachomatis* has emerged as a major causative agent in reactive arthritis. In earlier studies, 50% to 80% of all patients with reactive arthritis were positive in polymerase chain reaction (PCR)-based assays for chromosomal DNA from that organism.[12] Other studies have identified a somewhat different prevalence of *C trachomatis* compared with those of the ACR-specified enteric organisms.[2,13]

Classic reactive arthritis includes a mono- or oligoarthritis that most often involves joints of the lower extremities and includes enthesitis.[9–11] Approximately half of all patients with the disease suffer significant lower back pain. Reactive arthritis is associated with inflammatory changes such as increased leukocyte counts in joint effusions and inflammation of the synovium. In many cases, episodes of active arthritis last weeks to months but finally result in remission. Approximately half of patients who develop acute reactive arthritis progress to chronicity and, in these patients, the disease frequently assumes a relapsing-remitting phenotype, often without evidence of reinfection by the associated or other officially specified organisms. Patients with reactive arthritis often have extra-articular features, including iritis, uveitis, cervicitis, and several types of dermatitis, but most clinicians agree that these additional features are not intrinsic to diagnosis.[9–11,14,15] The general spectrum of reactive arthritis is probably significantly larger than that suggested by the strict official definition above. For example, up to 80% of patients seen in an early arthritis clinic had unexplained oligoarthritis, and occasionally polyarthritis, that closely resembled classic reactive arthritis, but no documented history of antecedent infection.[10] Currently, such patients are given a diagnosis of undifferentiated oligo- or polyarthritis.[16,17] Moreover, published[18] and unpublished data (Gérard, Carter, Hudson, and colleagues) indicate that a significant portion of patients diagnosed with undifferentiated inflammatory arthritis are PCR-positive for DNA from C trachomatis.

REACTIVE ARTHRITIS INDUCED BY GASTROINTESTINAL PATHOGENS

Reactive arthritis can follow infection by any of several species of gram-negative enteric pathogens, including those subsumed under the genera Yersinia, Campylobacter, Shigella, Salmonella, and others. Arthritis attributed to Klebsiella spp, E coli, and other normal gut bacterial species is rarer, as is synovial disease subsequent to infections with Neisseria gonorrhea, various Mycoplasma spp, Ureaplasma urealyticum, and others.[2,14,19] The official ACR clinical definition of reactive arthritis describes it as a sterile seronegative inflammatory disease.[11] This seems to be the case for synovial disease due to gastrointestinal infections with the canonical enteric species mentioned or others. With the possible exceptions of Yersinia and Shigella, available data indicate that the generation of synovial inflammation following infection with any of the relevant enteric pathogens does not involve metabolically active, or even viable, organisms in the joint.[2,20,21] It only requires that bacterial antigens reach the joint to induce the immunopathogenic response. Precisely how those antigens get to the joint, and the detailed mechanisms by which they engender inflammation, remain to be fully elucidated, although several interesting and plausible mechanisms have been proposed.[22]

It is clear that C trachomatis and C pneumoniae are not only viable when they reach the joint from their sites of primary infection; they remain viable and metabolically active throughout the duration of their synovial residence. However, these organisms infect the joint in an unusual biologic state designated "persistence." In contrast to the other canonical enteric pathogens that have been firmly associated with elicitation of reactive arthritis, some evidence suggests that Yersinia may also undergo some sort of persistent infection of the synovium. Specifically, Yersinia chromosomal DNA has been identified by PCR assay in synovial materials from at least a few patients with postenteric reactive arthritis, as has DNA from Shigella.[20,23,24] It is not clear whether these organisms are viable in the synovium, and if so whether they are transcriptionally and translationally active at that site. More study is required to assess this issue, because the molecular genetic or molecular biologic details of synovial infection by Yersinia may suggest strategies to treat or cure the resulting inflammatory arthritis.

Several studies have examined the incidence and prevalence of postenteric reactive arthritis, and many of these studies are from Scandinavian sources.[25-27] These generally have found the incidence to fall around the standard level of a few percent of those having diagnosed infections with the various bacterial pathogens. In some reports, species of particular bacterial genera were examined in terms of arthritigenic potential. In one report, S sonnei was identified as the predominant species of Shigella to elicit reactive arthritis.[25] Because Campylobacter has become the single most common bacterial infection to cause enteritis in developed nations, reactive arthritis due to this organism probably is now, and for the foreseeable future will remain, the primary causative agent for postenteric inflammatory joint disease.[28]

CHLAMYDIAL BIOLOGY

Nine species are currently recognized in the order *Chlamydiales*. All species are obligate intracellular parasites of eukaryotic cells, and all are pathogenic to their various hosts. *C trachomatis* is the etiologic agent for trachoma, a disease that remains the leading cause of preventable or treatable blindness worldwide.[29] This organism also is the most prevalent sexually-transmitted bacterial pathogen in the United States and other developed nations. *C pneumoniae* is a respiratory pathogen[30] and is an important etiologic agent in acute respiratory infections, including community-acquired pneumonia, sinusitis, and bronchiti.[31] Other chlamydial species are animal pathogens and are not relevant here.

According to standard microbiological description, all chlamydial species undergo a biphasic developmental cycle.[32] In the first phase, the infectious extracellular form of the organism, the elementary body, locates and attaches to an appropriate eukaryotic host cell. These latter are usually epithelial, or epithelia-like, cells, but many other cell types can be infected. The authors recently identified the low-density lipoprotein receptor family as the primary, but not exclusive, receptors to which chlamydiae attach on host cells. Following attachment, the elementary body is brought into a membrane-bound cytoplasmic inclusion, within which it reorganizes into the metabolically active form, the reticulate body. These latter undergo several rounds of cell division, at the termination of which most dividing reticulate bodies reorganize back to the elementary body form. The newly formed elementary bodies are released from the host cell by way of lysis or exocytosis to propagate infection further. This standard view of the developmental cycle was derived primarily from in vitro studies using infected host cell types that permit active chlamydial growth by way of complete passage through the developmental cycle. *C trachomatis* infecting HeLa or HEp-2 cells requires approximately 48 hours to complete the developmental cycle; *C pneumoniae* requires approximately 72 hours for that passage through the same cell types. It is clear, from results published by the authors and others, that under some circumstances or within certain host cell types, *C trachomatis* and *C pneumoniae* can alter their biologic state to generate persistent infections. Many studies indicate that it is in this persistent state that these organisms engender acute and chronic reactive arthritis.[29,33]

INITIAL STUDIES OF *CHLAMYDIA*-INDUCED ARTHRITIS

Early studies relating genital infection by *C trachomatis* with subsequent development of inflammatory arthritis were primarily correlational in nature. For example, one electron microscopic study of patients with early reactive arthritis provided evidence for *Chlamydia* in synovial mononuclear cells;[34] another report demonstrated elementary and reticulate bodies within synovial macrophages, also in a patient diagnosed with reactive arthritis.[35] A group in the UK identified elementary bodies in synovial tissue or synovial fluid of patients; none of the control patients gave evidence of the organism.[36,37] Light and electron microscopic research using synovial materials located objects that resembled chlamydiae in 75% of individuals early in the disease process.[38] The observation was confirmed in some samples by use of anti-*Chlamydia* antibodies. Culture of *C trachomatis* from relevant synovial samples has been problematic, although the reasons for this difficulty are now largely understood. Early studies reported culture of the organism from synovial tissue or fluid from of several individuals with reactive arthritis, while all samples from controls were negative;[39,40] another report also indicated successful culture of the organism from synovial fluid or tissue from a few patients with reactive arthritis.[41] Other workers reported isolation of the organism from several reactive arthritis patients but warned that contamination must be considered.[42,43] Most groups that have attempted culture of *C trachomatis* from synovial samples have failed in the attempt.[37,44] Thus, while microscopic studies had identified what appeared to be intact *Chlamydia* or antigens from the organism in synovial samples from patients with documented prior infection with the organism, most attempts to show viability of the bacteria via culture have not been successful. These negative culture results for *C trachomatis* from synovial materials engendered the current ACR definition of reactive arthritis, including the *Chlamydia*-induced disease, as a sterile inflammatory process of the synovium. It is now clear that synovial chlamydiae are viable and metabolically active; and the reason for the culture-negativity of synovial samples for this organism is understood. The ACR definition, however, has not been modified regarding *Chlamydia*-associated arthritis.

DISSEMINATION OF CHLAMYDIAE, SYNOVIAL HOST CELLS IN REACTIVE ARTHRITIS

Whereas *Campylobacter* is the most common cause of bacterial enteritis, *C trachomatis* is by far the most prevalent sexually-transmitted bacterial pathogen in the United States and in most other developed nations.[45] Recent data from the Centers for Disease Control and Prevention indicate more than 3 million new cases are reported each year, with a stable population of *Chlamydia*-infected individuals in excess of 6 million.[45] *C trachomatis* and *C pneumoniae* have been detected in synovial tissues by PCR and other means.[46–50] Inbred mice exhibited metabolically active, viable organism in the joint following either ocular or genital infection with ocular and genital serovars of *C trachomatis* (C and K serovars, respectively).[51] Studies in animal models of *C pneumoniae*-induced atherogenesis have demonstrated dissemination of the organism in macrophages to distant sites following intranasal or intraperitoneal infection. Unfortunately, synovial materials were not examined in most of these studies.[52] Regardless, the ability to disseminate clearly is not limiting for either chlamydial species at issue, nor is that ability constrained to any specific initial infection site or any host species. The synovium is a favored and stable end-point residence for disseminated chlamydiae.

Chlamydiae of all species are mucosal pathogens, and their primary target host cell type during initial infection is epithelial or epithelial-like cells.[32] However, *C trachomatis* and *C pneumoniae* have been shown to infect many other cell types, including vascular endothelial cells, smooth muscle cells, monocytic cells, and others.[53,54] Electron microscopic studies of synovial tissue from patients with *Chlamydia*-induced inflammatory arthritis indicated that the primary, although probably not the sole, host cell type for *C trachomatis* in the joint is the monocyte/macrophage.[38,55] This observation is consistent with those from other groups demonstrating that the vehicle of dissemination for chlamydiae from their primary site of infection is the monocytic cell.[52] Chlamydiae presumably reach the joint by way of extravasated infected monocytic cells originating at the site of initial infection. As mentioned, the joint is a site of stable long-term residence for disseminated chlamydiae. However, the reasons underlying homing of the organism to the synovium are not understood; and the basis for that long-term stability of residence is not known. These are areas that merit a significant research effort, because obviation of long-term residence of chlamydiae in the joint should eliminate the chronic form of the arthritis, and subverting homing of the organism to the joint could prevent the acute and chronic forms of the disease.

CHLAMYDOPHILA PNEUMONIA IN THE JOINT

While enteric pathogens and *C trachomatis* have long been associated with genesis of reactive arthritis, many groups have reported DNA from *C pneumoniae* in synovial tissues from a small but significant number of patients with various arthritides.[49,56,57] PCR-based screening showed that about 13% of synovial biopsies from nearly 200 patients with various arthritides were positive for *C pneumoniae* DNA.[50] No samples from control individuals were positive in parallel assays. Reverse transcription-PCR (RT-PCR) assays targeting primary transcripts from the ribosomal RNA operons of the organism, along with other methods, indicated that *C pneumoniae* is viable and metabolically active in joint materials from such patients.[58] Similar assays earlier had documented that *C trachomatis* was metabolically active during its synovial tenure.[59] It is well documented that *C pneumoniae* can induce a powerful inflammatory response at sites of its residence.[60,61] Most physicians now accept that this organism can elicit an inflammatory arthritis similar to that engendered by *C trachomatis*. Unlike the case for *C trachomatis*-induced arthritis, a clear and consistent pattern of extra-articular clinical features was difficult to specify in patients PCR-positive for *C pneumoniae* in synovial materials.[50] Patients with inflammatory arthritis due to *C pneumoniae* have a far higher prevalence of the ε4 allele type at the *APOE* locus on chromosome 19 than does the general population,[62] and this is a direct result of the enhancement of attachment of *C pneumoniae* to its host cells in individuals that express this allele type.[63] Epidemiologic data indicate that infection with *C pneumoniae* is virtually ubiquitous in adult populations studied to date.[8] An interesting and important question, therefore, is why the overall prevalence of this organism in synovial tissue is so much lower than that of *C trachomatis* in patients with inflammatory arthritis. It may be the case that the immune system can clear *C pneumoniae* from the joint more efficiently than it does *C trachomatis*. Alternatively, the former organism may be less likely to reach the joint, or if it does reach that site, it may be less likely to remain there to elicit inflammation than *C trachomatis*. These are significant issues for future research.

CHLAMYDIAL PERSISTENCE

Under some circumstances, including those relevant to synovial infections, the chlamydial developmental cycle can be arrested, obviating production and release of new elementary bodies. This state of arrested development under certain growth conditions or within certain host cell types has been designated "persistence."[33] The arrest in the cycle which engenders this state is transcriptionally governed. Much of the initial study of chlamydial persistence was done by the Byrne laboratory, based on studies of *C trachomatis* infection of HeLa cells treated first with penicillin, later with low levels of interferon-γ (IFN-γ).[64,65] In those studies, *Chlamydia*-infected cultures so treated contained reticulate body-like forms displaying aberrant morphology; supernatants from treated cultures contained no, or extremely low levels of, new infectious elementary bodies.[64,66] The Byrne group also showed that aberrant chlamydial forms accumulate replicated or segregated copies of the bacterial chromosome in the absence of cell division. Removing IFNγ from the medium releases *Chlamydia* from the block in completion of the cycle, resulting in return to normal morphology and elementary body production.[64–66] A similar effect on aberrant chlamydial forms was reported after amino acid deprivation or antibiotic treatment (**Fig. 1**).[67,68]

Studies on synovial tissues from patients with *Chlamydia*-induced reactive arthritis indicated that the primary synovial host cell for *C trachomatis* is the monocyte/macrophage.[69,70] These, plus electron- and immunoelectron-microscopic studies, identified only aberrant, intracellular chlamydial forms similar to those described by the Byrne group in their IFNγ-related studies, in those tissue preparations.[38,70] Combined with

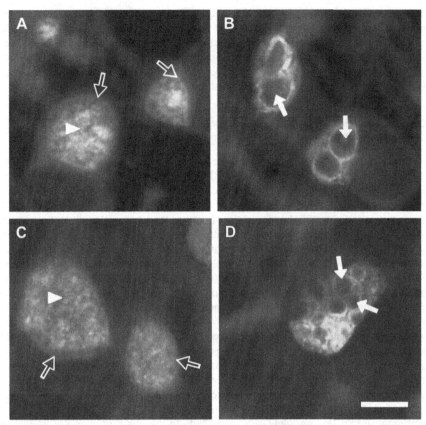

Fig. 1. *Chlamydia trachomatis* infected HEp-2 cells. Acutely (*A, C*) and persistently (*B, D*) infected cells are shown after fixation at 36 or 48 hours postinfection. Cells were stained with Pathfinder FITC-labeled anti-chlamydial LPS antibody (Bio-Rad, Woodinville, Washington). Persistent infection was induced by exposure to Penicillin G (PenG) beginning at 12 hrs (*B,* T12) or at 24 hrs (*D,* T24) after infection. Open arrows indicate normal reticulate bodies; solid arrows in B and D indicate aberrant reticulate bodies induced by PenG addition. Arrowheads indicate elementary bodies in the center of the inclusions in A and C. Bar = 10 μm. (Original magnification for all images ×40. Images collected by B. Hanson.)

the culture negativity of synovial tissue for *C trachomatis*, these data indicated that *Chlamydia*-induced inflammatory arthritis involves persistent, rather than actively-growing, organisms in the synovium. If *Chlamydia*-induced arthritis involves organisms in the persistent state, then understanding of the critical details underlying joint pathogenesis must be derived from knowledge of the molecular and biochemical behavior of the organism in that state, and how that behavior influences, and is influenced by, host processes.

Several in vitro model systems have been developed for study of chlamydial persistence. The system most closely resembling the in vivo realities of the infected joint involves use of normal human monocytic cells in culture infected at low multiplicity with chlamydial elementary bodies. Space does not permit discussion of development of this model, but that information is available.[53,71–73] Control studies with this model system showed that neither the donor source of monocytes nor the specific chlamydial strain or serovar matters in terms of the characteristics of chlamydial persistence. To date all data indicate that persistence of *C trachomatis* in human peripheral monocytic cells is a function of host cell type rather than of any specific aspect of host genetic background. Much of our current understanding of the molecular biologic or molecular genetic characteristics of chlamydial persistence, as a biologic phenomenon and in relation to synovial pathogenesis in reactive arthritis have been derived from study of this in vitro system.

MOLECULAR BIOLOGY AND GENETICS OF CHLAMYDIAL PERSISTENCE IN INFLAMMATORY ARTHRITIS

Transcriptional analyses of persistent *C trachomatis* in the in vitro monocyte model, and in synovial samples from patients with *Chlamydia*-induced arthritis, have revealed unusual biochemical and molecular genetic characteristics that distinguish this state from that characterizing normal passage through the developmental cycle. PCR-based studies indicated that synovial tissue, rather than synovial fluid, is the primary site of residence for the organism in chronic *Chlamydia*-induced arthritis.[48] Additionally, RT-PCR analyses targeting primary transcripts from the bacterial ribosomal RNA operons, and various short-lived chlamydial messengers, indicated that persistently-infecting *C trachomatis* cells are viable and metabolically active in the monocyte model system and in relevant synovial biopsy samples.[59,73] This was also shown for synovial *C pneumoniae*.[58] However, in each context the organisms show a highly unusual profile of gene expression. Early studies showed that during persistent infection either in vitro in human monocytic cells or in vivo in the joint, *C trachomatis* attenuates the expression of *omp1*, the gene encoding the chlamydial major outer membrane protein.[59] This explains the observed negativity of many synovial tissue samples from patients with *Chlamydia*-associated arthritis in standard direct fluorescence antibody analyses, because the monoclonal antibody used in those assays targets an epitope on that protein. Highly attenuated production of the major outer membrane protein also certainly must contribute to the aberrant shape of persistent chlamydiae.

Many transcriptional differences have now been reported between actively growing and persistent *C trachomatis* cells (**Table 1**). For example, genes encoding products involved in DNA replication and partition (*dnaA, polA, minD,* and *mutS*) are expressed during active growth and persistence, but transcription of genes whose products are required for the subsequent cytokinesis process (*ftsK* and *ftsW*) is severely attenuated during the latter state in the in vitro model of chlamydial persistence and in synovial tissue samples from patients with chronic *Chlamydia*-associated arthritis.[74] Again, this attenuation of expression from genes encoding products required for cytokinesis also has been demonstrated for persistently-infecting *C pneumoniae*.[75] These observations provide an explanation for the lack of new elementary body production by persistently-infecting chlamydiae in the in vitro model system and in vivo in the synovium, because the developmental cycle of the organism is arrested at the point of cell division. This lack of new infectious organism explains the culture negativity of synovial materials from individuals with *Chlamydia*-induced arthritis. Further, the results are consistent with an earlier observation that persistent *C trachomatis* cells accumulate fully replicated and segregated copies of the bacterial chromosome but do not undergo the cell division required for terminal elementary body production.[66]

The *C trachomatis* chromosome encodes enzymes for the glycolytic and pentose phosphate pathways, providing a means for the organism to produce its own ATP.[76] The several chlamydial genes encoding enzymes for these pathways are

Table 1
Selected *Chlamydia trachomatis* genes transcriptionally affected during persistent infection

Gene	Function	Transcriptional Effect	Reference
omp1	Major outer membrane protein	Severely down-regulated	59,73
ftsK	Protein required for cytokinesis	Severely down-regulated	74
ftsw	Protein required for cytokinesis	Severely down-regulated	74
pyk	Pyruvate kinase	Severely down-regulated	78
gap	Glyceraldehyde-3-phosphate dehydrogenase	Severely down-regulated	78
tal	Transaldolase	Severely down-regulated	78
cydB	Cytochrome oxidase subunit	Severely down-regulated	78
groEL	Heat shock protein 60 (authentic)	Attenuated	83
ct604	Hsp60 paralog	Strongly up-regulated	83
ct755	Hsp60 paralog	Severely down-regulated	83
zntA/cadA	Cation-transporting ATPase	Strongly up-regulated	92
proS	Proline tRNA synthetase	Strongly up-regulated	92
fabG	3-oxyacyl reductase	Up-regulated	92
ct868	Unknown protein	Down-regulated	92

As assessed by RT-PCR or real time RT-PCR in normal human monocytic cells in culture, infected with *C trachomatis* serovar K.[53,73]

expressed during active growth, and the translation products from those messengers are functional.[77] In *C trachomatis*-infected human monocytes in culture, expression of glycolysis and pentose phosphate pathway genes terminates by 3 days postinfection, the time at which the organism has transited to the persistent state. In contrast, *adt1*, a gene encoding an important ATP-ADP exchange protein, is expressed continuously and at high level during active and persistent infection. Assays targeting chlamydial transcripts encoding glycolytic and pentose phosphate pathway enzymes in synovial tissues from patients with *Chlamydia*-induced arthritis reflected those of the monocyte model.[78] Thus, *C trachomatis* is partly an energy parasite on its host in active infection, but it is reliant on its host cell for ATP during persistence. Further, *C trachomatis* shows a metabolic rate one to two orders of magnitude lower than that in infected HEp-2 cells at the same times postinfection.[78] Such a severe attenuation of metabolic rate also may contribute importantly to the lack of response to antibiotic treatment seen in patients with *Chlamydia*-induced arthritis.[79]

The *C trachomatis* and *C pneumoniae* genomes each specify three hsp60 protein-encoding genes.[76,80] In the former, the authentic hsp60 gene, *groEL*, is designated Ct110 in the genome sequence, and the two additional paralogs are designated Ct604 and Ct755. The *groEL* hsp60 protein is believed to be important in synovial pathogenesis.[81,82] Each of the three *C trachomatis* hsp60 genes is transcribed independently during active and persistent infection in in vitro models of these two states.[83] In actively-infected cells, Ct604 and Ct755 are expressed at higher level than is *groEL* (Ct110). Expression of the latter gene and Ct755 is attenuated during persistence in the monocyte model, whereas transcript levels from Ct604 are increased significantly in this state, suggesting that the product of Ct604 functions to engender or maintain persistence. The Ct755 gene product functions only during active chlamydial infection and may be a negative modulator of entry into the persistent state. Analyses of synovial biopsy samples from patients with *Chlamydia*-induced arthritis showed high mRNA levels from Ct604 and extremely low levels from Ct755, as in the monocyte model. However, transcript levels from the *groEL* gene were high in patient samples.[83] A recent study from this laboratory has demonstrated that some of the transcriptional and other details that characterize persistent *C pneumoniae* are not fully congruent with those that characterize *C trachomatis*. That study also showed that some molecular genetic aspects of chlamydial persistence in vitro are strongly dependent on the culture model system employed for the study.[84] How this reflects the situation in the synovium remains to be established fully.

The chlamydial *hrcA* gene product acts as a repressor at the CIRCE element upstream of *groELS*.[85] Real time RT-PCR experiments indicate that the noncongruity for expression of *groEL* between the in vitro persistence model and patient materials is a function of differential expression of the chlamydial *hrcA* gene in those two contexts. For example, in the model where *groEL* transcript levels are low, *hrcA* is highly expressed while in patient samples where *groEL* is expressed at high level, *hrcA* expression is attenuated (Gérard and Hudson, unpublished observations, 2005). Neither Ct604 nor Ct755 have this control element in their 5′ noncoding regions. The genome sequencing project identified three genes encoding σ factors on the *C trachomatis* chromosome, and these genes have been shown to be somewhat differentially expressed during the normal, active developmental cycle of the organism.[76,86] Chlamydiae must have some mechanism by which they govern the differential transcription of selected genes in persistent versus active infection summarized here. However, studies from several groups have indicated that differential expression of one or more σ factor-encoding genes does not fulfill this role. Research must be done in this area.

In the authors' view, *Chlamydia*-induced synovial pathogenesis probably is not a simple or straightforward function of the biology of chlamydial persistence alone. Critical aspects of that pathogenesis process must be a function of modification by other, uninfected neighboring synovial cells of the monocytic host cell-pathogen interactions that generate and maintain the persistent infection state. The challenge is to define the means by which readjustment in chlamydial gene expression is accomplished in response to input from its host monocyte and from uninfected neighboring cells, and how the alteration in chlamydial biochemistry and physiology elicits disease.

OTHER MOLECULAR GENETIC STUDIES CONCERNING CHLAMYDIAL PERSISTENCE

Pathogens other than chlamydiae undergo persistent infection.[87] For example, *Mycobacterium tuberculosis* undergoes persistent infection, and its primary host cell type, like that of persistent chlamydiae in the joint, is the monocytic cell. One report identified nearly 200 genes whose expression is required for *M tuberculosis* growth and persistence in an animal model, and most of these are not expressed, or are expressed at only a low level, during normal growth of the organism.[88] More than half of those genes encode proteins of unknown function on the *M tuberculosis* chromosome.[89] The genes encoding known proteins involved in *M tuberculosis* growth and persistence fall into categories similar to those identified in the study of IFNγ induced persistence of *C trachomatis*; that is, gene products required for lipid metabolism, translation, DNA repair and recombination, and others.[88–93] Unlike the large mycobacterial genome, the *C trachomatis* chromosome specifies only about 900 coding sequences[76,80] and all of them are expressed at one time or another during normal, active growth of the organism.[90,91] This means that, unlike *M tuberculosis*, *C trachomatis* does not have a gene or gene set whose sole function is the genesis or maintenance of the persistent state.[92] Thus, whereas mycobacterial persistence seems to be a function of expression of a specific set of genes, persistence for *C trachomatis* must result from a readjustment of transcript levels from genes already being expressed, as suggested by the transcript data outlined briefly in previous sections. Comparison of every gene identified as being involved in or required for *M tuberculosis* persistence to the *C trachomatis* and *C pneumoniae* genomes indicated that about 40% of the former have orthologs with reasonable to high similarity in DNA sequence in the chlamydial genomes. The remainder show poor or no similarity to any gene on either chlamydial chromosome; and each of these encodes a protein of currently unknown function.[92]

Given these initial observations, and the complete transcriptome analyses recently published for *C trachomatis* and *C pneumoniae,* it is of significant interest to define the complete transcriptional profile of persistent *C trachomatis* in the monocyte model system *versus* that in the in vivo synovial context, because this information should give insight into the synovial pathogenesis process.[90–94] The authors recently finished a complete transcriptome analyses for *C trachomatis* as a function of time postinfection in the in vitro monocyte model of persistence, and whereas analyses are not yet complete, initial analyses of the data indicate that several genes encoding products of currently unknown function are required for the transition from normal active growth to persistence (Gérard and Hudson, unpublished observations, 2008). A method for the genetic manipulation of *C psittaci,* a bird pathogen, was published recently.[95] If that method proves generally usable for all chlamydial species, it will allow definition of the functions of those currently unspecified gene products.

RELEVANT ASPECTS OF HOST-PATHOGEN INTERACTION

Establishment and maintenance of the persistent state for chlamydiae, and thus aspects of immunopathogenesis, must result from interaction between bacterium and host cell. Several host-directed microarray-based studies relevant to chlamydial infection have appeared over the last few years. One analyzed expression of some 1200 host genes on an array using RNA from *C trachomatis* and mock-infected HeLa cells.[96] Transcription of only 18 genes was up-regulated by chlamydial infection, including IL-11, MIP-2α, several transcription factors such as *c-jun*, various adhesion molecules, and genes specifying apoptosis-related products. Another group reported host transcript changes in 2 hour- *versus* 16 hour-*C trachomatis*–infected HeLa cells.[97] At 2 hours postinfection, only 13 of the 15,000 coding sequences on the array showed differences in transcript levels. These included two transcription factors, *junB*, a tumor-associated antigen, and a few others. At 16 hours postinfection, 130 genes showed differences in expression, including transcription factors (none of them identified in[96]), several immune system genes, genes encoding metabolism-related products, cancer-related genes, and others. In analyses relating to *C pneumoniae*, differences in mRNA levels for 268 genes were examined in infected endothelial cells, which showed that expression of 8% of them was affected.[98] Up-regulated genes included those specifying cytokines and chemokines, growth factors, and a few others.[99] Yet another report compared gene expression up-regulated by infection of THP-1 cells with *C trachomatis* (L2 biovar) with *Coxiella burnetii* at 36 hr postinfection.[100] Expression of more than 500 host genes was increased, whereas only about 300 responded similarly to *C burnetii.* Many genes specifying cytokines and chemokines were similarly up-regulated by both. Genes up-regulated only in response to *C trachomatis* included several related to apoptosis and lymphocyte activation. Another study showed that the panel of host (HeLa cell) genes whose expression is up-regulated by infection with *C trachomatis* and *C pneumoniae* is generally comparable for the two pathogens, although the level of up-regulation elicited by the latter was lower than that elicited by the former.[101] Another study of persistence in *C pneumoniae* induced in vitro by sequestration of iron suggested that the transit to persistence from active passage through the developmental cycle is a midcycle attenuation event rather than a specific program of gene expression supporting that transit.[94] In each of these reports, host genes not previously studied or even considered in relation to active chlamydial infection were affected by the intracellular presence of chlamydiae, suggesting a more extensive interplay between host and pathogen than originally envisioned. Host-directed array analyses similar to those described here, but using nucleic acid preparations from monocytic host cells infected with *C trachomatis* (and *C pneumoniae*) during the transit from active to persistent infection, and during established persistence must be undertaken. That determination was done in the time course-based experiments for transcriptome analyses of *C trachomatis* gene expression in the monocyte model of persistence (Gérard and Hudson, unpublished observations, 2008). Data from that study have not been fully analyzed. Studies from other groups have demonstrated manipulation of host cell processes by chlamydiae, including production of a chlamydial protease that degrades the host transcription factor RFX5,[102] and production of another chlamydial protein that interacts with host cell death receptors.[103] A protein designated pgp3, encoded on the 7 kbp plasmid found in *C trachomatis*, was recently demonstrated to be secreted from the infected organism into the cytoplasm of the host cell.[104] The precise function of this protein in manipulation of host cell processes remains to be elucidated, but evidence indicates that it is involved in pathogenesis. More study of these and other chlamydial gene products will be required before the molecular genetics of host-pathogen interaction leading to synovial inflammation are fully understood.

SUMMARY

The observations outlined briefly demonstrate that some understanding of meaningful details concerning the *Chlamydia*-induced synovial pathogenesis process in reactive arthritis has emerged from research efforts over the last 20 years. However, many important questions remain, several of which center on issues of host-pathogen interaction. It has never been clear why only a subset of the many individuals who acquire a genital infection by *C trachomatis*, or the minority of individuals who are *C pneumoniae*-infected, develop the acute inflammatory arthritis, nor is it clear why only about half of those who do develop the acute disease progress to chronicity. The authors contend that this must be an issue of differential host-pathogen interplay as dictated by host genetic background, and by the genetic component of the infecting chlamydial strain or serovar. At this point, however, there is virtually no understanding regarding the specific aspects of host genetic complement that contribute to disease development or progression. Recent data from this group has indicated that synovial inflammation in patients with reactive arthritis is a function of ocular (trachoma) strains of *C trachomatis* in the joint acquired by way of genital infection, rather than by standard genital strains as expected.[105] (Gérard, Carter, and Hudson, unpublished observations, 2008). This surprising observation must be confirmed. If it is, analysis of the gene products, or their pattern of expression during active and persistent infection, encoded by the genomes of those ocular strains or serovars should provide important clues regarding the molecular genetic basis of arthritogenicity. Because genital infections by ocular *C trachomatis* strains are rare, these results may also explain in part the low incidence of reactive arthritis among individuals with a genital chlamydial infection. Further, for those patients who develop the acute arthritis but do not progress to chronic disease following a genital chlamydial infection, it is not known whether the organism is actually cleared from the joint or whether it remains at that site as a low-level, subclinical infection. It is not understood why in some patients with chronic *Chlamydia*-induced arthritis the disease cycles between quiescence and active arthritis. Again, this latter phenotype must certainly result from on-going and dynamic host-pathogen interaction, but the detailed nature of those interactions remains to be elucidated.

All currently available data indicate that persistent chlamydial infection of the synovium is a central facet of the arthritogenic process. Whereas there are the beginnings of an understanding of the biology of persistence for *C trachomatis*, and to a lesser extent for *C pneumoniae*, there is little information concerning how that infection state is elicited within monocytic cells. Understanding is beginning concerning the molecular interactions occurring within *Chlamydia*-infected monocytes that engender the persistent state, as opposed to those obtaining in epithelial cells that do not. Data from this group and others indicate that inflammatory arthritis elicited by *C pneumoniae* is significantly less common than is the congruent *C trachomatis*-induced disease. This is surprising given the high prevalence of infection with this respiratory pathogen in essentially all adult populations studied to date. Moreover, arthritis elicited by *C pneumoniae* does not seem to include the same coherent suite of extra-articular features, unlike arthritis elicited by *C trachomatis*. To date, however, most studies targeting *Chlamydia*-induced arthritis, and the role of persistence in engendering or maintaining the disease, have focused on *C trachomatis*. In the authors' view, a coherent and systematic investigation of *C pneumoniae*-induced inflammatory arthritis must be done, because it should reveal important details of how this organism elicits pathogenesis, as opposed to the means used by its related species. Such a research program also would provide insight into whether details relating to persistence differ between these two human pathogens. Moreover, it is clear that synovial materials from some patients show polymicrobial infection.[106] However, it is not known whether and, if so, how those additional bacterial species contribute to joint pathogenesis. Investigation of the role that other bacterial species play in engendering, maintaining, or exacerbating synovial inflammation will prove valuable.

Studies from many groups have provided evidence that conventional antibiotic therapy is generally ineffective for the treatment of *Chlamydia*-induced arthritis once it has developed (see a related article by Carter and Hudson in this issue). A few reports indicate that treatment with some particular antibiotics may be counterproductive.[79,107] Thus (in addition to vigilant identification and treatment of urogenital infections with *C trachomatis*, and pulmonary infections with *C pneumoniae*, to obviate subsequent *Chlamydia*-induced arthritis) it will be critical to develop new therapeutic strategies to treat reactive arthritis in its acute form and, more importantly, in its chronic form. One avenue that might be explored centers on determination of some means for "reactivating" persistent infection. That is, finding a mechanism by which the transcriptional and other blocks that underlie the persistent form of the organisms can be reversed, thus returning the organisms to full passage through the developmental cycle where antibiotics treatments can be effective. Information provided in another article in this issue strongly indicates that combination antibiotic therapy may be an effective means of treating *Chlamydia*-induced arthritis.[108] For further discussion, see the article by Carter and Hudson elsewhere in this issue.

REFERENCES

1. Reiter H. Über einer bisher unerkannte Spirochäteninfektion (spirochaetosis arthritica). Dtsche Med Wschr 1916;42:1535–6.

2. Leirisalo-Repo M. Reactive arthritis. Scand J Rheumatol 2005;34:251–9.
3. Sieper J, Kingsley G. Recent advances in the pathogenesis of reactive arthritis. Immunol Today 1996;17:160–3.
4. Inman RD, Whittum-Hudson JA, Schumacher HR, et al. Chlamydia-associated arthritis. Curr Opin Rheumatol 2000;12:254–62.
5. Zeidler H, Kuipers JG, Köhler L. Chlamydia-induced arthritis. Curr Opin Rheumatol 2004;16:380–92.
6. Gérard HC, Whittum-Hudson JA, Schumacher HR, et al. Chlamydia and inflammatory arthritis. In: Columbus F, editor. Focus on arthritis research. New York: Nova Science Publishers; 2005. p. 175–99.
7. Whittum-Hudson JA, Gérard HC, Schumacher HR, et al. Pathogenesis of Chlamydia-associated arthritis. In: Bavoil P, Wyrick P, editors. Chlamydia—genomics and pathogenesis. Norwich (UK): Horizon Bioscience;; 2007. p. 475–504.
8. Leinonen M. Pathogenetic mechanisms and epidemiology of Chlamydia pneumoniae. Eur Heart J 1993;14:57–61.
9. Schumacher HR. Evaluating inflammatory arthritis. Intern Med 1995;3:3–6.
10. Schumacher HR. Chlamydia-associated arthritis. Isr Med Assoc J 2000;2:532–5.
11. Klippel JH. Primer on the rheumatic diseases. 12th edition. Atlanta: Arthritis Foundation Press; 2007.
12. Schumacher HR, Arayssi T, Branigan PJ, et al. Surveying for evidence of synovial Chlamydia trachomatis by PCR. A study of 411 synovial biopsies and synovial fluids. Arthritis Rheum 1997;40(Suppl):S270.
13. Fendler C, Laitko S, Sorensen H, et al. Frequency of triggering bacteria in patients with reactive arthritis and undifferentiated oligoarthritis and the relative importance of the tests used for diagnosis. Ann Rheum Dis 2001;60:337–43.
14. Sieper J, Rudwaleit M, Khan MA, et al. Concepts and epidemiology of spondyloarthritis. Best Prac Res Clin Rheumatol 2006;20:401–17.
15. Carter JD. Reactive arthritis: defined etiologies, emerging pathophysiology, and unresolved treatments. Infect Dis Clin North Am 2006;20:827–47.
16. Zeidler H, Werdier D, Klauder A, et al. Undifferentiated arthritis and spondyloarthropathy as a challenge for prospective follow-up. Clin Rheumatol 1987; 6(Suppl 2):112–20.
17. Carter JD, Gerard HC, Espinoza L, et al. Chlamydiae as etiologic agents for chronic undifferentiated spondyloarthropathy. Arthritis Rheum, in press.
18. Schnarr S, Putschky N, Jendro MC, et al. Chlamydia and Borrelia DNA in synovial fluid of patients with early undifferentiated oligoarthritis: results of a prospective study. Arthritis Rheum 2001;44:2679–85.
19. Rohekar S, Tsui FW, Tsui HW, et al. Symptomatic acute reactive arthritis after an outbreak of Salmonella. J Rheumatol 2008;35:1599–602.
20. Braun J, Tuszewski M, Eggens U, et al. Nested polymerase chain reaction strategy simultaneously targeting DNA sequences of multiple bacterial species in inflammatory joint diseases. I. Screening of synovial fluid samples of patients with spondyloarthropathies and other arthritides. J Rheumatol 1997;24: 1092–100.
21. Granfors K, Jalkanen S, Toivanen P, et al. Bacterial lipopolysaccharide in synovial fluid cells in Shigella triggered reactive arthritis. J Rheumatol 1992; 19:500.
22. Hill Gaston JS, Lillicrap MS. Arthritis associated with enteric infection. Best Prac Res Clin Rheumatol 2003;17:219–39.
23. Wilkinson NZ, Kingsley GH, Jones HW, et al. Detection of DNA from a range of bacterial species in the joints of patients with a variety of arthritides using

a nested, broad-range polymerase chain reaction. Rheumatology 1999;38: 260–6.

24. Hill Gaston JS, Cox C, Granfors K. Clinical and experimental evidence for persistent Yersinia infection in reactive arthritis. Arthritis Rheum 1999;42:2239–42.

25. Hannu T, Mattila L, Siitonen A, et al. Reactive arthritis due to *Shigella* infection: a clinical and epidemiological nationwide study. Ann Rheum Dis 2005;64:594–8.

26. Söderlin MK, Börjesson O, Kautiainen H, et al. Annual incidence of inflammatory joint diseases in a population-based study in southern Sweden. Ann Rheum Dis 2002;61:911–5.

27. Savolainen E, Kaipiainen-Seppänen O, Kröger L, et al. Total incidence and distribution of inflammatory joint diseases in a defined population: results from the Kuopio 2000 arthritis survey. J Rheumatol 2003;30:2460–8.

28. Pope JE, Krizova A, Garg AX, et al. *Campylobacter* reactive arthritis: a systematic review. Semin Arthritis Rheum 2007;37:48–55.

29. Whittum-Hudson JA, Hudson AP. Human chlamydial infections: persistence, prevalence, and prospects for the future. Nat Sci Soc 2005;13:371–82.

30. Campbell LA, Kuo CC. *Chlamydia pneumoniae* pathogenesis. J Med Microbiol 2002;51:623–5.

31. Hahn DL, Dodge RW, Golubjatnikov R. Association of *C pneumoniae* (strain TWAR) infection with wheezing, asthmatic bronchitis, adult-onset asthma. JAMA 1991;266:225–30.

32. Hackstadt T. Cell biology. In: Stephens RS, editor. *Chlamydia*—intracellular biology, pathogenesis, and immunity. Washington, DC: ASM Press; 1999. p. 101–38.

33. Hogan RJ, Mathews SA, Mukhopadhyay S, et al. Chlamydial persistence: beyond the biphasic paradigm. Infect Immun 2004;72:1843–55.

34. Norton WL, Lewis D, Ziff M. Light and electron microscopic observation on the synovitis of Reiter's disease. Arthritis Rheum 1966;9:747–57.

35. Ishikawa H, Ohno O, Yamasaki K, et al. Arthritis presumably caused by *Chlamydia* in Reiter's syndrome. Case report with electron microscopic studies. J Bone Joint Surg AM 1986;68:777–9.

36. Keat AC. *Chlamydia trachomatis* infection in human arthritis. In: Oriel D, Ridgway G, Schachter J, editors. Chlamydial infections. New York: Cambridge University Press; 1986. p. 269–79.

37. Keat A, Thomas B, Dixey J, et al. *Chlamydia trachomatis* and reactive arthritis: the missing link. Lancet 1987;1:72–4.

38. Schumacher HR, Magge S, Cherian PV, et al. Light and electron microscopic studies on the synovial membrane in Reiter's syndrome. Immunocytochemical identification of chlamydial antigen in patients with early disease. Arthritis Rheum 1988;31:937–46.

39. Schachter J, Barnes D, Jones JP, et al. Isolation of Bedsoniae from the joint of patients with Reiter's syndrome. Proc Soc Exp Biol Med 1966;122:283–5.

40. Schachter J. Isolation of Bedsoniae from human arthritis and abortion tissues. Am J Ophthalmol 1967;63(Suppl):1082–6.

41. Engleman EP, Schachter J, Gilbert RJ, et al. *Bedsonia* and Reiter's syndrome: a progress report. Arthritis Rheum 1969;12(Suppl):292.

42. Dunlop EM, Freedman A, Garland JA, et al. Infection by Bedsoniae and the possibility of spurious isolation: 2. Genital infection, disease of the eye, Reiter's disease. Am J Ophthalmol 1967;63(Suppl):1073–81.

43. Dunlop EM, Harper IA, Jones BR. Seronegative polyarthritis: the Bedsonia (*Chlamydia*) group of agents and Reiter's disease. Ann Rheum Dis 1968;27: 234–40.

44. Gordon FB, Quan AL, Steinman TI, et al. Chlamydial isolates from Reiter's syndrome. Br J Vener Dis 1973;49:376–8.
45. Centers for Disease Control and Prevention. Chlamydia. Available at: see. www.cdc.gov/std/stats07/chlamydia.htm. Accessed in 2008.
46. Bas S, Griffais R, Kvien TK, et al. Amplification of plasmid and chromosome Chlamydia DNA in synovial fluid of patients with reactive arthritis and undifferentiated seronegative oligoarthropathies. Arthritis Rheum 1995;38:1005–13.
47. Bas S, Scieux C, Vischer TL. Different humoral immune response to Chlamydia trachomatis major outer membrane protein variable domains I and IV in Chlamydia-infected patients with or without reactive arthritis. Arthritis Rheum 1999;42:942–7.
48. Branigan PJ, Gérard HC, Hudson AP, et al. Comparison of synovial tissue and fluid as sources for nucleic acids for detection of C trachomatis by polymerase chain reaction. Arthritis Rheum 1996;39:1740–6.
49. Braun J, Laitko S, Treharne J, et al. Chlamydia pneumoniae—a new causative agent of reactive arthritis and undifferentiated oligoarthritis. Ann Rheum Dis 1994;53:100–5.
50. Schumacher HR, Gérard HC, Arayssi TK, et al. Chlamydia pneumoniae is present in synovial tissue of arthritis patients with lower prevalence than that of C trachomatis. Arthritis Rheum 1999;42:1889–93.
51. Whittum-Hudson JA, Gérard HC, Clayburne G, et al. A non-invasive murine model of Chlamydia-induced reactive arthritis. Rev de Rheum Engl Ed 1999; 66(Suppl):50S–6S.
52. Moazed TC, Kuo CC, Grayston JT, et al. Evidence of systemic dissemination of Chlamydia pneumoniae via macrophages in the mouse. J Infect Dis 1998;177: 1322–5.
53. Köhler L, Nettelnbreker E, Hudson AP, et al. Ultrastructural and molecular analysis of the persistence of Chlamydia trachomatis (serovar K) in human monocytes. Microb Pathog 1997;22:133–42.
54. Dreses-Werringloer U, Gérard HC, Whittum-Hudson JA, et al. C pneumoniae infection of human astrocytes and microglial cells in culture displays an active, rather than a persistent, growth phenotype. Am J Med Sci 2006;332:168–74.
55. Nanagara R, Li F, Beutler AM, et al. Alteration of C trachomatis biological behavior in synovial membranes: suppression of surface antigen production in reactive arthritis and Reiter's syndrome. Arthritis Rheum 1995;38:1410–7.
56. Cascina A, Marone BA, Mangiarotti P, et al. Cutaneous vasculitis and reactive arthritis following respiratory infection due to C pneumoniae: report of a case. Clin Exp Rheumatol 2002;20:845–7.
57. Hannu T, Puolakkainen M, Leirisalo-Repo M. Chlamydia pneumoniae as a triggering agent in reactive arthritis. Rheumatology 1999;38:411–4.
58. Gérard HC, Schumacher HR, El-Gabalawy H, et al. Chlamydia pneumoniae infecting the human synovium are viable and metabolically active. Microb Pathog 2000;29:17–24.
59. Gérard HC, Branigan PJ, Schumacher HR, et al. Synovial C trachomatis in patients with reactive arthritis are viable but show aberrant gene expression. J Rheumatol 1998;25:734–42.
60. Saikku P. C pneumoniae—clinical spectrum. In: Stephens R, Byrne G, Christiansen G, et al, editors. Human chlamydial infections. San Francisco: International Chlamydia Symposium; 1998. p. 145–54.
61. Ward ME. Mechanisms of Chlamydia-induced disease. In: Stephens RS, editor. Chlamydia—intracellular biology, pathogenesis, and immunity. Washington, DC: ASM Press; 1999. p. 171–210.

62. Gérard HC, Wang GF, Balin GJ, et al. Frequency of apolipoprotein E (APOE) allele types in patients with Chlamydia-associated arthritis and other arthritides. Microb Pathog 1999;26:35–43.

63. Gérard HC, Fomicheva E, Whittum-Hudson JA, et al. Apolipoprotein E4 enhances attachment of C pneumoniae elementary bodies to host cells. Microb Pathog 2008;44:279–85.

64. Beatty WL, Byrne GI, Morrison RP. Morphologic and antigenic characterization of interferon gamma mediated persistent C trachomatis infection. Proc Natl Acad Sci U S A 1993;90:3998–4002.

65. Beatty WL, Morrison RP, Byrne GI. Persistent chlamydiae, from cell culture to a paradigm for chlamydial pathogenesis. Microbiol Rev 1995;58:685–99.

66. Beatty WL, Morrison RP, Byrne GI. Reactivation of persistent Chlamydia trachomatis infection in cell culture. Infect Immun 1995;63:199–205.

67. Jones ML, Gaston JS, Pearce JH. Induction of abnormal C trachomatis by exposure to interferon-gamma or amino acid deprivation and comparative antigenic analysis. Microb Pathog 2001;30:299–309.

68. Harper A, Pogson CI, Pearce JH. Amino acid transport into cultured McCoy cells infected with Chlamydia trachomatis. Infect Immun 2000;68:5439–42.

69. Beutler AM, Whittum-Hudson JA, Nanagara R, et al. Intracellular location of inapparently-infecting Chlamydia in synovial tissue from patients with Reiter's syndrome. Immunol Res 1994;13:163–71.

70. Beutler AM, Schumacher HR, Whittum-Hudson JA, et al. In situ hybridization for detection of inapparent infection with C trachomatis in synovial tissue of a patient with Reiter's syndrome. Am J Med Sci 1995;310:206–13.

71. Schmitz E, Nettelnbreker E, Zeidler H, et al. Intracellular persistence of chlamydial major outer membrane protein, lipopolysaccharide and ribosomal RNA after non-productive infection of human monocytes with Chlamydia trachomatis serovar K. J Med Micrbiol 1993;38:278–85.

72. Rothermel CD, Schachter J, Lavrich P, et al. Chlamydia trachomatis-induced production of interleukin-1 by human monocytes. Infect Immun 1989;57:2705–11.

73. Gérard HC, Köhler L, Branigan PJ, et al. Viability and gene expression in Chlamydia trachomatis during persistent infection of cultured human monocytes. Med Microbiol Immunol 1998;187:115–20.

74. Gérard HC, Krauße-Opatz B, Rudy D, et al. Expression of Chlamydia trachomatis genes required for DNA synthesis and cell division in active vs. persistent infection. Mol Microbiol 2001;41:731–41.

75. Byrne GI, Ouellette SP, Wang Z, et al. C pneumoniae expresses genes required for DNA replication but not cytokinesis during persistent infection of Hep-2 cells. Infect Immun 2001;69:5423–9.

76. Stephens RS, Kalman S, Lammel C, et al. Genome sequence of an obligate intracellular pathogen of humans: Chlamydia trachomatis. Science 1998;282:754–9.

77. Iliffe-Lee ER, McClarty G. Glucose metabolism in Chlamydia trachomatis: the 'energy parasite' hypothesis revisited. Mol Microbiol 1999;33:177–87.

78. Gérard HC, Freise J, Rudy D, et al. C trachomatis genes whose products are related to energy metabolism are expressed differentially in active vs. persistent infection. Microbes Infect 2002;4:13–22.

79. Balaban HQ, Merrin J, Chait R, et al. Bacterial persistence as a phenotypic switch. Science 2004;305:1622–5.

80. Read TD, Brunham RC, Shen C, et al. Genome sequences of Chlamydia trachomatis MoPn and Chlamydia pneumoniae AR39. Nucleic Acids Res 2000;28:1397–406.

81. Campbell F, Birkelund S, Ward ME, et al. *Chlamydia trachomatis* protein antigens stimulate synovial fluid-derived T cell clones from reactive arthritis patients. In: Stary A, editor. Proceeding of the European Society for *Chlamydia* Research. Bologna (Italy): Societa Editrice Esculapio; 1996. p. 78.

82. Hill Gaston JS, Deane KHO, Jecock RM, et al. Identification of two *C trachomatis* antigens recognized by synovial fluid T cells from patients with *Chlamydia*-induced reactive arthritis. J Rheumatol 1996;79:513–9.

83. Gérard HC, Whittum-Hudson JA, Schumacher HR, et al. Differential expression of the three *Chlamydia trachomatis* hsp60-encoding genes in active vs persistent infection. Microb Pathog 2004;36:35–9.

84. Klos A, Thalmann J, Peters J, et al. The transcript profile of persistent C pneumoniae in vitro depends on the means by which persistence is induced. FEMS Microbiol Lett 2008;29:120–6.

85. Wilson AC, Tan M. Stress response gene regulation in *Chlamydia* is dependent on HrcA-CIRCE interactions. J Bacteriol 2004;186:3384–91.

86. Mathews SA, Volp KM, Timms P. Development of a quantitative gene expression assay for *Chlamydia trachomatis* identified temporal expression of sigma factors. FEBS Lett 1999;458:354–8.

87. Rhen M, Erikssonm S, Clements M, et al. The basis of persistent bacterial infection. Trends Microbiol 2003;11:80–6.

88. Sassetti CM, Rubin EJ. Genetic requirements for mycobacterial survival during infection. Proc Natl Acad Sci U S A 2003;100:12989–94.

89. Cole ST, Eiglmeier K, Parkhill J, et al. Deciphering the biology of *Mycobacterium tuberculosis* from the complete genome sequence. Nature 1998;393:537–44.

90. Belland RJ, Zhong G, Cran DD, et al. Genomic transcriptional profiling of the developmental cycle of *Chlamydia trachomatis*. Proc Natl Acad Sci U S A 2003;100:8478–83.

91. Nicholson TL, Olinger L, Chong K, et al. Global stage-specific gene regulation during the developmental cycle of *Chlamydia trachomatis*. J Bacteriol 2003; 185:3179–89.

92. Gérard HC, Whittum-Hudson JA, Schumacher HR, et al. Synovial *C trachomatis* up-regulates expression of a panel of genes similar to that transcribed by *M tuberculosis* during persistent infection. Ann Rheum Dis 2007;65:321–7.

93. Belland RJ, Nelson DE, Virok D, et al. Transcriptome analysis of chlamydial growth during IFNγ-mediated persistence and reactivation. Proc Natl Acad Sci U S A 2003;100:15971–6.

94. Mäurer AP, Mehlitz A, Mollenhopf HJ, et al. Gene profiles of *Chlamydophila pneumoniae* during the developmental cycle and iron depletion-mediated persistence. PLoS Pathog 2007;3:752–79.

95. Binet R, Maurelli AT. Transformation and isolation of allelic exchange mutants of *C psittaci* using recombinant DNA introduced by electroporation. Proc Natl Acad Sci U S A 2009;106:292–7.

96. Hess S, Rheinheimer C, Tidow F, et al. The reprogrammed host: *Chlamydia trachomatis*-induced up-regulation of glycoprotein 130, cytokines, transcription factors, and anti-apoptotic genes. Arthritis Rheum 2001;44:2392–401.

97. Minsheng X, Bumgarner RE, Lampe MF, et al. *Chlamydia trachomatis* infection alters host cell transcription in diverse cellular pathways. J Infect Dis 2003; 187:424–34.

98. Coombes BK, Mahony JB. cDNA array analysis of altered gene expression in human endothelial cells in response to *Chlamydia pneumoniae* infection. Infect Immun 2001;69:1420–7.

99. Dessus-Babus S, Knight ST, Wyrick PB. Chlamydial infection of polarized HeLa cells induces PMN chemotaxis but the cytokine profile varies between disseminating and non-disseminating strains. Cell Microbiol 2000;2:317–27.

100. Ren Q, Robertson SJ, Howe D, et al. Comparative DNA microarray analysis of host cell transcriptional responses to infection by *Coxiella burnetii* or *Chlamydia trachomatis*. Ann NY Acad Sci 2003;990:701–13.

101. Hess S, Peters J, Bartling G, et al. More than just innate immunity: comparative analysis of *C pneumoniae* and *C trachomatis* effects on host-cell gene regulation. Cell Microbiol 2003;5:785–95.

102. Fan PI, Don F, Huang Y, et al. *Chlamydia pneumoniae* secretion of a protease-like activity factor for degrading host cell transcription factor required for major histocompatibility complex antigen expression. Infect Immun 2002;70:345–9.

103. Stenner-Liewen F, Liewen H, Zapata JM, et al. CADD, a *Chlamydia* protein that interacts with death receptors. J Biol Chem 2002;277:9633–6.

104. Li Z, Chen D, Zhong Y, et al. The chlamydial plasmid-encoded protein pgp3 is secreted into the cytosol of *Chlamydia*-infected host cells. Infect Immun 2008; 76:3415–28.

105. Hudson AP, Schumacher HR, Whittum-Hudson JA, et al. Patients infected with *Chlamydia trachomatis* frequently have ocular, not genital, serovars of the organism in synovial tissue. Arthritis Rheum 2007;56(Suppl):S169.

106. Gérard HC, Wang Z, Wang GF, et al. Chromosomal DNA from a variety of bacterial species is present in synovial tissue in patients with various forms of arthritis. Arthritis Rheum 2001;44:1689–97.

107. Dreses-Werringloer U, Köhler L, Hudson AP. Detection of nucleotide variability in rpoB in rifampin-sensitive and rifampin-resistant isolates of *C trachomatis*. Antimicrob Agents Chemother 2003;47:2316–8.

108. Carter JD, Valeriano J, Vasey FB. Doxycycline vs doxycycline and rifampin in undifferentiated spondyloarthropathy, with special reference to *Chlamydia*-induced arthritis. A prospective, randomized 9-month comparison. J Rheumatol 2004;31:1773–80.

Reactive Arthritis: Clinical Aspects and Medical Management

John D. Carter, MD[a],*, Alan P. Hudson, PhD[b]

KEYWORDS

• Reactive arthritis • Chlamydia • Salmonella • Shigella
• Campylobacter • Yersinia

Reactive arthritis (ReA) is an inflammatory arthritis that arises after certain types of gastrointestinal or genitourinary infections, representing the classic interplay of host and environment. It belongs to the group of arthritidies known as the spondyloarthropathies (SpAs). The classic syndrome is a triad of symptoms, including the urethra, conjunctiva, and synovium; however, the majority of patients do not present with this classic triad.[1] In general, there are two forms of ReA, postvenereal (*Chlamydia trachomatis* [Ct]) and postdysentery (*Salmonella, Shigella, Campylobacter,* and *Yersinia*), but several other bacteria have been implicated as potential causes. Epidemiologic and prospective studies have been difficult to perform on ReA for several reasons. The disease description and definition has been clouded by over-reliance on the complete classic triad of symptoms and the many different terms and eponyms used to describe the condition. Diagnostic criteria for ReA exist, including that of the American College of Rheumatology[2] and the Third International Workshop on Reactive Arthritis in 1995,[3] but data in this review suggest new criteria are needed. Although the postvenereal and postdysentery forms of the condition are clinically indistinct, these subtypes could have different long-term prognoses or treatment implications.

HISTORY OF REACTIVE ARTHRITIS

Considering the many terms and eponyms used in the literature to describe this condition, a brief review of the history of ReA is warranted. Although many attribute the earliest description of ReA to Hans Reiter in 1916, when he described the clinical triad of arthritis, nongonococcal urethritis, and conjunctivitis in a German soldier after an episode of bloody diarrhea,[4] the syndrome also was described by two French physicians (Fiessinger and Leroy) in that same year.[5] Therefore, it often was dubbed

---

[a] Department of Internal Medicine, Division of Rheumatology, University of South Florida, 12901 Bruce B. Downs Boulevard, MDC 81, Tampa, FL 33612, USA
[b] Department of Microbiology and Immunology, Wayne State University, Detroit, MI, USA
* Corresponding author.
E-mail address: jocarter@health.usf.edu (J.D. Carter).

Rheum Dis Clin N Am 35 (2009) 21–44
doi:10.1016/j.rdc.2009.03.010
0889-857X/09/$ – see front matter © 2009 Elsevier Inc. All rights reserved.

Reiter's syndrome, but Fiessinger-Leroy syndrome also has been used. The literature, however, clearly describes cases of ReA many years before Reiter or Fiessinger and Leroy. The earliest description of ReA may date back to approximately 460 BC, when Hippocrates wrote, "A youth does not suffer from gout until sexual intercourse."[6] Although the term, *gout*, was used indiscriminately at the time to describe inflammatory arthritis,[7] it is difficult to know whether or not this is a true description of ReA because it is not implicitly stated that the condition was preceded by a venereal infection. It has been speculated that Christopher Columbus developed ReA in 1494, when he developed fever and severe arthritis of the lower extremities after a case of dysentery (possibly *Shigella flexneri*).[7] In 1498, Columbus had a flare of his articular inflammation that was accompanied by eye "hemorrhage and pain"; and in 1504 he was "paralyzed and bedridden" because of "gout." Several others have described similar cases in the literature, including Pierre van Forest's description of a case of "secondary arthritis and urethritis" in 1507,[8] Thomas Sydenham's association of arthritis with diarrhea in 1686,[9] Stoll's documentation of arthritis following dysentery in 1776,[10] and Yvan's description of a French captain who developed "ophthalmia" and inflammatory arthritis primarily of the lower extremities 15 days after a venereal infection.[11] There were two clear descriptions of the classic triad of ReA; the first was in 1818 by Brodie and his documentation of five patients who had urethritis, arthritis, and conjunctivitis,[12] and the second was in 1897 with Launois' distinction of septic from aseptic arthritis, the latter occasionally developing cutaneous lesions on the plantar surface of the feet (keratoderma blenorrhagicum).[13] During this same time period in 1824, Cooper proposed the concept of the relationship between venereal infection and arthritis, particularly of the lower extremities.[14]

Baron Yvan was the surgeon-in-ordinary to Napolean I. His description more than 200 years ago of a patient who had probable ReA was as follows:

> *40 year old invalid captain with a weak constitution entered the infirmary...to be treated for a gonorrhea he had caught 15 days previously. On the 12th day, the patient was immediately affected with intense ophthalmia in both eyes. He was very sensitive to light and the engorgement of the conjunctiva was extreme...On the 21st the patient suffered pains in the right foot joint. The pain was accompanied by a slight tumefaction which grew day by day; the knee joint as well as the right arm and forearm became painful.[11]*

Sir Benjamin Brodie, an English physiologist and surgeon who pioneered research in joint disease, described five patients who had classic ReA in his treatise, *Pathologic and Surgical Observations on the Diseases of the Joints*. He recognized the similar "train of symptoms" that all five patients experienced and clearly noted the relapsing course in the few who developed chronic disease:

> *A gentleman, 45 years of age, in the middle of June 1817, became affected with...a purulent discharge from the urethra...On the 23d of June he first experienced some degree of pain in his feet...June 25th, the pain in his feet was more severe; the tunica conjunctivae of his eyes were much inflamed, with a profuse discharge of pus...On the 27th of June the left knee became painful...exceedingly distended...The inflammation in his eyes and urethra was somewhat abated.[12]*

This patient's symptoms resolved nearly completely in December 1817, but then he developed exacerbations that were similar in nature, including "inflammation seated in the tunicks of the eye." Brodie recognized that these recurrent symptoms were related to the initial episode; his treatment of choice was vinum colchici seminis (wine of the Colchicum seed).

In 1942, the symptoms of ReA again were recognized as a syndrome by two Harvard researchers (Bauer and Engelmann) and in their review of the literature they realized that Reiter had described this same syndrome in 1916, so they coined the term, *Reiter's syndrome*.[15] A more thorough search might have revealed that Reiter was only one in a long line of previous physicians who described this postinfectious arthritis. Hans Reiter, however, did take the notion of ReA having an infectious etiology one step further, when he surmised that this condition was caused specifically by a spirochete. His terminology for the condition was "spirochetosis arthritica."[4] This supposition is now understood to be incorrect. The term, Reiter's syndrome, has been widely used, although in recent years its use has been in decline.[16] During World War II, Hans Reiter authorized medical experiments on concentration camp prisoners. Because of this, some have correctly argued against the use of the Reiter eponym.[17,18] Because Hans Reiter was not the first to describe the syndrome, because many clinicians are reluctant to diagnose this condition in those who do not display the complete triad of symptoms, thereby missing the majority of cases, and because ReA is a more descriptive term, the term ReA has become the appropriate terminology for this disease process regardless of whether or not the symptoms involve the three classic organ systems.

EPIDEMIOLOGY

The lack of a disease definition or specific diagnostic criteria for ReA makes epidemiologic studies problematic.[19,20] An epidemiologic discussion of ReA not only should include the typical analyses of incidence and prevalence but also an analysis of attack rate, which is of equal importance. Because only a percentage of subjects exposed to the known causative organisms of ReA develop the disease, the attack rate refers to that percentage. The incidence, prevalence, and attack rate of ReA vary widely among different studies. The variability of genetic background, including different prevalence of human leukocyte antigen-B27 (HLA-B27) in the various communities studied, might be a partial explanation. Local environmental factors also play a role in the apparent variable attack rate of ReA. For example, infection with one of the causative organisms, *Yersinia enterocolitica*, is uncommon in the United States but reported more commonly in Europe.[21] As a further complication, infections with the same organisms in the same community can vary over time.[22] An example was the recent outbreak of *Salmonella* in 2008 that affected approximately 1500 people in the United States and Canada. It also is likely that different species from the same genus of the triggering bacteria vary in their arthritogenic propensity. *Salmonella Saint Paul* was responsible for this recent outbreak in the United States and Canada. Although this is a less common *Salmonella* species, it had not previously been implicated as a cause of ReA. Other *Salmonella* species (eg, *S typhimurium* and *S enteritidis*) are well-documented causes of ReA. Finally, it is possible that local differences in the microbes themselves and that increased recognition and improved treatment of the causative organisms also may affect the incidence, prevalence, and attack rate of ReA.

Bacteria that commonly cause ReA are *Salmonella*, *Shigella*, *Campylobacter*, *Yersinia*, and Ct. Ct is the most common etiologic agent causing ReA in the United States.[23,24] Despite the obvious difference of initial route of infection (ie, gastrointestinal versus genitourinary), another distinction exists. The postdysentery form of ReA is preceded by a symptomatic infection, and recent data suggest that the more severe the initial gastrointestinal infectio, the more likely ReA develops.[25–27] An initial Ct infection, however, often is asymptomatic.[28–30] Data described later suggest that many cases of postchlamydial ReA follow an asymptomatic infection. Several published studies also indicate that Chlamydophila (Chlamydia) pneumoniae (Cpn), a related respiratory pathogen, is another causative agent in ReA, albeit at a lower frequency.[31–33]

The postdysentery form of ReA affects men and women with the same frequency, whereas the postvenereal form occurs at a male-to-female ratio of 9:1. Adults are more likely to develop ReA than children.[22,34] The attack rate of postdysentery ReA generally ranges from 1.5%[35] to approximately 30%[36] depending on the study and causative organism; however one recent self-reported questionnaire study suggested that as many as 63% of patients experience symptoms consistent with ReA after an acute Salmonella infection.[37] ReA is believed to occur in approximately 5% of individuals who develop an acute Ct infection.[38]

It is likely that clinicians are under-diagnosing ReA. This contention is borne out by looking, specifically, at postchlamydial ReA. New genital infections with Ct must be reported to the Centers for Disease Control and Prevention, and that institution has estimated that as many as 3 million new cases per year occur in the United States, with as many as 4 to 6 million cases active at any one time.[39,40] As discussed previously, data indicate that approximately 5% of patients develop objective features consistent with ReA after a Ct infection.[38] By using an attack rate of 5%, as many as 150,000 cases of acute Chlamydia-induced ReA would occur in the united States each year (3 million × 0.05). This is a low estimate representing half or fewer of the total cases, because it does not include those cases that result from the postdysentery organisms. For comparison, the estimated annual incidence of rheumatoid arthritis (RA) in the United States is 44.6 per 100,000.[41] If the population is approximately 281 million (2000 census figure), approximately 125,000 new cases of RA per year occur. A 2002 study in Sweden found the annual incidence of ReA higher than that of RA.[42] Thus, ReA represents a considerable burden on the United States health care system and that of other nations, and its impact on those systems well may be significantly under-recognized.

Data suggest that the incidence of certain types of ReA, specifically Ct-induced[43] and Yersinia-induced ReA,[44] might be in decline. The reasons for this are not entirely clear, but they may relate to better prevention and treatment of the causative organisms. There also are data that suggest that the use of antibiotics that are active against Ct, when patients present for treatment of their venereal disease, reduces the risk for postvenereal ReA.[45] Data also suggest, however, that other types (eg, ReA secondary to Campylobacter and Salmonella) are on the rise.[44] It has been demonstrated that the use of proton pump inhibitors increases the risk for developing ReA after a Campylobacter or Salmonella infection.[46]

A final issue complicating epidemiologic studies of ReA is the variable disease course. Patients' initial features of ReA can range from fulminant to mild. Also, a significant percentage of patients' disease course remits spontaneously in weeks to a few months. Generally, if the ReA symptoms last longer than 6 months, then the disease is considered chronic. Patients who progress to chronic ReA can display varying disease symptoms and, in some, disease features can relapse and remit.

CLINICAL FEATURES

The clinical features of ReA are well described and generally congruent for the postvenereal and the postenteric forms. The acute and chronic symptoms can include articular, tendon, mucosal, cutaneous, ocular, and occasionally cardiac manifestations (Table 1) or systemic features (fever, malaise, and weight loss); the latter usually are confined to the acute stage. Symptoms typically start within 1 to 4 weeks of the

Table 1
Clinical manifestations of reactive arthritis

Acute symptoms
Articular
Most commonly present with oligoarthritis but also can present with polyarthritis or monoarthritis
Axial
Frequently involved
Sacroiliac joints
Lumbar spine
Occasionally involved
Thoracic spine (usually seen in chronic ReA)
Cervical spine (usually seen in chronic ReA)
Cartilagenous joints (symphysis pubis; sternoclavicular and costosternal joints)
Peripheral
Frequently involved
Large joints of the lower extremities (especially knees)
Dactylitis (sausage digit)
Very specific for a spondyloarthropathy
Enthesitis
Hallmark feature
Inflammation at the transitional zone where collagenous structures, such as tendons and ligaments insert into bone
Common sites: plantar fasciitis and Achilles tendonitis but any enthesis can be involved
Mucosal
Oral ulcers (generally painless)
Sterile dysuria (occurs with both postvenereal and postdysentery forms)
Cutaneous
Keratoderma blenorrhagicum
Pustular or plaque-like rash on the soles or palms
Grossly and histologically indistguishable from pustular psoriasis
Also can involve nails (onycholysis, subungual keratosis, or nail pits), scalp, extremities
Circinate balanitis
Erythema or plaque-like lesions on the shaft or glans of penis
Ocular
Conjunctivitis: typically during acute stages only
Anterior uveitis (iritis): often recurrent
Rarely described: scleritis, pars planitis, iridocyclitis, and others
Cardiac
Pericarditis (uncommon)
Chronic symptoms (>6 months)
Articular
Axial
Sacroiliac joints
Lumbar spine
Thoracic spine

(continued on next page)

Table 1 (continued)
Cervical spine
Cartilagenous joints (symphysis pubis; sternoclavicular joints)
Peripheral
Large joints of the lower extremities (especially knees)
Dactylitis (sausage digit)
Very specific for a spondyloarthropathy
Enthesitis
Chronic inflammation can cause collagen fibers to undergo metaplasia forming fibrous bone
Chronic enthesitis leads to radiographic findings
Plantar/Achilles spurs
Periostitis
Nonmarginal syndesmophytes
Syndesmoses of the sacroiliac joints
Mucosal
Sterile dysuria
Cutaneous
Keratoderma blennorrhagicum
Circinate balanitis
Ocular
Anterior uveitis (iritis): often recurrent
Rarely described: scleritis, pars planitis, iridocyclitis, and others
Cardiac
Aortic regurgitation
Valvular pathologies

From Carter JD. Reactive arthritis: defined etiologies, emerging pathophysiology, and elusive treatment. Infect Dis Clin N Am 2006;20(4):827–47; with permission.

initial infection. As in the case of chlamydiae, however, the inciting infection could be asymptomatic; therefore, reliance on a symptomatic triggering infection results in underdiagnosis or misdiagnosis. Reports vary widely, but it generally is believed that approximately 30% to 50% of patients who develop ReA experience chronic symptoms. One study suggested the true figure might be as high as 63%.[20] Patients who have chronic ReA often exhibit a relapsing disease course.

Enthesitis deserves special mention. Enthesitis is inflammation at the transitional zone in which collagenous structures, such as tendons and ligaments, insert into bone. This is a hallmark feature of any of the SpAs, including ReA. Common types of enthesitis in ReA are Achilles tendonitis and plantar fasciitis, but inflammation can occur at any enthesis. Sacroiliitis, a major feature of all SpAs, represents a combination of synovitis and enthesitis.[47] A recent report of more than 6000 cases of culture-confirmed infections with bacterial enteric pathogens revealed that enthesitis was the most common finding in those individuals who developed ReA, and arthritis was less frequent.[27]

TRIGGERING MICROBES

The triggering microbes of ReA are gram-negative bacteria with a lipopolysaccharide (LPS) component of their cell walls. All of these bacteria, or their bacterial products, have been demonstrated in the synovial tissue or fluid of patients who have ReA.

This has been demonstrated in several studies involving many different laboratories.[48–56] It is apparent that the entire bacteria or bacterial components traffic to the joints of patients who have ReA. Once these bacteria are in the synovium and other affected organs, their roles in the pathophysiology are less clear.

Chlamydiae

Ct is a common pathogen and believed the most common cause of ReA.[23,24] Ct has been demonstrated in 50% of patients who have had a preceding symptomatic urogenital infection and who developed ReA.[57] The routine presence of Ct has been demonstrated by polymerase chain reaction (PCR) in the synovial tissue of patients who have had ReA.[50,58] These chlamydiae are viable, albeit in an aberrant state.[50] These persistently infecting, viable chlamydiae have been demonstrated years after the initial infection.[50,59] Similar PCR studies have demonstrated Cpn in the synovial tissue of patients who have had ReA, although it is detected less commonly.[51] Ct and Cpn, however, occasionally have been demonstrated in the synovial tissue of patients who have had other types of arthritis or even asymptomatic individuals.[60,61]

Data exist corroborating the notion that chlamydial-induced ReA is vastly underdiagnosed. The explanation for this likely is twofold: the triggering chlamydial infection often might be asymptomatic, and clinical triad is expressed incompletely in most patients. In one study, 78% of subjects who developed ReA features after Ct or nongonococcal infections had an asymptomatic initial infection.[38] The term, *undifferentiated SpAs (uSpAs)*, is used to designate patients who have clinical and radiographic features consistent with the SpAs but who do not fulfill the classification criteria for any of the established disease categories. Because ReA is a type of SpA and the majority of patients who have ReA do not present with the classic triad of symptoms,[1] the contention that Ct could function etiologically to engender uSpA is reasonable. It has been argued that uSpA is a forme fruste of ReA.[62] A recent study analyzed the PCR positivity for chlamydiae in the synovial tissue of patients diagnosed with uSpA.[59] These data demonstrated that the rate of PCR positivity from patients who had uSpA (62%) was significantly higher than that found in synovial tissue from subjects who had osteoarthritis (12%), suggesting that chlamydial infection may be etiologic for uSpA in many patients. Among subjects who had a PCR-positive synovial tissue assay for Ct, 88% had an asymptomatic initial infection; this mirrors the data previous discussed.[38] These, in part, could explain the disconnect between the expected and observed number of diagnosed cases of ReA.

The different chlamydial species also could have an additive or synergistic effect in determining ReA attack rate or incidence. Given that Cpn is a common infection, previous exposure to Cpn could have an effect on a subsequent response to a Ct infection or vice versa. Reports have demonstrated that prior Cpn infection primes a Th1 T-cell response to Ct antigens.[63]

Salmonella

Salmonella is a rod-shaped, motile bacterium widespread in animals and environmental sources. It is one of the most common enteric infections in the United States and is the most frequently studied enteric bacteria associated with ReA. Cases of ReA secondary to ReA seem to be on the rise.[44] After salmonellosis, individuals of Caucasian descent may be more likely than those of Asian descent to develop ReA;[64] and children may be less susceptible than adults.[34] The attack rate of *Salmonella*-induced ReA has ranged between 6% and 30%.[36,65] As with the other causative organisms, efforts have been made to detect *Salmonella* in synovial tissue or fluid. *Salmonella* bacterial degradation products have been detected in the synovial fluid from patients who have *Salmonella*-induced ReA, but no viable organisms have been detected.[54]

There have been large outbreaks of *S typhimurium* and *S enteritidis* with rheumatologic follow-up of affected individuals. Regarding the outbreaks of *S typhimurium*, these occurred in three different countries and the attack rate of ReA ranged from 6% to 15% with the HLA-B27 prevalence ranging from 17% to 50% of these individuals.[65–68] The attack rate of ReA ranged from 7% to 29% with four different outbreaks of *S enteritidis* in four different countries.[36,69,70] A HLA-B27 prevalence of 33% affected individuals was reported in one of these outbreaks.[70] A large study in Denmark comparing the different enteric pathogens known to cause ReA suggested that *Salmonella* was the second most common triggering infection (behind *Campylobacter*) and the second most arthritogenic, after *Yersinia*.[25] There also has been one outbreak of *S bovismorbificans* that resulted in 12% of individuals developing ReA, of whom 45% were HLA-B27 positive.[71]

Shigella

All four of the species of *Shigella* (*S flexneri, S dysenteriae, S sonnei*, and *S boydii*) can cause ReA. In 1944, *Shigella* was the first bacteria to be implicated directly as a cause of ReA.[72] *Shigella*, however, is the least common of the gastrointestinal-inducing organisms that are associated with ReA in developed countries.[73] This is in large part due to the rarity of this organism in these communities. Previous data suggested that *S flexneri* and *S dysenteriae* are the most common causes, and *S sonnei* is a rare cause worldwide.[73] A study in 2005 from Finland, however, revealed cases of ReA to *S sonnei, S flexneri*, and *S dysenteriae*, with *S sonnei* the most common cause.[74] The overall attack rate of *Shigella*-induced ReA in this study was 7% and another 2% had other reactive musculoskeletal symptoms including enthesitis. Of the subjects who developed ReA, 36% were HLA-B27 positive.

Shigella is phylogenetically indistinguishable from *Escherichia coli*, sharing all but 175 of 3235 open reading frames,[73] and recent reports have suggested that *E coli* might be an infrequent cause of ReA.[25–27] Despite these similarities, they behave differently. *Shigella* is a motile organism with the ability to invade human enterocytes, lyse intracellular vacuoles to enter the cytoplasm, and move from cell to cell. *E coli* can do none of these.[73] These capabilities likely are critical to the propensity to cause ReA. Similar to Ct and Cpn, bacterial DNA from *Shigella* has been demonstrated in the synovial tissue of patients who have ReA. In contrast, there have been no studies to detect viable organisms, only bacterial fragments.[48,52]

Campylobacter

Campylobacter jejuni infections are the leading cause of bacterial gastroenteritis reported in the United States.[75] It is estimated that 2.1 to 2.4 million cases of human campylobacter infections occur in the United States each year. The arthritis that develops usually is an oligo- or polyarticular arthritis, and it tends to be mild.[76] In contrasting to other types of ReA, inflammatory back pain is believed uncommon.[77]

A study in Finland in 2002 of 870 patients who had *Campylobacter*-positive stool cultures found that 7% of these individuals developed ReA.[76] The development of ReA was not associated with HLA-B27 in this study. Fourteen percent of affected individuals were HLA-B27 positive (similar to the background prevalence in Finland). The majority of cases were associated with *C jejuni* but *C coli* was another cause. Similar to patients who had *Salmonella* infection, children were far less likely to develop ReA after a *Campylobacter* infection. A recent systematic review suggested an attack rate of 1% to 5% of ReA after a *Campylobacter* infection and no significant association with HLA-B27.[77]

Yersinia

There are three species in the genus *Yersinia*, but only *Y enterocolitica* and *Y pseudotuberculosis* cause gastroenteritis. *Y enterocolitica* and *Y pseudotuberculosis* have been associated with ReA. Although *Yersinia* infections are not as common as some of the other enteric pathogens, some data suggest that *Yersinia* is particularly arthritogenic. A follow-up study in Denmark suggests that it was the most likely to cause ReA, with an attack rate of 23%.[25] In 1998, two different outbreaks of *Y pseudotuberculosis* were reported.[78,79] One occurred in Finland (serotype O:3) and resulted in 12% of affected individuals developing ReA.[78] The other occurred in Canada (serotype Ib) and 12% reported "joint pain" after their infection.[79]

As with the majority of the other known triggering microbes, two studies have attempted to localize *Yersinia* in the synovial tissue or fluid of affected individuals. Although both studies demonstrated that *Yersinia* does traffic to the joints,[49,53] one suggested that these *Yerisinae* are metabolically active[49] and the other demonstrated only bacterial degradation products.[53]

Other Possible Triggering Microbes

Many other organisms have been implicated as potential causes of ReA. These include *Ureaplasma urealyticum*, *Helicobacter pylori*, and various intestinal parasites. The majority of these are of single cases or small series. Because of the limited numbers, the pathophysiology is not well studied with these other organisms. Reports of ReA secondary to *E coli*,[25–27] *Clostridium difficile*,[80] and intravesicular bacille Calmette-Guérin[81] have garnered recent recognition.

PATHOPHYSIOLOGY
Triggering Microbes Persist

The triggering microbes and their associated molecular biology in relation to arthritis, specifically ReA, are discussed elsewhere in this issue in the article by Gerard and colleagues. A brief review is warranted. PCR technology occasionally has demonstrated the presence of chromosomal DNA from the known triggers in the synovial tissue of patients who have the postdysentery form of ReA.[48,52–54] Recent studies from many laboratories have demonstrated that Ct and Cpn, such as *Mycobacterium tuberculosis*, can undergo long-term, persistent infections,[50,51,58,59] and the role persistent Ct infections play in the genesis of ReA has been established. The role of bacterial persistence in chronic ReA is less well established. One difference is that these chlamydiae exist in a persistent metabolically active state whereas the postenteric organisms do not, with the possible exception of *Yersinia*.[49]

The causative bacteria (or bacterial fragments) of ReA occasionally have been demonstrated in the synovial tissue of who have with various types of arthritis, so the importance of this finding has been questioned.[82–84] Furthermore, bacterial DNA from various pathogens not associated with ReA have been discovered in synovial tissue.[60,85] Even viable chlamydial infections have been documented in the synovial tissue of patients who have osteoarthritis and asymptomatic volunteers, albeit to a much lower degree; background PCR positivity rates of approximately 5% to 20% for Ct in synovial samples have been reported.[59,61,86]

The importance of host genetic variability and host tolerance is highlighted by a certain percentage of the population harboring bacterial DNA from the enteric organisms or persistently viable chlamydial infections in their synovium. Various hosts might respond differently to the same pathogen, thereby manifesting different phenotypic expressions to these same organisms. Furthermore, in the case of Ct, there are several different serovars; these different serovars may portend diverse prognoses that include variable pathogenic sequelae. Despite this background PCR-positivity rate, data suggest these other groups of patients are far less likely to be positive for these organisms. A study comparing synovial tissue chlamydial PCR-positivity in patients who have suspected chlamydial-induced ReA versus an osteoarthritis control population demonstrated that the ReA subjects were significantly more likely to be positive for Ct or Cpn.[59]

The pattern of gene expression associated with persistently viable chlamydiae is significantly different from that seen during normal active infections. For example, during the persistent state, expression of the major outer membrane protein (omp1) gene and several genes required for the cell division process is severely down-regulated; this is coupled with an up-regulation of heat shock proteins (HSPs). HSPs in general are paramount to the persistent state of Ct and Cpn because they provide many functions involved with cell survival. Under stressful conditions, HSPs allow cells to survive lethal assaults by preventing protein denaturation.[87,88] The HSP-60 molecule, specifically, has many functions that seem important to the pathophysiology of ReA. HSP-60 has been shown to be pivotal in the inability of chlamydial-infected cells to undergo apoptosis.[89] These same molecules also are believed to play a role in antibiotic resistance[87] and potentially be immunogenic.[90] Despite HSPs' important role in the pathophysiology of Chlamydia-induced ReA, there are differences even within the Chlamydia genus. In the case of Ct, specifically, the persistent state is characterized by the differential up-regulation of three paralog HSP-60 genes (Ct110, Ct604, and Ct755).[91] There also are differences in cytokine and chemokine mRNA profiles demonstrated in human synovial tissue chronically infected with Ct versus Cpn.[58] Regardless of these differences, elimination of the HSPs likely is important in abrogating the pathogenic sequelae of Chlamydia-induced ReA or ReA in general. Such an accomplishment eliminates the immunogenic nidus itself or renders the infected cell more susceptible to apoptosis or therapy.

Host Response

The causative bacteria of ReA are incorporated intracellularly, in part or in whole, then taken from the site of initial infection and trafficked to the synovium. That which governs this process, however, is not yet evident. It also is not clear if their presence in the affected organs represents a trigger for an autoimmune response or if these organisms are the source of the inflammatory process. It seems that this phenomenon of host tolerance is multifactorial in nature.

Cellular Uptake

The causative organisms of ReA are incorporated into peripheral blood mononuclear cells (PBMCs) and persist intracellularly in synovial cells (primarily macrophages). How this process of intracellular uptake occurs is less apparent. Chlamydial infection, specifically, is initiated when the elementary body (EB) binds to the target eukaryotic cell. Intriguing recent evidence suggests that apolipoprotein E (ApoE4) that is adherent to the surface of Cpn EBs attaches to the host cell low-density lipoprotein receptor family carrying the EB with it; this is not true for Ct.[92] This could represent a truly remarkable adaptation of chlamydiae using a basic cellular function involving cell homeostasis as its pathway to host cell attachment and uptake.

Toll-like Receptors

The Toll-like receptors (TLRs) recognize extracellular pathogens and activate immune cell responses as part of the innate immune system. TLR-4 recognizes LPS, thereby potentially playing a role in the pathophysiology of ReA. TLR-4 deficient mice exposed to *Salmonella* demonstrate dramatically increased bacterial growth and demise.[93] Other animal data have shown that effective host clearance of Ct depends on appropriate TLR-4 expression by neutrophils.[94] TLR-4 functions as a coreceptor with CD14 for the detection of bacterial LPS.[95] PBMCs from eight patients who had *Salmonella* infections (four who had and four who did not have ReA) have been analyzed in the acute and recovery phases of the infection.[96] During the recovery phase, the patients who had ReA demonstrated down-regulation of CD14 whereas the response of those who did not have ReA was similar to that of healthy controls. Despite these animal and in vitro human studies implicating TLR-4 in the pathophysiology of ReA, in vivo human data suggest that genetic variants of TLR-2, but not TLR-4, are important in the development of ReA after a *S enteritidis* infection.[97]

Th1 Versus Th2 Response

Although the Th1 cytokines, such as tumor necrosis factor (TNF)-α, play a role in the clinical manifestations of ReA, their importance seems less important than that in other types of inflammatory arthritis.[98–100] This might be true particularly for chronic ReA. Data suggest that a Th2 cytokine profile is more typical. Compared with patients who have RA, patients who have ReA demonstrated significantly lower levels of TNF-α in their peripheral blood, and patients who had disease duration of greater than 6 months secreted significantly less TNF-α.[98] Similar findings have been demonstrated in the joints of patients who have ReA (ie, higher levels of interleukin 10 and lower levels of TNF-α and interferon (IFN)-γ, favoring a Th2 profile).[99,100]

Temporal relationships of these different Th1 and Th2 cytokines or blunting of initial cytokine response also might be important in disease manifestations and maintenance. Slight changes in the Th1/Th2 balance may explain the relapsing course frequently seen in chronic ReA. Alterations in the initial Th1/Th2 balance also may predispose to disease initiation. Animal data have demonstrated a lesser initial TNF-α, IFN-γ, and interleukin 4 response to chlamydial infection leading to decreased bacterial clearance.[101] Therefore, lower initial responses of these Th1 cytokines may increase the likelihood of developing ReA compared with those patients who are exposed to the causative organism, exhibit a more robust initial Th1 response, and do not develop ReA. Along these same lines, background cytokine levels favoring a Th2 response might contribute to bacterial persistence; in vitro data reveal that low levels of TNF-α and IFN-γ help promote the persistent state of Ct and Cpn.[102–104] Other data suggest a role for the Th3 response with expression of transforming growth factor $\beta2$ and granulocyte monocyte-colony stimulating factor.[105]

HLA-B27

The host factor associated most notably with the pathogenesis of the SpAs in general, and which has been associated with ReA, has an equally mysterious role as that of the entire host response. There are many theories regarding the precise role of HLA-B27, but none are proved. Because HLA-B27 is a class I histocompatability antigen, it has been postulated that HLA-B27 presents arthritogenic microbial peptides to T cells, stimulating an autoimmune response, so-called molecular mimicry.[106] Conversely, B27 itself may serve as the autoantigen that is targeted by the immune system.[107] It also is possible that exposure to the triggering bacteria may subvert self-tolerance to the B27 antigen, and animal data exist to support this notion.[108] Another theory suggests that the role of HLA-B27 may be to enhance invasion of the causative organisms, specifically *Salmonella*, into human intestinal epithelial cells.[109] It also has been suggested that *Salmonella* invasion leads to significant recognizable changes in the B27-bound peptide repertoire.[110] A similar study, however, found only minimal changes in the peptide repertoire.[111] Intracellular uptake of chlamydiae may not be altered by HLA-B27, but intracellular replication and formation of inclusion bodies might be suppressed by the cytoplasmic tail of this antigen.[112] If true, this could predispose the cell to chlamydial persistence. Conversely, it has been suggested that HLA-B27 has no influence on invasion or replication of Ct serovar L2 within cell lines.[113]

HLA-B27 has multiple alleles that could influence host response and disease susceptibility. Few studies have analyzed the specific HLA-B27 alleles in the setting of ReA. One recent study suggests that although HLA-B*2705 is the most common allele observed in B27 positive ReA patients, this allele is seen less frequently than in the other SpAs and in B27 healthy controls.[114] Another study suggests that HLA-B*5703 increases the risk for the classic triad of symptoms of ReA in a specific population.[115]

HLA-B27 is believed to increase susceptibility to ReA, but the data suggest there is too much emphasis placed on this HLA haplotype. The literature often states a HLA-B27 prevalence of 75% to 85% in ReA. A thorough search, however, reveals a reported range of 0% to 88%,[116,117] with the majority of the data suggesting an HLA-B27 prevalence of 30% to 50%.[67,70,71,74,76,118–120] Recent reports dictate that HLA-B27 has no role in determining postenteric ReA susceptibility;[27,37,76,77] the same likely is true for postchlamydial ReA.

Rather than truly increasing disease susceptibility, HLA-B27 might portend a different prognostication. Several large studies are in agreement that patients who are HLA-B27 positive have more severe symptoms, thereby making the condition more clinically apparent.[25,121] This haplotype also might increase risk for developing the complete triad of symptoms.[122] Therefore, HLA-B27 actually could function as a diagnostic bias rather than a true genetic susceptibility locus. This requires further study.

DIAGNOSTIC TESTS

There are diagnostic criteria available, but these are broad and rely on clinical symptoms only. The American College of Rheumatology criteria, published in 1981, require the presence of a peripheral arthritis occurring in association with urethritis or cervicitis.[2] The Third International Workshop on Reactive Arthritis in 1995 requires a peripheral arthritis with sacroiliac involvement and a preceding gastrointestinal or genitourinary infection.[3] The current American College of Rheumatology definition might be too limited in scope and the latter's reliance on a preceding infection could lead to underdiagnosis. Difficulties with these diagnostic criteria have been raised.[19] The traditional disease definition also suggests that ReA represents a sterile inflammatory arthritis, but data presented herein, specifically pertaining to chlamydiae, call this into question.

Although not pathognomonic for the condition, the documentation of the DNA presence of one of the causative organisms by PCR in synovial tissue or fluid of patients who fulfill the clinical criteria for ReA represents the most accurate means of diagnosing the condition. The contention that the synovium yields the most accurate results is supported by studies comparing the PCR results from synovial tissue and

PBMC in patients who have ReA. These data suggest that only a small minority of patients who are PCR positive for Ct in synovium were PCR positive in their PBMC.[59,123] Unfortunately, such synovial tissue analysis is not readily available for the majority of clinicians. Even when synovial tissue or fluid is obtained, the concordance rate of PCR results between PCR testing laboratories is low, suggesting it is a learned science.[124] It has been suggested that chlamydial IgG or IgA titers are useful at diagnosing patients who have persistent chlamydia infections.[125,126] The majority of these data, however, apply only to Cpn in disease states other than ReA. There also is cross-reactivity between chlamydial serotypes, so their usefulness has been questioned. Recent data advocate that serology positive for anti–HSP-60 IgG might be diagnostic of Ct-induced ReA,[124] but HSP is a conserved molecule with high potential for false-positive results. This contention merits further study. Stool and urogenital sampling for the causative organisms in patients who have chronic disease have been analyzed, but many patients test negative, limiting the usefulness of this approach.[127,128] Because more than half of affected patients are HLA-B27 negative and recent reports cited suggest it has no role in disease predilection, HLA-B27 should not be used as a diagnostic tool. Therefore, currently there is no practical diagnostic test.

ReA can follow two disease courses. The first is an acute syndrome occurring shortly after the triggering infection followed by gradual resolution of the symptoms; the second begins in a similar fashion yet can progress to chronicity, sometimes years. During the acute stage, individuals often display elevated acute phase reactants, such as an elevated erythrocyte sedimentation rate or C-reactive protein level. Conversely, patients who have chronic ReA typically display normal levels. Patients in the acute phase also might display other indicators of inflammatory response, including leukocytosis or thrombocytosis.

The radiographic features of ReA include sacroiliitis, periostitis, nonmarginal syndesmophytes, periosteal new bone formation, joint erosions, and joint space narrowing. These findings are apparent only on plain radiographs, however, with chronic disease. Syndesmophytes and sacroiliitis are more common in patients who have postvenereal ReA rather than in those who have postenteric ReA, but radiologic findings in lumbosacral spine radiographs are characteristically similar.[129] There may be a role for MRI or ultrasound (of the sacroiliac or other joints) to detect earlier changes, but neither has been formally studied in ReA.

TREATMENT
Nonsteroidal Anti-Inflammatory Drugs

A breadth of clinical experience suggests that nonsteroidal anti-inflammatory drugs (NSAIDs) help with the inflammatory arthritis associated with ReA, but there are no well-designed prospective trials analyzing their efficacy for this indication. Although helpful for the articular symptoms, they are not believed efficacious for the potential extra-articular symptoms of ReA. Data suggest that continuous use of NSAIDs might reduce radiographic progression for other types of SpAs, in particular ankylosing spondylitis;[130] however, it is not clear if the same might be true for chronic ReA.

Corticosteroids

Corticosteroids have limited benefit for the axial symptoms and may be more effective for the peripheral arthritis of ReA.[22] Local corticosteroid injections into affected joints may provide short-term relief. Topical corticosteroids also seem helpful for some of the extra-articular manifestations, such as iritis, circinate balanitis, and keratoderma blenorrhagicum. Because bacterial persistence is a hallmark pathophysiologic feature of ReA, there could be theoretic concerns with the use of systemic corticosteroids in ReA, particularly early in the disease course. There are no data, however, to distinguish whether or not corticosteroids have any impact on the long-term outcome of ReA.

Disease Modifying Antirheumatic Drugs

DMARDs have been used as treatments in patients who have chronic ReA because these patients can develop radiographic abnormalities with subsequent joint deformities if left untreated. The best-studied DMARD in the setting of ReA is sulfasalazine (SSZ). A placebo-controlled prospective trial of 134 subjects demonstrated a trend toward improvement with 62% of the participants on SSZ versus 47% on placebo demonstrating overall response (P = .089).[131] There were no significant improvements, however, in any of the individual clinical measures followed compared with placebo, including swollen and tender joint counts. Because SSZ is a treatment of inflammatory bowel disease and 67% of patients who have ReA have histologic evidence consistent with IBD on bowel biopsies,[132] this medication might be a good therapeutic option for patients who have chronic disease, particularly of the postenteric variety. Methotrexate, azathioprine, and cyclosporine have been advocated as potential treatments for ReA but never formally evaluated in a prospective trial.

Tumor Necrosis Factor Antagonists

The TNF-α antagonists have demonstrated great success in the treatment of other types of SpAs. There are potential theoretic concerns, however, regarding TNF-α antagonism in ReA. As discussed previously, lower levels of TNF-α have been demonstrated in ReA compared with other types of inflammatory arthritis and ReA is believed more of a Th2-driven disease.[98–100] Also, chlamydiae are the most common trigger of ReA[23,24] and might be a common cause of uSpA;[59] in vitro data suggest that persistent Ct and Cpn levels are inversely associated with TNF-α levels.[102–104] Conversely, patients who have ReA exhibit higher serum levels of TNF-α levels compared with normal controls,[105] so this might suggest that these patients would benefit from TNF-α antagonists.

There are no randomized trials in ReA to accurately assess the efficacy of anti-TNF therapy. Several case reports and a small open-label study suggest clinical benefit with these drugs in the treatment of ReA;[133–135] however, one patient in the small open-label trial required total knee replacement 6 months after beginning therapy.[133] In this same open-label study of etanercept, synovial PCR positivity for chlamydiae was followed with equivocal results, including two patients who became positive for this organism on treatment.[133] In preliminary experiments, the relative bacterial load in paired synovial tissue samples from a patient who had Ct -induced arthritis was assessed before and after several months of treatment with etanercept. Real-time PCR analyses demonstrated that the second biopsy sample held a bacterial load that was several-fold higher than that of the initial, pretreatment sample (A.P. Hudson, unpublished data, 2008). These initial observations support the contention that anti–TNF-α therapy may not be appropriate for extended use in patients who have chronic Chlamydia-induced arthritis. The general lack of viability of the postenteric organisms in the setting of ReA suggests that anti-TNF therapy might have more of a role in these patients. The usefulness of TNF-α antagonists in the treatment of ReA is unanswered.

Antibiotics

Because ReA clearly is triggered by bacteria and because, in the case of *Chlamydia*-induced ReA, the synovial-based long-term viability of the organism has been demonstrated, a potential role for antibiotics is suggested. Similar to the results with the TNF-antagonists, treatment of ReA with antibiotics has produced equivocal results, although these data are more abundant. The majority of the studies have proved antibiotic therapy ineffective, but some studies suggest benefit. Potential explanations for these apparent discordant results are discussed.

Studies assessing the long-term administration of doxycycline, ciprofloxacin, and azithromycin in ReA failed to show benefit.[120,136–138] There was no effort to separate postenteric from postvenereal patients in these trials, however. A trial assessing 3 months of treatment with lymecycline showed no benefit in patients who had postdysentery ReA, whereas there was improvement in patients who had *Chlamydia*-induced ReA.[139] A subgroup analysis of another trial demonstrating that ciprofloxacin had no benefit as a treatment for ReA suggested improvement in postchlamydial patients.[140] A follow-up of one of the aforementioned "negative" ciprofloxacin trials suggested that this antibiotic significantly improved long-term prognosis.[141] Finally, another study suggested significant improvement in patients who had postchlamydial ReA with a combination of knee synovectomy and 3 months of azithromycin.[142] Therefore, it seems that there may be benefit in the postchlamydial form but not ReA that is secondary to the postdysentery organisms.

Such inconsistent outcomes sometimes derive from the particular antibiotic used in a given study, because not all such drugs have equal efficacy against the triggering bacteria. To date little meaningful information is available relating to the synovial accessibility of antibiotics after standard oral administration. In general practice, the efficacy of antibiotic treatment for Ct or Cpn is assayed using in vitro systems during the acute chlamydial life cycle. Individuals who have *Chlamydia*-induced ReA, however, harbor persistent organisms with an attenuated life cycle, thus equivocating the validity of the standard means of testing for drug efficacy. The in vitro effect of standard concentrations of ciprofloxacin, ofloxacin, doxycycline, or azithromycin induced the persistent state rather than clearing the organism.[143–146] These same in vitro data suggest synergistic eradication of the persistent chlamydial infection with a combination of azithromycin and rifampin.[144] Furthermore, a 2004 study revealed significant improvement in patients who had presumed *Chlamydia*-induced ReA after 9 months of a combination of rifampin and doxycycline compared with doxycycline monotherapy; however, there was no placebo control.[118] Therefore, it is possible that a prolonged combination of antibiotics may eradicate the persistent state of chlamydiae along with its pathogenic sequelae, but more studies are needed.

SUMMARY

Although environmental exposures have been implicated as potential causes for nearly all chronic diseases, ReA is one of the few with a known bacterial trigger. This insight into disease initiation has led to significant advances in the pathophysiology of this condition. As disease pathophysiology often stays one step ahead of science, however, many of the mysteries that surrounded ReA remain unsolved, including the clinical implications of bacterial persistence. In similar fashion, HLA-B27 is believed important in determining disease susceptibility, yet recent data downplay its importance and suggest it might be a better predictor of disease severity. Although bacteria are known to trigger ReA, the role of antibiotics remains ill defined, although recent studies lend hope for combination antibiotics. Anti-TNF therapy has proved efficacious in the other SpAs, but sufficient data are lacking and theoretic concerns with their use remain. Just as epidemiologic studies have been hampered by an incomplete historical review resulting in multiple eponyms for ReA, it is likely that the pathophysiology that surrounds disease initiation needs to be targeted in hopes of finding a definitive treatment.

REFERENCES

1. Parker CT, Thomas D. Reiter's syndrome and reactive arthritis. J Am Osteopath 2000;100(2):101–4.
2. Willkens RF, Arnett FC, Bitter T, et al. Reiter's syndrome: evaluation of preliminary criteria for definite disease. Arthritis Rheum 1981;24:844–9.
3. Kingsley G, Sieper J. Third International Workshop on Reactive Arthritis. 23–26 September 1995, Berlin, Germany. Ann Rheum Dis 1996;55:564–84.
4. Reiter H. Uber eine bisher unerkannate Spirochateninfektion (Spirochetosis arthritica). Dtsch Med Wochenschr 1916;42:1535–6.
5. Fiessinger M, Leroy E. Contribution a l'etude d'une epidemie de dysenterie dans le somme. Bull Mem Soc Med Hop Paris 1916;40:2030–69.
6. Llydce. Hippocratic writing. New York: Pelican Books; 1978. p. 229.
7. Allison DJ. Christopher Columbus: the first case of Reiter's disease in the old world? Lancet 1980;2:1309.
8. Sharp JT. Reiter's syndrome. In: Hollander JH, McCarthy DJ, editors. Arthritis and allied conditions. 8th edition. Philadelphia: Lea and Febiger; 1979. p. 1223–9.
9. Sydenham T. The works of Thomas Sydenham, M.D. Translated by RG Latham. London: Sydenham Society, II; 1848. p. 257–9.
10. Stoll M. De l'arthrite dysenterique. Arch Med Gen Trop 1869;14:29–30.
11. Yvan AU. Observation sur une metastase de gonorrhee. Ann Soc Med Prat de Montpellier 1806;119–25.
12. Brodie BC. Pathological and surgical observations on diseases of the joints. London: Longman; 1818. p. 54.
13. Launois MPE. Arthropaties recidivantes amythrophie generalize troubles trophiques multiples. D'origine blennofthalmique. Bull Mem Soc Med Hop Paris 1897; 14:93–104.
14. Cooper A. On gonorrhoeal rheumatism. On gonorrhoeal ophthalmia. Lancet 1824;2:273–4.
15. Bauer W, Engelmann EP. Syndrome of unknown aetiology characterized by urethritis, conjunctivitis, and arthritis (so-called Reiter's Disease). Trans Assoc Am Physicians 1942;57:307–8.
16. Lu DW, Katz KA. Declining use of the eponym "Reiter's Syndrome" in the medical literature, 1998–2003. J Am Acad Dermatol 2005;53(4):720–3.
17. Wallace DJ, Weisman M. Should a war criminal be rewarded with eponymous distinction? The double life of Hans Reiter (1881–1969). J Clin Rheumatol 2000;6(1):49–54.
18. Panush RS, Wallace DJ, Dorff RE, et al. Retraction of the suggestion to use the term "Reiter's syndrome" sixty-five years later: the legacy of Reiter, a war criminal, should not be eponymic honor but rather condemnation. Arthritis Rheum 2007;56(2):693–4.
19. Braun J, Kingsley G, van der Heijde D, et al. On the difficulties of establishing a consensus on the definition of and diagnostic investigations of reactive arthritis. Results and discussion of a questionnaire prepared for the 4th

International Workshop on Reactive Arthritis, Berlin, Germany, July 3–6, 1999. J Rheumatol 2000;27:2185–92.

20. Michet CJ, Machado EB, Ballard DJ, et al. Epidemiology of Reiter's syndrome in Rochester, Minnesota 1950-1980. Arthritis Rheum 1988;31(3):428–32.
21. Leirisalo-Repo M, Suoranta H. Ten-year follow-up study on patients with Yersinia arthritis. Arthritis Rheum 1988;31:533–7.
22. Flores D, Marquez J, Garza M, et al. Reactive arthritis: newer developments. Rheum Dis Clin North Am 2003;29(1):37–59.
23. Barth WF, Segal K. Reactive arthritis (Reiter's syndrome). Am Fam Physician 1999;60(2):499–503, 507.
24. Carter JD. Reactive arthritis: defined etiologies, emerging pathophysiology, and unresolved treatment. Infect Dis Clin North Am 2006;20(4):827–47.
25. Schiellerup P, Krogfelt KA, Locht H. A comparison of self-reported joint symptoms following infection with different enteric pathogens: effect of HLA-B27. J Rheumatol 2008;35(3):480–7 [Epub 2008 Jan 15].
26. Garg AX, Marshall J, Salvadori M, et al. Walkerton Health Study Investigators. A gradient of acute gastroenteritis was characterized, to assess risk of long-term health sequelae after drinking bacterial-contaminated water. J Clin Epidemiol 2006;59(4):421–8 [Epub 2006 Jan 27].
27. Townes JM, Deodhar AA, Laine ES, et al. Reactive arthritis following culture-confirmed infections with bacterial enteric pathogens in Minnesota and Oregon: a population-based study. Ann Rheum Dis 2008;67(12):1689–96 [Epub 2008 Feb 13].
28. Nelson HD, Helfand M. Screening for chlamydial infection. Am J Prev Med 2001; 20(3 Suppl):95–107.
29. Manavi K. A review on infection with Chlamydia trachomatis. Best Pract Res Clin Obstet Gynaecol 2006;20(6):941–51.
30. Stamm WE. Chlamydia trachomatis infections: progress and problems. J Infect Dis 1999;179(Suppl 2):380–3.
31. Saario R, Toivanen A. Chlamydia pneumonia as a cause of reactive arthritis. Br J Rheumatol 1993;32(12):1112.
32. Braun J, Laitko S, Treharne J, et al. Chlamydia pneumonia—a new causitive agent of reactive arthritis and undifferentiated oligoarthritis. Ann Rheum Dis 1994;53(2):100–5.
33. Hannu T, Puolakkainen M, Leirisalo-Repo M. Chlamydia pneumoniae as a triggering infection in reactive arthritis. Rheumatology (Oxford) 1999; 38(5):411–4.
34. Rudwaleit M, Richter S, Braun J, et al. Low incidence of reactive arthritis in children following a salmonella outbreak. Ann Rheum Dis 2001;60(11):1055–7.
35. Eastmond CJ, Rennie JA, Reid TM. An outbreak of Campylobacter enteritis— a rheumatological followup survey. J Rheumatol 1983;10(1):107–8.
36. Dworkin MS, Shoemaker PC, Goldoft MJ, et al. Reactive arthritis and Reiter's syndrome following and outbreak of gastroenteritis caused by Salmonella enteritidis. Clin Infect Dis 2001;33(7):1010–4.
37. Rohekar S, Tsui FW, Tsui HW, et al. Symptomatic acute reactive arthritis after an outbreak of salmonella. J Rheumatol 2008;35(8):1599–602 [Epub 2008 Jun 1].
38. Rich E, Hook EW 3rd, Alarcon GS, et al. Reactive arthritis in patients attending and urban sexually transmitted disease clinic. Arthritis Rheum 1996;39(7): 1172–7.
39. Whittum-Hudson JA, Hudson AP. Human chlamydial infections: persistence, prevalence, and prospects for the future. Nat Sci et Soc 2005;13:371–82.

40. Groseclose SL, Zaidi AA, Delisle SJ, et al. Estimated incidence and prevalence of genital *Chlamydia trachomatis* infections in the United States, 1996. Sex Transm Dis 1999;26(6):339–44.

41. Doran MF, Pond GR, Crowson CS, et al. Trends in incidence and morality in rheumatoid arthritis in Rochester, Minnesota, over a forty-year period. Arthritis Rheum 2002;46(3):625–31.

42. Soderlin MK, Borjesson O, Kautiainen H, et al. Annual incidence of inflammatory joint disease in a population based study in southern Sweden. Ann Rheum Dis 2002;61(10):911–5.

43. Iliopoulos A, Karras D, Ioakimidis D, et al. Change in the epidemiology of Reiter's syndrome (reactive arthritis) in the post-AIDS era? An analysis of cases appearing in the Greek Army. J Rheumatol 1995;22(2):252–4.

44. Leirisalo-Repo M, Hannu T, Mattila L. Microbial factors in spondyloarthropathies: insights from population studies. Curr Opin Rheumatol 2003;15(4):408–12.

45. Bardin T, Enel C, Cornelis F, et al. Antibiotic treatment of venereal disease and Reiter's syndrome in a Greenland population. Arthritis Rheum 1992;35(2): 190–4.

46. Doorduyn Y, Van Pelt W, Siezen CL, et al. Novel insight in the association between salmonellosis or campylobacteriosis and chronic illness, and the role of host genetics in susceptibility to these diseases. Epidemiol Infect 2008; 136(9):1225–34 [Epub 2007 Dec 7].

47. François RJ, Gardner DL, Degrave EJ, et al. Histopathologic evidence that sacroiliitis in ankylosing spondylitis is not merely enthesitis. Arthritis Rheum 2000; 43(9):2011–24.

48. Braun J, Tuszewski M, Eggens U, et al. Nested polymerase chain reaction strategy simultaneously targeting DNA sequences of multiple bacterial species in inflammatory joint diseases. I. Screening of synovial fluid samples of patients with spondyloarthropathies and other arthritides. J Rheumatol 1997;24(6): 1092–100.

49. Gaston JS, Cox C, Granfors K. Clinical and experimental evidence for persistent Yersinia infection in reactive arthritis. Arthritis Rheum 1999;42(10):2239–42.

50. Gerard HC, Branigan PJ, Schumacher HR Jr, et al. Synovial Chlamydia trachomatis in patients with reactive arthritis/Reiter's syndrome are viable but show aberrant gene expression. J Rheumatol 1998;25(4):734–42.

51. Gerard HC, Schumacher HR, El-Gabalawy H, et al. *Chlamydia pneumoniae* present in the human synovium are viable and metabolically active. Microb Pathog 2000;29(1):17–24.

52. Granfors K, Jalkanen S, Toivanen P, et al. Bacterial lipopolysaccharide in synovial fluid cells in Shigella triggered reactive arthritis 1992;19(3):500.

53. Nikkari S, Merilahti-Palo R, Saario R, et al. Yersinia-triggered reactive arthritis. Use of polymerase chain reaction and immunocytochemical in the detection of bacterial components from synovial specimens. Arthritis Rheum 1992;35(6): 682–7.

54. Nikkari S, Rantakokko K, Ekman P, et al. Salmonella-triggered reactive arthritis: use of polymerase chain reaction, immunocytochemical staining, and gas-chromatography-mass spectrometry in the detection of bacterial components from synovial fluid. Arthritis Rheum 1999;42(1):84–9.

55. Taylor-Robinson D, Gilroy CB, Thomas BJ, et al. Detection of *Chlamydia trachomatis* DNA in joints of reactive arthritis patients by polymerase chain reaction. Lancet 1992;340(8811):81–2.

56. Viitanen AM, Arstila TP, Lahesmaa R, et al. Application of the polymerase chain reaction and immunoflourescence to the detection of bacteria in Yersinia-triggered reactive arthritis. Arthritis Rheum 1991;34(1):89–96.

57. Rahman MU, Hudson AP, Schumacher HR. Chlamydia and Reiter's syndrome (reactive arthritis). Rheum Dis Clin North Am 1992;18:67–79.

58. Gerard HC, Wang Z, Whittum-Hudson JA, et al. Cytokine and chemokine mRNA produced in synovial tissue chronically infected with *Chlamydia trachomatis* and *C. pneumoniae*. J Rheumatol 2002;29(9):1827–35.

59. Carter JD, Gerard HC, Espinoza LR, et al. An analysis of Chlamydial infections as the etiology of chronic undifferentiated spondyloarthropathy. Arthritis Rheum 2008;58(9 Suppl):S2049 [abstract].

60. Gerard HC, Wang Z, Wang GF, et al. Chromosomal DNA from a variety of bacterial species is present in synovial tissue from patients with various forms of arthritis. Arthritis Rheum 2001;44(7):1689–97.

61. Schumacher HR Jr, Arayssi T, Crane M, et al. *Chlamydia trachomatis* nucleic acids can be found in the synovium of some asymptomatic subjects. Arthritis Rheum 1999;42(6):1281–4.

62. Aggarwal A, Misra R, Chandrasekhar S, et al. Is undifferentiated seronegative spondyloarthropathy a forme fruste of reactive arthritis? Br J Rheumatol 1997;36(9):1001–4.

63. Telyatnikova N, Hill Gaston JS. Prior exposure to infection with *Chlamydia pneumoniae* can influence the T-cell-mediated response to *Chlamydia trachomatis*. FEMS Immunol Med Microbiol 2006;47(2):190–8.

64. McColl GJ, Diviney MB, Holdswaorth RF, et al. HLA-B27 expression and reactive arthritis susceptibility in two patient cohorts infected with *Salmonella typhimurium*. Aust N Z J Med 2000;30(1):28–32.

65. Buxton JA, Fyfe M, Berger S, et al. Reactive arthritis and other sequelae following sporadic *Salmonella typhimurium* infection in British Columbia, Canada: a case control study. J Rheumatol 2002;29(10):2154–8.

66. Hannu T, Mattila L, Siitonen A, et al. Reactive arthritis following an outbreak of *Salmonella typhimuriom* phage type 193 infection. Ann Rheum Dis 2002;61(3):264–6.

67. Inman RD, Johnston ME, Hodge M, et al. Postdysenteric reactive arthritis. A clinical and immunogenetic study following an outbreak of salmonellosis. Arthritis Rheum 1988;31(11):1377–83.

68. Lee AT, Hall RG, Pile KD. Reactive joint symptoms following an outbreak of *Salmonella typhimurium* phage tyoe 135a. J Rheumatol 2005;32(3):524–7.

69. Locht H, Kihlstrom E, Lindstrom FD. Reactive arthritis after Salmonella among medical doctors—study of an outbreak. J Rheumatol 1993;20(5):845–8.

70. Mattila L, Leirisalo-Repo M, Koskimies S, et al. Reactive arthritis following an outbreak of Salmonella infection in Finland. Br J Rheumatol 1994;33(12):1136–41.

71. Mattila L, Leirisalo-Repo M, Pelkonene P, et al. Reactive arthritis following an outbreak of Salmonella Bovismorbificans infection. J Infect 1998;36(3):289–95.

72. Paronen J. Reiter's disease: a study of 344 cases observed in Finland. Acta Med Scand 1948;131(Suppl 212):1–112.

73. Gaston JS. Shigella induced reactive arthritis. Ann Rheum Dis 2005;64:517–8.

74. Hannu T, Mattila L, Siitonen A, et al. Reactive arthritis attributable to Shigella infection: a clinical and epidemiological nationwide study. Ann Rheum Dis 2005;64(4):594–8.

75. Altekruse SF, Stern NJ, Fields PI, et al. *Campylobacter jejuni*—an emerging foodborne pathogen. Emerg Infect Dis 1999;5(1):28–35.
76. Hannu T, Mattila L, Rautelin H, et al. Campylobacter-triggered reactive arthritis: a population-based study. Rheumatology 2002;41:312–8.
77. Pope JE, Krizova A, Garg AX, et al. Campylobacter reactive arthritis: a systematic review. Semin Arthritis Rheum 2007;37(1):48–55 [Epub 2007 Mar 13].
78. Hannu T, Mattila L, Nuorti JP, et al. Reactive arthritis after an outbreak of *Yersinia pseudotuberculosis* serotype O:3 infection. Ann Rheum Dis 2003;62(9): 866–9.
79. Press N, Fyfe M, Bowie W, et al. Clinical and microbiological follow-up of an outbreak of *Yersinia pseudotuberculosis* serotype Ib. Scand J Infect Dis 2001; 33(7):523–6.
80. Birnbaum J, Bartlett JG, Gelber AC. Clostridium difficile: an under-recognized cause of reactive arthritis? Clin Rheumatol 2008;27(2):253–5 [Epub 2007 Sep 28].
81. Tinazzi E, Ficarra V, Simeoni S, et al. Reactive arthritis following BCG immunotherapy for urinary bladder carcinoma: a systematic review. Rheumatol Int 2006;26(6):481–8.
82. Cox CJ, Kempsell KE, Gaston JS. Investigation of infectious agents associated with arthritis by reverse transcription PCR of bacterial rRNA. Arthritis Res Ther 2003;5(1):R1–8.
83. Cuchacovich R, Japa S, Huang WQ, et al. Detection of bacterial DNA in Latin American patients with reactive arthritis by polymerase chain reaction and sequencing analysis. J Rheumatol 2002;29(7):1426–9.
84. Wilkinson NZ, Kingsley GH, Jones HW, et al. The detection of DNA from a range of bacterial species in the joints of patients with a variety of arthritidies using a nested, broad-range polymerase chain reaction. Rheumatology 1999;38(3): 260–6.
85. Siala M, Jaulhac B, Gdoura R, et al. Analysis of bacterial DNA in synovial tissue of Tunisian patients with reactive and undifferentiated arthritis by broad-range PCR, cloning and sequencing. Arthritis Res Ther 2008;10(2):R40 [Epub 2008 Apr 14].
86. Olmez N, Wang GF, Li Y, et al. Chlamydial nucleic acids in synovium in osteoarthritis: what are the implications? J Rheumatol 2001;28(8):1874–80.
87. Zugel U, Kaufmann SH. Role of heat shock proteins in protection from and pathogenesis of infectious diseases. Clin Microbiol Rev 1999;12(1):19–39.
88. Zugel U, Kaufmann SH. Immune response against heat shock proteins in infectious diseases. Immunobiology 1999;201(1):22–35.
89. Dean D, Powers VC. Persistent *Chlamydia trachomatis* infections resist apoptotic stimuli. Infect Immun 2001;69(4):2442–7.
90. Curry AJ, Portig I, Goodall JC, et al. T lymphocyte lines isolated from atheromatous plaque contain cells capable of responding to Chlamydia antigens. Clin Exp Immunol 2000;121(2):261–9.
91. Gerard HC, Whittum-Hudson JA, Schumacher HR, et al. Differential expression of three *Chlamydia trachomatis* hsp60-encoding genes in active vs. persistent infections. Microb Pathog 2004;36(1):35–9.
92. Gérard HC, Fomicheva E, Whittum-Hudson JA, et al. Apolipoprotein E4 enhances attachment of *Chlamydophila* (*Chlamydia*) *pneumoniae* elementary bodies to host cells. Microb Pathog 2008;44(4):279–85 [Epub 2007 Oct 18].
93. Vazquez-Torres A, Vallance BA, Bergman MA, et al. Toll-like receptor 4 dependence of innate and adaptive immunity to Salmonella: importance of the Kupffer cell network. J Immunol 2004;172(10):6202–8.

94. Zhang X, Glogauer M, Zhu F, et al. Innate immunity and arthritis: neutrophil Rac and toll-like receptor 4 expression define outcomes in infection-triggered arthritis. Arthritis Rheum 2005;52(4):1297–304.
95. Rallabhandi P, Bell J, Boukhvalova MS, et al. Analysis of TLR4 polymorphic variants: new insigths itno TLR4/MD-2/CD14 stoichiometry, structure, and signaling. J Immunol 2006;177(1):322–32.
96. Kirveskari J, He Q, Holmstrom T, et al. Modulation of peripheral blood mononuclear cell activation status during Salmonella-triggered reactive arthritis. Arthritis Rheum 1999;42(10):2045–54.
97. Tsui FW, Xi N, Rohekar S, et al. Toll-like receptor 2 variants are associated with acute reactive arthritis. Arthritis Rheum 2008;58(11):3436–8.
98. Braun J, Yin Z, Spiller I, et al. Low secretion of tumor necrosis factor alpha, but no other Th1 or Th2 cytokines, by peripheral blood mononuclear cells correlates with chronicity in reactive arthritis. Arthritis Rheum 1999;42(10):2039–44.
99. Thiel A, Wu P, Lauster R, et al. Analysis of the antigen-specific T cell response in reactive arthritis by flow cytometry. Arthritis Rheum 2000;43(12):2834–42.
100. Yin Z, Braun J, Neure L, et al. Crucial role of interleukin-10/interleukin-12 balance in the regulation of the type 2 T helper cytokine response in reactive arthritis. Arthritis Rheum 1997;40(10):1788–97.
101. Inman RD, Chiu B. Early cytokine profiles in the joint define pathogen clearance and severity of arthritis in Chlamydia-induced arthritis in rats. Arthritis Rheum 2006;54(2):499–507.
102. Ishihara T, Aga M, Hino K, et al. Inhibition of chlamydia trachomatis growth by human interferon-alpha: mechanisms and synergistic effect with interferon-gamma and tumor necrosis factor-alpha. Biomed Res 2005;26(4):179–85.
103. Perry LL, Feilzer K, Caldwell HD. Immunity to Chlamydia trachomatis is mediated by T helper 1 cells through IFN-gamma-dependent and –independent pathways. J Immunol 1997;158(7):3344–52.
104. Takano R, Yamaguchi H, Sugimoto S, et al. Cytokine response of lymphocytes persistent infected with Chlamydia pneumoniae. Curr Microbiol 2005;50(3):160–6.
105. Rihl M, Gu J, Baeten D, et al. Alpha beta but not gamma delta T cell clones in synovial fluids of patients with reactive arthritis show active transcription of tumour necrosis factor alpha and interferon gamma. Ann Rheum Dis 2004;63(12):1673–6.
106. Dulphy N, Peyrat MA, Tieng V, et al. Common intra-articular T cell expansions in patients with reactive arthritis: identical beta-chain junctional sequences and cytotoxicity toward HLA-B27. J Immunol 1999;162(7):3830–9.
107. Kuon W, Kuhne M, Busch DH, et al. Identification of novel human aggrecan T cell epitopes in HLA-B27 transgenic mice associated with spondyloarthropathy. J Immunol 2004;173(8):4859–66.
108. Popov I, Dela Cruz CS, Barber BH, et al. Breakdown of CTL tolerance to self HLA-B*2705 induced by exposure to Chlamydia trachomatis. J Immunol 2002;169(7):4033–8.
109. Saarinen M, Ekman P, Ikeda M, et al. Invasion of Salmonella into human intestinal epithelial cells is modulated by HLA-B27. Rheumatology (Oxford) 2002;41(6):651–7.
110. Maksymowych WP, Ikawa T, Yamaguchi A, et al. Invasion by Salmonella typhimurium induces increased expression of the LMP, MECL, and PA28 proteasome genes and changes in the peptide repertoire of HLA-B27. Infect Immun 1998;66(10):4624–32.

111. Ramos M, Alvarez I, Garcia-del-Portillo F, et al. Minimal alterations in the HLA-B27-bound peptide repertoire induced upon infection of lymphoid cells with *Salmonella typhimurium*. Arthritis Rheum 2001;44(7):1677–88.

112. Kuipers JG, Bialowons A, Dollmann P, et al. The modulation of chlamydial replication by HLA-B27 depends on the cytoplasmic domain of HLA-B27. Clin Exp Rheumatol 2001;19(1):47–52.

113. Young JL, Smith L, Matyszak MK, et al. HLA-B27 expression does not modulate intracellular *Chlamydia trachomatis* infection of cell lines. Infect Immun 2001; 69(11):6670–5.

114. Sampaio-Barros PD, Conde RA, Donadi EA, et al. Frequency of HLA-B27 and its alleles in patients with Reiter syndrome: comparison with the frequency in other spondyloarthropathies and a healthy control population. Rheumatol Int 2008; 28(5):483–6 [Epub 2007 Aug 24].

115. Díaz-Peña R, Blanco-Gelaz MA, Njobvu P, et al. Influence of HLA-B*5703 and HLA-B*1403 on susceptibility to spondyloarthropathies in the Zambian population. J Rheumatol 2008;35(11):2236–40 [Epub 2008 Oct 15].

116. Thomson GT, Chiu B, De Rubeis D, et al. Immunoepidemiology of post-Salmonella reactive arthritis in a cohort of women. Clin Immunol Immunopathol 1992; 64(3):227–32.

117. Leirisalo-Repo M, Helenius P, Hannu T, et al. Long-term prognosis of reactive salmonella arthritis. Ann Rheum Dis 1997;56(9):516–20.

118. Carter JD, Valeriano J, Vasey FB. A prospective, randomized 9-month comparison of doxycycline vs. doxycycline and rifampin in undifferentiated spondyloarthritis—with special reference to Chlamydia-induced arthritis. J Rheumatol 2004;31(10):1973–80.

119. Hannu T, Kauppi M, Tuomala M, et al. Reactive arthritis following an outbreak of *Campylobacter jejuni* infection. J Rheumatol 2004;31(3):528–30.

120. Kvien TK, Gaston JS, Bardin T, et al. Three-month treatment of reactive arthritis with azithromycin: A EULAR double-blind, placebo-controlled study. Ann Rheum Dis 2004;63(9):1113–9.

121. Sonkar GK, Usha. Role of HLA B27 in diagnosis of seronegative spondyloarthropathies. Indian J Pathol Microbiol 2007;50(4):908–13.

122. Girschick HJ, Guilherme L, Inman RD, et al. Bacterial triggers and autoimmune rheumatic diseases. Clin Exp Rheumatol 2008;26(1 Suppl 48):S12–7.

123. Jendro MC, Raum E, Schnarr S, et al. Cytokine profile in serum and synovial fluid of arthritis patients with *Chlamydia trachomatis* infection. Rheumatol Int 2005; 25(1):37–41 [Epub 2003 Oct 31].

124. Kuipers JG, Sibilia J, Bas S, et al. Reactive and undifferentiated arthritis in North Africa: use of PCR for detection of *Chlamydia trachomatis*. Clin Rheumatol 2009; 28(1):11–6 [Epub 2008 Aug 8].

125. den Hartog JE, Land JA, Stassen FR, et al. Serological markers of persistent *C. trachomatis* infections in women with tubal factor subfertility. Hum Reprod 2005; 20(4):986–90.

126. Huittinen T, Leinonen M, Tenkanen L, et al. Synergistic effect of persistent *Chlamydia pneumoniae* infection, autoimmunity, and inflammation on coronary risk. Circulation 2003;107(20):2566–70.

127. Schnarr S, Putschky N, Jendro MC, et al. Chlamydia and Borrelia DNA in synovial fluid of patients with early undifferentiated oligoarthritis: results of a prospective study. Arthritis Rheum 2001;44(11):2679–85.

128. Wollenhaupt J, Schnarr S, Kuipers JG. Bacterial antigens in reactive arthritis and spondarthritis. Rational use of laboratory testing in diagnosis and follow-up. Baillieres Clin Rheumatol 1998;12(4):627–47.
129. Mannoja A, Pekkola J, Hämäläinen M, et al. Lumbosacral radiographic signs in patients with previous enteroarthritis or uroarthritis. Ann Rheum Dis 2005;64(6): 936–9 [Epub 2004 Nov 11].
130. Wanders A, Heijde D, Landewé R, et al. Nonsteroidal antiinflammatory drugs reduce radiographic progression in patients with ankylosing spondylitis: a randomized clinical trial. Arthritis Rheum 2005;52(6):1756–65.
131. Clegg DO, Reda DJ, Weisman MH, et al. Comparison of sulfasalazine and placebo in the treatment of reactive arthritis (Reiter's syndrome). A Department of Veterans Affairs Cooperative Study. Arthritis Rheum 1996;39(12):2021–7.
132. Cuvelier C, Barbatis C, Mielants H, et al. Histopathology of intestinal inflammation related to reactive arthritis. Gut 1987;28(4):394–401.
133. Flagg SD, Meador R, Hsia E, et al. Decreased pain and synovial inflammation after etanercept therapy in patients with reactive and undifferentiated arthritis: an open-label trial. Arthritis Rheum 2005;53(4):613–7.
134. Haibel H, Brandt J, Rudawaleit M, et al. Therapy of chronic enteral reactive arthritis with infliximab [abstract]. Ann Rheum Dis 2003;62:AB0380.
135. Oili KS, Niinisalo H, Korpilahde T, et al. Treatment of reactive arthritis with infliximab. Scand J Rheumatol 2003;32(2):122–4.
136. Smieja M, MacPherson DW, Kean W, et al. Randomised, blinded, placebo controlled trial of doxycycline for chronic seronegative arthritis. Ann Rheum Dis 2001;60(12):1088–94.
137. Wakefield D, McCluskey P, Verma M, et al. Ciprofloxacin treatment does not influence course or relapse rate of reactive arthritis and anterior uveitis. Arthritis Rheum 1999;42(9):1894–7.
138. Yli-Kerttula T, Luukkainen R, Yli-Kerttula U, et al. Effect of a three month course of ciprofloxacin on the outcome of reactive arthritis. Ann Rheum Dis 2000;59(7): 565–70.
139. Lauhio A, Leirisalo-Repo M, Lahdevirta J, et al. Double-blind, placebo-controlled study of three-month treatment with lymecycline in reactive arthritis, with special reference to Chlamydia arthritis. Arthritis Rheum 1991;34(1):6–14.
140. Sieper J, Fendler C, Laitko S, et al. No benefit of long-term ciprofloxacin in patients with reactive arthritis and undifferentiated oligoarthritis: a three-month, multicenter, double-blind, randomized, placebo-controlled study. Arthritis Rheum 1999;42(7):1386–96.
141. Yli-Kerttula T, Luukkainen R, Yli-Kerttula U, et al. Effect of three month course of ciprofloxacin on the late prognosis of reactive arthritis. Ann Rheum Dis 2003; 62(9):880–4.
142. Pavlica L, Nikolic D, Magic Z, et al. Successful treatment of postvenereal reactive arthritis with synovectomy and 3 months' azithromycin. J Clin Rheumatol 2005;11(5):257–63.
143. Dreses-Werringloer U, Padubrin I, Jurgens-Saathoff B, et al. Persistence of *Chlamydia trachomatis* is induced by ciprofloxacin and ofloxacin in vitro. Antimicrob Agents Chemother 2000;44(12):3288–97.
144. Dreses-Werringloer U, Padubrin I, Zeidler H, et al. Effects of azithromycin and rifampin on *Chlamydia trachomatis* infection in vitro. Antimicrob Agents Chemother 2001;45(11):3001–8.

145. Morrissey I, Salman H, Bakker S, et al. Serial passage of *Chlamydia* spp. In sub-inhibitory fluoroquinolone concentrations. J Antimicrob Chemother 2002;49(5): 757–61.
146. Suchland RJ, Geisler WM, Stamm WE. Methodologies and cell lines used for antimicrobial susceptibility testing of *Chlamydia* spp. Antimicrob Agents Chemother 2003;47(2):636–42.

Soft Tissue Infections

Karina D. Torralba, MD*, Francisco P. Quismorio, Jr., MD

KEYWORDS

- Tenosynovitis • Bursitis • Pyomyositis • Necrotizing fasciitis
- Soft tissue infections • Ultrasonography

Infections are a leading cause of morbidity and mortality among patients who have rheumatic diseases.[1] Short-term outcomes were poor for patients who had rheumatic diseases admitted to the ICU, especially for those who had infections.[2] Several risk factors, including inherent immunologic abnormalities, genetics, and use of medications, such as corticosteroids and biologics, have been associated with the development of infections in patients who have rheumatic diseases.[3–5] Regardless of which agent is used, it has been found that 20.5% of patients who have rheumatoid arthritis (RA) treated with tumor necrosis factor inhibitors are at risk for developing serious skin and soft tissue infections.[6] This article reviews clinical features and challenges in the diagnosis and management of necrotizing fasciitis, septic tenosynovitis, septic bursitis, and pyomyositis, especially in relation to patients who have rheumatic diseases.

NECROTIZING FASCIITIS

Necrotizing fasciitis is a rare but life-threatening rapidly progressive bacterial infection of subcutaneous tissue and superficial fascia that is potentially fatal if appropriate treatment measures are not instituted quickly. Usually occurring after compromised skin integrity because of infection or trauma, necrotizing fasciitis is manifested by flagrant inflammatory features at the site of infection that may be accompanied by hemorrhagic bullae, necrosis, and crepitus, often unresponsive to antibiotic therapy.[7] Systemic septic features may arise. Overall mortality rate in patients who have rheumatic diseases is 27.8%.[8] Diabetes mellitus, surgery, trauma, and peripheral vascular disease are predisposing conditions.[7] Necrotizing fasciitis frequently affects the lower limbs, although any site may be involved, including the head and neck.

Necrotizing fasciitis can be a polymicrobial infection with a mixture of Gram-positive and Gram-negative aerobes and anaerobes (Type I) or it can be monomicrobial (Type II) with group A streptococcus being the most common isolate.[7,9] Infections associated with methicillin-resistant *Staphylococcus aureus* (MRSA) are a major problem.[10] Clinical assessments have been developed using a skin staging system[11]

Division of Rheumatology, Department of Internal Medicine, Keck School of Medicine, University of Southern California, 2011 Zonal Avenue, HMR 711, Los Angeles, CA 90033, USA
* Corresponding author.
E-mail address: ktorrabl@usc.edu (K.D. Torralba).

Rheum Dis Clin N Am 35 (2009) 45–62
doi:10.1016/j.rdc.2009.03.002
0889-857X/09/$ – see front matter © 2009 Elsevier Inc. All rights reserved.
rheumatic.theclinics.com

and laboratory parameters.[12] Early diagnosis and aggressive therapy with antibiotics and effective surgical debridement are essential for a favorable outcome.[7,13] CT and ultrasonography (US) may show changes in fascia, subcutaneous fat, and muscle, although more histopathologic diagnosis is still needed.[14,15] Debridement also serves a diagnostic purpose, with tissue sampling and culture results allowing identification of optimal antibiotic therapy. The use of hyperbaric oxygen remains controversial; however, it may be a useful adjunct in clostridial infection.[16]

Necrotizing fasciitis in patients who have rheumatic disease has been reported; however, it is not clear whether the incidence is higher in this patient group when compared with that of the general population.[8] Several reports of necrotizing fasciitis occurring in patients who have systemic lupus erythematosus (SLE) have been reported.[8,17–21] Kamran and colleagues[20] found eight cases of necrotizing fasciitis in a cohort of 449 patients who had SLE followed between 1994 and 2007. Although no direct associations could be established, the presence of hypo-albuminemia, lymphopenia, active disease, nephritis, prior history of significant infections, and use of immunosuppressives (especially corticosteroids) were noted in their patients. Fatal necrotizing fasciitis due to *Streptococcus pneumoniae* was reported in a newly diagnosed patient who had SLE who was on no immunosuppressive therapy.[21]

Necrotizing fasciitis has also been reported in patients who have polymyositis,[22,23] antisynthetase syndrome,[24] and dermatomyositis.[25] Group A β-hemolytic streptococcus,[22,23] and *Streptococcus pyogenes*[23] and *Staphylococcus aureus*[25] were isolated.

Isolated cases of necrotizing fasciitis in association with Still disease, RA,[26–34] and mixed connective tissue disease[35] have been reported. As in other patient groups, the lower extremities were most commonly involved. Periorbital necrotizing fasciitis has been observed in RA[28] and in dermatomyositis.[23] One case was preceded by diverticulitis[27] and another case had profound thrombocytopenia.[36] Fifteen patients who had gout complicated by necrotizing fasciitis had a severe course with septic shock, limb amputation, and a high mortality rate.[37] Cutaneous polyarteritis nodosa developed in a patient 6 weeks following a bout of necrotizing fasciitis attributable to group A β-hemolytic streptococcus.[38]

Necrotizing fasciitis has been reported to develop in patients on biologic agents for RA[26,34] and for dermatomyositis[25] and after intramuscular (IM) injection of nonsteroidal anti-inflammatory drugs (NSAIDs). There are several published reports linking the use of IM NSAIDs and necrotizing fasciitis.[39–43] In two cases, IM diclofenac and tenoxicam into the thigh were given to two elderly people for gout and osteoarthritis, respectively, followed 2 days later by fulminant course of necrotizing fasciitis complicated by septic shock due to *Streptococcus pneumoniae* infection; one case resulted in multiple organ failure and death. It is suggested that IM injections can cause tissue trauma and can serve as a portal of infection even when done properly,[41] and that NSAIDs, through their anti-inflammatory activity, impair host defense by disrupting leukocyte function in producing cytokines and other soluble mediators.[40] A critical analysis of published reports on necrotizing fasciitis caused by group A streptococci concluded that although retrospective studies suggest that NSAIDs used to relieve the early nonspecific symptoms delay diagnosis and treatment, five prospective studies do not support NSAIDs as a risk factor, nor do they worsen established disease.[40] A recent case-control study found no independent association between NSAIDs and invasive group A streptococcal disease.[44]

Necrotizing fasciitis has also been reported following orthopedic procedures, such as rotator cuff repair[45] and anterior cruciate ligament construction.[46]

PYOMYOSITIS

Pyomyositis, known by numerous other names, including tropical myositis, temperate myositis, pyogenic myositis, suppurative myositis, myositis purulenta tropica, and epidemic abscess, is a relatively rare pyogenic infection of skeletal muscle. Delays in diagnosis are not uncommon. It can be misdiagnosed as thrombophlebitis, osteomyelitis, septic arthritis, neoplasm, hematoma, peritonitis, and muscle strain.[47,48] Complications, such as compartment syndrome, contiguous osteomyelitis, sepsis, and death, can occur.[49]

The pathogenesis of pyomyositis needs further clarification, although it is largely believed to involve bacteremia and muscle damage due to trauma or injury,[50,51] Conditions causing skin compromise, such as local injections, infections, and chronic inflammatory skin diseases, are believed to be predisposing risk factors. In most cases, the mechanism of disease is unknown. Bacteremia is noted in up to 35% of temperate cases and in 10% of tropical cases.[50] Intravenous drug use with or without endocarditis, and injection sites, both local and distant, have been noted.[50] Usually affecting the lower extremity and pelvic girdle muscles, the quadriceps is the most commonly affected muscle followed by the gluteal and iliopsoas muscles.[49,52] Less commonly affected sites include the abdominal wall,[53] chest wall, splenius capitis,[54] paraspinal,[55] and pelvic muscles. Multisite involvement is noted in 16% of cases.[49]

The clinical course is divided into three stages: invasive, suppurative, and sepsis. Fever, anorexia, and mild local symptoms, including nonspecific crampy muscle pain, are present during the first 2 weeks. Pain on weight-bearing along with restricted active and passive range of motion may be present.[56,57] Diagnosis is often made during the suppurative stage when high fever, chills, muscle swelling, fluctuance, and skin erythema are noted. Leukocytosis with neutrophilia and elevated markers of inflammation are nonspecific features. Serum creatine kinase may be normal. Left untreated, systemic toxicity unfolds over a few weeks.[50]

Pyomyositis was originally called tropical myositis because initial descriptions came from Africa, Asia, and other tropical areas; subsequent reports from temperate regions appeared. Tropical myositis has been described in all age groups, although there is a predominance of children and immunocompetent adults.[51] In temperate regions, pyomyositis is most prevalent among young adults and in those who have a history of immunosuppression, which probably accounts for the increasing incidence of cases in the United States.[49–51,58] There is a male predominance in both temperate and tropical cases. Trauma, including strenuous exercise, is noted in 30% and 50% of cases of tropical and temperate myositis, respectively. HIV infection increases risk for pyomyositis because of neutrophil dysfunction and other mechanisms.[51,59] Among HIV-infected people, pyomyositis usually occurred in those who had end-stage AIDS.[59] In a review of 246 HIV-negative cases, 119 (48%) had a comorbid medical condition, including diabetes mellitus (19%) and malignancy (10.6%), whereas a rheumatologic disorder was noted in 14 (5.7%) patients.[59] Pyomyositis involving lower extremity muscle groups has been reported in a patient who had RA[60] and relapsing Henoch-Schönlein nephritis.[56] Salmonella pyomyositis has been reported in a patient who had SLE.[61] Anterior tibial compartment syndrome as a complication has been reported in a patient who had RA.[62]

Staphylococcus aureus is the most common pathogen seen in up to 90% of cases,[48] followed by group A streptococcus and other organisms, including groups B, C, G streptococci, *Haemophilus influenza, Aeromonas hydrophila, Fusobacterium* sp, *Bartonella* sp, *Klebsiella pneumoniae* and other Gram-negative bacilli, anaerobes, *Salmonella* sp, *Candida* sp, *Cryptococcus*, and tuberculous and atypical mycobacteria.[50,63-68] Panton-Valentine leucocidin (PVL), a virulence factor associated with *Staphylococcus aureus*, has been implicated in a case of pyomyositis predated by recurrent furunculosis.[69] Among diabetic subjects who have thigh pyomyositis, oxacillin-resistant *Staphylococcus aureus* is an emerging offending organism.[70] PVL and SCCmec type in *Staphylococcus aureus* soft tissue infections seems to be related overall to a higher incidence of abscesses and mortality,[71] with PVL positivity present in most cases of infection due to MRSA.[71]

Diagnosis is established by cultures of specimens obtained during surgery or by imaging-guided aspiration.[72] Office-based US-guided aspiration of pus has been used.[65] US was useful in the early diagnosis of biceps pyomyositis in a patient who had Behçet disease receiving infliximab.[57] Specific radiographic changes may not be noted early in the disease.[48] US can show hyperechogenicity indicative of increased muscle swelling with edema, with areas of hypoechogenicity that can indicate muscle necrosis.[14] CT detects muscle swelling and fluid attenuation with rim enhancement.[15] MRI is notably more sensitive and is the preferred imaging technique of choice in early disease. MRI can define the location and extent of muscle damage.[47,48,73,74] Pathologic analysis has shown edematous separation of muscle fibrils and fibers, interfiber lymphocyte and plasma cell infiltration, followed by disintegration of myofibers.[50]

Effective treatment involves prompt institution of antibiotics coupled with surgical incision and drainage, especially in cases affecting deeper muscles. The mortality rate varies between 0.89% and 10%,[47] with sepsis as the main cause of death.[75] Gram-negative bacterial infections, bacteremia, and higher mortality rates have been noted in patients who have comorbidities.[76] APACHE II scoring at diagnosis has been suggested as an independent prognostic factor for mortality.[76]

Tuberculous Pyomyositis

Tuberculous pyomyositis is a rare manifestation of extrapulmonary tuberculosis and has been reported in immunocompromised and immunocompetent subjects.[77,78] Tuberculous pyomyositis alone without bone infection is noted to be rare.[79] This condition has been reported in a patient who had ankylosing spondylitis who developed sternocleidomastoid myositis after adalimumab therapy and successfully responded to antibiotics.[80] A retrospective study from an endemic area found that 1.8% of all culture-positive and histology-proven tuberculosis cases had muscle involvement either from contiguous or hematogenous spread or by traumatic inoculation.[81] Chest wall and paraspinal muscles were typically infected by contiguous spread, whereas hematogenous seeding involved multiple muscles of the limbs.[81]

SEPTIC TENOSYNOVITIS

Septic tenosynovitis can occur at any site; however, the flexor tendons and tendon sheaths of the digits of the hands are the most frequent sites. An outer parietal layer and an inner visceral layer with an intervening fluid-filled synovial space defines the tendon sheath. With pus accumulation, pressure increases in this sheath leading to tissue ischemia, necrosis, and tendon rupture.[82] The retinacular system of the flexors is contributory to the greater morbidity involved in septic flexor tenosynovitis.

The four cardinal signs of septic flexor hand tenosynovitis as originally described by Kanavel are: (a) uniform symmetric finger swelling, (b) digit held in partial flexion at rest, (c) tenderness, and (d) pain along the tendon sheath especially with passive digit extension.[83] Acute carpal tunnel syndrome is a rare presenting feature of pyogenic flexor tenosynovitis compressing the median nerve.[84,85] Septic tenosynovitis can present within hours to days of initial exposure. A history of trauma or a puncture wound, especially at flexor creases where the tendon sheath is most superficial to the skin, can be recalled by most patients. A history of animal or human bite, illicit drug use, or venereal disease exposure may help determine the causative organism. *Staphylococcus aureus*, *Staphylococcus epidermidis*, streptococci, enterococci, and Gram-negative organisms are the most commonly reported isolates.[50] Bite wounds typically involve more than one pathogen. In the absence of trauma, hematogenous spread should be considered, as in *Neisseria gonorrhea* infection. Tenosynovitis is seen in up to 68% of disseminated gonococcal infection and involves multiple sites, especially the extensor tendons in the wrists, fingers, toes, and ankles.[86–88] The presence of papules, hemorrhagic pustules, or vesicles in a patient who has tenosynovitis, especially in the wrists and dorsum of the hands, suggests a disseminated gonococcal infection.

The gold standard for the diagnosis of infectious tenosynovitis is a Gram stain and culture of synovial sheath fluid, obtained either by needle aspiration guided by imaging or at the time of surgery. US can demonstrate fluid collection and synovial thickening around the extensor tendon[14] and can be used to guide needle aspiration as noted in cases of infection due to *N gonorrhea*[88] and *Pasteurella multicoda*.[89] US is sensitive and specific in the evaluation of posterior tibial tendon tenosynovitis.[90] Timely empiric antibiotics should be started based on the nature of the injury and adjusted accordingly when results of diagnostic studies become available. For patients who have risk factors for infection with MRSA, such as intravenous drug use, recent hospitalization, or in geographic regions with high prevalence, therapy for this organism should be considered.[50] Surgery with open drainage or closed-catheter irrigation should not be delayed because of the potential for long-term morbidity.

Tuberculous and Atypical Mycobacterial Tenosynovitis

Tuberculous tenosynovitis, a rare manifestation of extrapulmonary tuberculosis, typically involves the flexor tendons of hand and wrist. The onset is insidious, with a slow-growing mass along the tendon followed later by pain and limitation of movement. An indolent clinical course and absence of systemic symptoms often contribute to delays in diagnosis.[91–93] Carpal tunnel syndrome may be a presenting complaint.[94] Risk factors include immunocompromised state, old age, and immigration from an endemic area; chronic diseases, including SLE and RA, may be present.[91,95–97] Tendons that are rarely involved include the tibialis anterior and Achilles tendons.[98–100] US and MRI may demonstrate minimal or no synovial fluid, in contrast to that seen in pyogenic tenosynovitis.[91] Tuberculin skin testing is often positive and a definitive diagnosis is confirmed by histopathology, culture, or polymerase chain reaction (PCR) test on tissue obtained at surgery.[101]

Nontuberculous mycobacteria (NTM) are nonmotile acid-fast bacilli that are ubiquitous in the soil and water. The global AIDS epidemic and the increasing use of immunosuppressive agents have in part led to the increasing frequency of infections by these organisms, including musculoskeletal and soft tissue infections. Tenosynovitis due to NTM is rare but shares clinical and pathologic features with tuberculous cases. The pathogenic organisms include *Mycobacterium marinum*, *M nonchromogenicum*, *M heckshornense*, *M scrofulaceum*, *M intracellulare*, *M kansasii*, and *M avium complex*.[102–114] *M marinum*, a natural pathogen of fish, infects humans by inoculation of skin abrasions or punctures following contact most commonly in a fish tank or swimming pool.[115] Infections due to NTM can be protracted and recurrent. Surgical debridement, tissue cultures, and histopathologic analysis are critical in establishing diagnosis.[116]

A considerable delay in diagnosis continues to be noted in reported cases of myco-bacterial and fungal tenosynovitis because of their chronic protracted course and lack of distinguishing clinical features. Additionally, certain caveats in mycobacterial inves-tigation include frequently negative acid-fast stains because of low bacterial burden and Lowenstein-Jensen cultures requiring up to 8 weeks because of the slow-growing nature of these organisms. Caseating granulomas on histopathology support the diag-nosis; however, studies on tuberculous arthritis revealed absence of granulomatous inflammation in 12% of cases, whereas in 27% noncaseating granulomas were seen.[117]

MRI may help differentiate tenosynovitis caused by inflammatory arthritis from tuberculous tenosynovitis in the wrist. Simple homogenous fluid signal in the tendon sheath is a typical finding in the former, whereas in the latter the MRI shows thickened synovium and heterogenous synovial fluid with scattered foci of low signal in the tendon sheath.[118,119] The presence of bone erosions, osteomyelitis, and median nerve encasement favor a diagnosis of tuberculous tenosynovitis.[119] Rice bodies can be seen in tuberculous and in nontuberculous tenosynovitis and bursitis by US and MRI.[120,121]

Tenosynovitis Due to Fungi and Other Pathogens

Localized tenosynovitis caused by *Histoplasma capsulatum* can occur in the absence of disseminated disease.[122] In endemic areas, histoplasma infection should be considered in the differential diagnosis of chronic tenosynovitis. *Cryptococcus neofor-mans* causing tenosynovitis has been reported in immunocompromised subjects, including a patient receiving adalimumab.[123,124] Other fungal organisms implicated in infectious tenosynovitis include *Blastomyces dermatitidis* and *Sporothrix schenckii*.[125,126]

Two rare human pathogens, *Cellulosimicrobium cellulans*, a Gram-positive bacte-rium, and *Prototheca* sp, an achlorophyllic algae, have recently been shown to cause septic tenosynovitis.[127,128]

Tenosynovitis of the extensor tendons of the hands can be a feature of leprosy.[129] The combination of tenosynovitis, thickened peripheral nerve, and inflammatory poly-arthritis in a patient from an endemic area should raise the possibility of leprosy even in the absence of skin lesions.[129]

Q fever, a worldwide zoonosis caused by *Coxiella burnetii*, rarely presents as an iso-lated osteoarticular infection, including chronic tenosynovitis. Granulomatous inflam-mation in the synovium must be differentiated from mycobacterial and fungal infections by specific Q fever serologic tests and by PCR test on the tissue specimen.[130]

SEPTIC BURSITIS

Routes of infection differ for deep bursae and superficial bursae. Superficial bursae, especially the olecranon and prepatellar bursae, become infected most commonly by direct traumatic percutaneous inoculation or by contiguous spread from an adja-cent infected site, such as cellulitis. Prepatellar septic bursitis is more common than olecranon septic bursitis in hospital-based studies, whereas other studies have reported a reversed frequency.[131] On the other hand, deep bursae, such as the sub-acromial bursa, are more likely to become infected by hematogenous spread or by inoculation attributable to previous local injection.[50,132,133] As part of the evaluation, a history of repetitive or acute trauma related to work, recreation, local injections, or even physical disabilities or other postural tendencies that cause restricted movement (such as wheelchair-bound individuals) should be elicited. Environmental exposures to pets or plants can also give clues to the cause of the disease. Chronic skin conditions and other comorbidities should be noted. Nonseptic bursitis due to gout, RA, seronegative spondyloarthropathies, and other inflammatory disorders, can become secondarily infected.

Clinical features include erythema, swelling, and pain with a point of maximal central tenderness. Fever, cellulitis, and other signs of skin compromise may be noted. *Staphylococcus aureus* is the most common isolate in more than 80% of cases.[50] Group B hemolytic streptococci are the next most common organism, followed by enterococci, Gram-negative organisms, and coagulase-negative staphylococci. In chronic bursitis, unusual organisms should be considered, including *M tuberculosis*, NTM, *Brucella* sp, fungi, or molds. *Prototheca* sp, an algae, has been reported to cause septic bursitis in patients who have malignancy.[134]

Because septic bursitis shares many clinical features with gouty and traumatic bursitis, bursal fluid aspiration and examination for crystals, Gram stain, and culture are essential. Imaging with US[14] and CT[15] can help in the diagnosis and localization of pathology. Although the sensitivity of the leukocyte count is limited and culture results are not immediately available, antibiotics should be initiated as soon as possible, initially targeting staphylococci and streptococci, and modified when results become available. Septic bursitis in immunosuppressed patients tends to be severe and more difficult to treat. Deep bursal infection requires more aggressive therapy than infected superficial bursae.[135] Bursal drainage may be needed in half of cases, either by incision or needle aspiration.[50] Bursectomy may be indicated in refractory cases.

Septic Olecranon Bursitis

A retrospective study of 118 patients who had septic olecranon bursitis in a Canadian home parenteral therapy program suggests that it is a common condition with an estimated populated-based incidence of 10 per 100,000 per year.[136] The majority of patients were males, mean age 44 years, employed in different occupations, including those that entail heavy physical work, and recalled a history of elbow injury. Comorbidities, including diabetes and liver cirrhosis, were noted in 30% of patients. Pain, swelling, and erythema over the olecranon bursa are the usual presenting features. Fever is noted in 20% to 86% of patients.[131,136] Septic olecranon bursitis may be mistaken for cellulitis, elbow arthritis, or nonseptic bursitis due to trauma, gout, RA, or other inflammatory arthritis. It can be accompanied by osteomyelitis[137] and cellulitis.[138] Reactive polyarthritis concomitant to septic olecranon bursitis due to *Staphylococcus aureus* has been described.[139] Direct invasion during traumatic skin injury is the usual route of infection. Aside from *Staphylococcus aureus* and streptococci, other organisms include *Brucella abortus*, *Haemophilus influenzae*, *Serratia marcescens*, and *Pseudomonas aeruginosa*. Rare causative organisms reported in immunocompromised hosts include molds *Paecilomyces lilacinus*[140] and *Exophiala oligosperma*,[141] and the algae *Prototheca wickerhamii*.[142] *Candida parapsilosis* was isolated in an immunocompetent subject who acquired the infection from a local steroid injection.[143]

Diagnosis is confirmed by pathogen isolation from bursal fluid culture. US can be useful in early stages to detect fluid collection and to guide needle aspiration.[144,145] Although MRI is valuable in excluding osteomyelitis or abscess, there is a significant overlap in findings associated with septic and nonseptic olecranon bursitis.[146] Septic olecranon bursitis can be adequately managed on an ambulatory basis in most cases with sequential intravenous followed by oral antibiotics, with surgery in refractory cases.[136]

Prepatellar and Infrapatellar Bursitis

Among several bursae around the knee, the prepatellar, infrapatellar, and deep patellar bursae seem to be more susceptible to infection than other bursae. Prepatellar septic bursitis occurs primarily in young and middle-aged males and occasionally in children.[147] Trauma is a significant predisposing factor as evident in its occurrence among carpet layers, college wrestlers, and other manual occupations.[131,148] Prepatellar bursitis due to *Staphylococcus aureus*, representing most probably a reactive process, has been reported in three patients who had 1-week duration of adjacent erysipelas.[149] The principal pathogenic organism is *Staphylococcus aureus*. Other pathogens recently reported include β-hemolytic streptococcus, *Sporothrix scheneckii*,[150] and *Brucella melitensis*.[151] Differential diagnoses include other peripatellar conditions causing pain and swelling, such as cellulitis and septic arthritis. Patellar osteomyelitis in children may be misdiagnosed as septic prepatellar bursitis.[152]

Infection of the deep patellar bursa, which is located deep to the patellar ligament and proximal to the insertion of the ligament to the tibial tubercle, is rarely reported. The characteristic physical findings include a protective stance in which the patient keeps the involved knee fully extended and resists passive motion. Maximal tenderness may be located centrally near the patellar ligament.[153] US and MRI are valuable in visualizing the deep patellar bursa.[154,155]

Staphylococcus aureus infection from the prepatellar bursa can spread to the deep patellar bursa, requiring surgical drainage.[156] Fungal infection of the infrapatellar bursa due to *Phialophora richardsiae* developed in a patient who previously received intrabursal corticosteroid injection for infrapatellar bursitis.[157]

Subacromial and Other Bursae

The subacromial bursa is located between the deep surface of the deltoid muscle, the superficial surface of the subscapularis, and the tendon of the long head of the biceps and is comprised of subacromial and subdeltoid portions. Although uncommon, septic subacromial bursitis is associated with more inflammatory bursal and systemic reaction. Infection with *Staphylococcus aureus*, the most common offending organism, is associated with immunocompromised states, trauma, intravenous drug abuse (**Fig. 1**), and chronic illness as risk factors. Infection may be due to hematogenous spread, by contiguous spread from an infected glenohumeral joint,[158] or by direct inoculation. Septic subacromial bursitis is a rare complication of intrabursal corticosteroid injection.[132] Isotretinoin therapy has been proposed as a risk factor for *Staphylococcus aureus* infections, including septic bursitis after percutaneous injection, primarily because of the high rates of colonization of the skin (50%) and anterior nares (70%) with this kind of treatment.[159] Candida infection has been reported in an immunocompetent elderly patient who showed no significant systemic symptoms after subacromial bursal steroid injections for shoulder impingement syndrome.[133] Similarly, septic arthritis is a rare complication of intra-articular steroid injection and pus can become localized in the subacromial bursa.[158]

Diagnosis based on clinical grounds is difficult to establish because of nonspecific features similar to those in septic arthritis, such as fever and other signs of local inflammation. MRI is useful in determination of extent of the bursal involvement and need for further aspiration or surgical intervention.[135] US-guided needle aspiration of bursal fluid is remarkably helpful.[160]

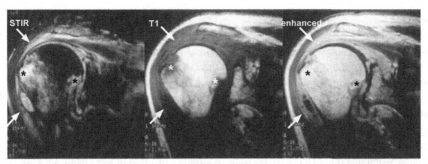

Fig. 1. *Staphylococcus aureus* cellulitis, bursitis, synovitis, and osteomyelitis. A 23-year-old female who has a history of intravenous drug abuse has right shoulder pain, swelling, erythema, and limited range of motion. Coronal STIR, T1, and enhanced T1 MRI demonstrates an enlarged, thickened, fluid-filled continuous subacromial-subdeltoid bursa (*arrows*). Edema and enhancement extend to the surrounding tissues and humeral head (*). (*Courtesy of* P. Colletti, MD, Los Angeles, CA.)

Tuberculous and Atypical Mycobacterial Bursitis

Tuberculous infection of the greater trochanter bursa is a rare but well-established manifestation of extrapulmonary tuberculosis.[161] A university-based referral center in Spain found that this condition composed more than 1% of musculoskeletal tuberculosis, with 50% of patients having evidence of lung or other musculoskeletal disease.[162] Less commonly, tuberculosis may involve other deep and superficial bursae, including the subacromial,[163] subdeltoid,[164] bicipitoradial,[165] olecranon, prepatellar, and ischiogluteal bursae.[166] The pathogenesis is unclear but hematogenous spread and direct extension from bone are important.[167] Diagnosis is often delayed because of its indolent course. Risk factors include chronic illness, immunocompromised state, and corticosteroid use.[168,169] CT and MRI can delineate the extent of infection and can guide the surgical approach.[166] Diagnosis is confirmed by histopathology, culture, or PCR test on the tissue specimen. Serial gallium scintigraphy is useful in monitoring response to therapy.[169] Reactivation of tuberculous greater trochanteric bursitis has been reported.[170]

Rice bodies, so called because of their resemblance to shiny rice grains, have been found attached to the synovial lining of a tuberculous subdeltoid bursa,[164] ulnar bursa, and flexor tendon sheath.[171] These consist of an inner amorphous core of eosinophilic material surrounded by collagen and fibrin. Found more commonly in rheumatoid arthritis and bursitis, the pathogenesis is unclear, although it has been suggested that they arise from synovial microinfarction leading to sloughing and encasement by fibrin from the synovial fluid.

Septic bursitis due to NTM is uncommon, primarily involves superficial bursae, and can develop in both immunocompromised and healthy subjects. Up to 38% of patients who have this condition have a chronic systemic illness and are often on immunosuppressive agents.[172] NTM infections among patients who have SLE have been noted to occur later in the disease course than mycobacterial infections.[173] The most common portals of entry for infection are through a minor skin abrasion contaminated with soil, or during local corticosteroid bursal injection. Clinical courses of olecranon bursitis due to *M gordonae*, *M avium complex*, and *M terrae* were marked by a chronicity and a delay in diagnosis up to several months.[172] Olecranon bursitis due to *M avium complex* developed in a patient receiving alefacept for psoriasis.[174] Management of olecranon bursitis caused by NTM is not standardized, although

---

Box 1
General guidelines in the evaluation and treatment of patients who have soft tissue infections

Histories of environmental exposures, repetitive or acute trauma, whether related to work, posture limitations, or recreation, should give clues to the causative organism.

History of comorbidities, use of immunosuppressive agents, risk factors for HIV infection can give clues to the potential severity of the underlying infection.

Microbiologic studies should be used to identify causative pathogen.

Musculoskeletal imaging, whenever possible, should be used to determine extent of infection, guide needle aspiration, and monitor treatment.

Empiric antibiotics should be started as soon as possible and adjusted accordingly once results of fluid culture and sensitivities are available.

Risk factors for antibiotic-resistant organisms (eg, intravenous drug abuse, MRSA) should be considered in antibiotic selection.

Aggressive surgery is indicated in necrotizing fasciitis and in other infections not responsive to antibiotic therapy.

---

most reported cases undergo bursal resection and treatment with at least two microbial agents for a variable period of time.

SUMMARY

Soft tissue infections are commonly reported in both immunocompetent and immunocompromised patients, including those who have rheumatic diseases. Use of immunomodulators, including biologic agents, seems to be associated with increased risk for these infections. Increased vigilance among physicians can facilitate timely diagnosis and treatment and therefore produce better outcomes (**Box 1**). The emergence of antibiotic-resistant pathogens needs to be considered. Musculoskeletal imaging, microbiology, and pathology techniques are collectively useful in establishing the diagnosis. US may be a viable tool, which rheumatologists themselves may be able to use even in clinic-based settings. Larger, controlled studies are needed to look at the underlying pathogenic processes, including genetic factors, that predispose patients to these kinds of infections, and to explore the efficacy of techniques in diagnosing these diseases.

REFERENCES

1. Juarez M, Misischia R, Alarcaon GS. Infections in systemic connective tissue diseases: systemic lupus erythematosus, scleroderma, and polymyositis/dermatomyositis. Rheum Dis Clin North Am 2003;29(4):163–84.
2. Godeau B, Mortier E, Roy PM, et al. Short and longterm outcomes for patients with systemic rheumatic diseases admitted to intensive care units: a prognostic study of 181 patients. J Rheumatol 1997;24(7):1317–23.
3. Bresnihan B, Cunnane G. Infection complications associated with the use of biologic agents. Rheum Dis Clin North Am 2003;29(1):185–202.
4. Dixon WG, Watson K, Lunt M, et al. Rates of serious infection, including site-specific and bacterial intracellular infection, in rheumatoid arthritis patients receiving anti-tumor necrosis factor therapy: results from the British Society for Rheumatologists. Arthritis Rheum 2006;54(8):2368–76.

5. Garred P, Madsen HO, Halberg P, et al. Mannose-binding lectin polymorphisms and susceptibility to infection in systemic lupus erythematosus. Arthritis Rheum 1999;42(10):2145–52.
6. Favalli EG, Desiati F, Atzeni F, et al. Serious infections during anti-TNF alpha treatment in rheumatoid arthritis patients. Autoimmun Rev 2009;8(3): 266–73.
7. Lopez FA, Lartchenko S. Skin and soft tissue infections. Infect Dis Clin North Am 2006;20:759–72.
8. Mok MY, Wong SY, Chan TM, et al. Necrotizing fasciitis in rheumatic diseases. Lupus 2006;15(6):380–3.
9. Wong CH, Chang HC, Pasupathy S, et al. Necrotizing fasciitis: clinical presentation, microbiology, and determinants of mortality. J Bone Joint Surg Am 2003; 85(8):1455–60.
10. Miller LG, Perdreau-Remington F, Rieg G, et al. Necrotizing fasciitis caused by community-associated methicillin-resistant Staphylococcus aureus in Los Angeles. N Engl J Med 2005;352(14):1445–53.
11. Wang YS, Wong CH, Tay YK. Stages of necrotizing fasciitis based on the evolving cutaneous features. Int J Dermatol 2007;46(10):1036–41.
12. Wong CH, Khin LW, Heng KS, et al. The LRINEC (Laboratory Risk Indicator for Necrotizing Fasciitis) score: a tool for distinguishing necrotizing fasciitis from other soft tissue infections. Crit Care Med 2004;32(7):1535–41.
13. Wong CH, Yam AK, Tan AB, et al. Approach to debridement in necrotizing fasciitis. Am J Surg 2008;196(3):e19–24.
14. Chau CLF, Griffith JF. Musculoskeletal infections: ultrasound appearances. Clin Radiol 2005;60(2):149–59.
15. Fayad LM, Carrino JA, Fishman EK. Musculoskeletal infection: role of CT in the emergency department. Radiographics 2007;27(6):1723–36.
16. Smeets L, Bous A, Heymans O. Necrotizing fasciitis: case report and review of literature. Acta Chir Belg 2007;107(1):29–36.
17. Mendez EA, Espinoza LM, Harris M, et al. Systemic lupus erythematosus complicated by necrotizing fasciitis. Lupus 1999;8(2):157–9.
18. Khawcharoenporn T, Apisarnthanarak A, Karatisin P, et al. Salmonella group C necrotizing fasciitis: a case report and review of the literature. Diagn Microbiol Infect Dis 2006;54(4):319–22.
19. Hashimoto N, Sugiyama H, Asagoe K, et al. Fulminant necrotizing fasciitis developing during long term corticosteroid treatment of systemic lupus erythematosus. Ann Rheum Dis 2002;61:848–9.
20. Kamran M, Wachs J, Putterman C. Necrotizing fasciitis in systemic lupus erythematosus. Semin Arthritis Rheum 2008;37(4):236–42.
21. Isik A, Koca SS. Necrotizing fasciitis resulting from Streptococcus pneumoniae in recently diagnosed systemic lupus erythematosus case: a case report. Clin Rheumatol 2007;26(6):999–1001.
22. Kaneita Y, Takata C, Itobayashi E, et al. Streptococcal toxic shock syndrome: report of two cases. Intern Med 1995;34(7):643–5.
23. Carruthers A, Carruthers J, Wright P. Necrotizing fasciitis with polymyositis. Br Med J 1975;3(5979):355–6.
24. Lateef A, Vasoo S, Boey ML. Soft tissue manifestations of mycobacterial infection in patients with rheumatic diseases. Ann Acad Med Singapore 2007; 36(2):152–3.
25. Choi KH, Yoo WH. Necrotizing fasciitis in a patient treated with etanercept for dermatomyositis. Rheumatol Int 2009;29(4):463–6.

26. Chan AT, Cleeve V, Daymond TJ. Necrotising fasciitis in a patient receiving infliximab for rheumatoid arthritis. Postgrad Med J 2002;78(915):47–8.
27. Piedra T, Martin-Cuesta L, Arnaiz J, et al. Necrotizing fasciitis secondary to diverticulitis. Emerg Radiol 2007;13(6):345–8.
28. Jensen SL, Amato JE, Hartstein ME, et al. Bilateral periorbital necrotizing fasciitis. Arch Dermatol 2004;140(6):664–6.
29. Jarrett P, Ha T, Oliver F. Necrotizing fasciitis complicating disseminated cutaneous *Herpes zoster*. Clin Exp Dermatol 1998;23(2):87–8.
30. McEntegart A, Capell HA. Necrotizing fasciitis in a patient with rheumatoid arthritis. Rheumatology 2002;41(7):828–9.
31. Chikkamuniyappa S. Streptococcal toxic shock syndrome and sepsis manifesting in a patient with chronic rheumatoid arthritis. Dermatol Online J 2004;10(1):7.
32. Sugimoto S, Nakazawa J, Yomodo M, et al. Necrotizing fasciitis resulting from *Escherichia coli* in a patient with chronic rheumatoid arthritis. J Clin Rheumatol 2001;7(2):83–5.
33. Suwannaroj S, Mootsikapun P, Vipulakorn K, et al. *Salmonella* group D septic arthritis and necrotizing fasciitis in a patient with rheumatoid arthritis and diabetes mellitus. J Clin Rheumatol 2001;7(2):83–5.
34. Baghai M, Osman DR, Wolk DM, et al. Fatal sepsis in a patient with rheumatoid arthritis treated with etanercept. Mayo Clin Proc 2001;76(6):653–6.
35. Yuhara T, Takemura H, Akama T, et al. Necrotizing fasciitis caused by *Streptococcus pneumoniae* in mixed connective tissue disease. Mod Rheumatol 2000;10(3):180–2.
36. Kusne S, Eibling DE, Yu VL, et al. Gangrenous cellulitis associated with Gram-negative *Bacilli* in pancytopenic patients: dilemma with respect to effective therapy. Am J Med 1988;85(4):490–4.
37. Yu KH, Ho HH, Chen JY, et al. Gout complicated with necrotizing fasciitis – report of 15 cases. Rheumatology 2004;43(4):518–21.
38. Stein RH, Phelps RG, Sapadin AN. Cutaneous polyarteritis nodosa after streptococcal necrotizing fasciitis. Mt Sinai J Med 2001;68(4–5):336–8.
39. Orlando A, Marrone C, Nicoli N, et al. Fatal necrotising fasciitis associated with intramuscular injection of nonsteroidal anti-inflammatory drugs after complicated endoscopic polypectomy. J Infect 2007;54(3):e145–8.
40. Aronoff DM, Bloch KC. Assessing the relationship between the use of nonsteroidal anti-inflammatory drugs and necrotizing fasciitis caused by group A *Streptococcus*. Medicine 2003;82(4):225–35.
41. Frick S, Cerny A. Necrotizing fasciitis due to *Streptococcus pneumoniae* after intramuscular injection of nonsteroidal anti-inflammatory drugs: report of 2 cases and review. Clin Infect Dis 2001;33(5):740–4.
42. Souyri C, Olivier P, Grolleau S. Severe necrotizing soft-tissue infections and nonsteroidal anti-inflammatory drugs. Clin Exp Dermatol 2007;33(3):249–55.
43. Okan G, Yavlaci S, Ince U, et al. Necrotizing fasciitis following intramuscular diclofenac injection. J Eur Acad Dermatol Venereol 2008;22(12):1521–2.
44. Factor SH, Levine OS, Schwartz B, et al. Invasive group A streptococcal disease: risk factors for adults. Emerg Infect Dis 2003;9(8):970–7.
45. Zani S, Babigian A. Necrotizing fasciitis of the shoulder following routine rotator cuff repair. J Bone Joint Surg Am 2008;90(5):1117–20.
46. Campion J, Allum R. Necrotising fasciitis following anterior cruciate ligament reconstruction. Knee 2006;13(1):51–3.
47. Drosos G. Pyomyositis, a literature review. Acta Orthop Belg 2005;71(1):9–16.

48. Theodorou SJ, Theodorou DJ, Resnick D. MR imaging findings of pyogenic bacterial myositis in patients with local muscle trauma: illustrative cases. Emerg Radiol 2007;14(2):89–96.
49. Bickels J, Ben-Sira L, Kessler A, et al. Primary pyomyositis. J Bone Joint Surg Am 2002;84(12):2277–86.
50. Small LN, Ross JJ. Tropical and temperate pyomyositis. Infect Dis Clin North Am 2005;19(4):981–9.
51. Crum-Cianflone NF. Bacterial, fungal, parasitic, and viral myositis. Clin Microbiol Rev 2008;21(3):473–94.
52. Chiedozi LC. Pyomyositis. Review of 205 cases in 112 patients. Am J Surg 1979; 137(2):255–9.
53. Kennedy CA, Mathisen G, Goetz MB. Tropical pyomyositis of the abdominal wall musculature mimicking acute abdomen. West J Med 1990;152(3):296–8.
54. John BM, Patnaik SK. Multifocal pyomyositis. Medical Journal of the Armed Forces of India 2007;63(4):191–2.
55. Hassan FOA, Shannak A. Primary pyomyositis of the paraspinal muscles: a case report and literature review. Eur Spine J 2008;17(Suppl 2):S239–42.
56. Gupta S, Grainger SJ, Wright M. Unusual cause of hip pain in a patient with relapsing Henoch-Schonlein nephritis. J R Coll Physicians Edinb 2007;37(2):110–1.
57. Kane D, Balint PV, Wood F, et al. Early diagnosis of pyomyositis using clinic-based ultrasonography in a patient receiving infliximab therapy for Behcet's disease. Rheumatology 2003;42(12):1564–79.
58. Hossain A, Reis ED, Soundararajan K, et al. Nontropical pyomyositis: analysis of eight patients in an urban center. Am Surg 2000;66(11):1064–6.
59. Crum NF. Bacterial pyomyositis in the United States. Am J Med 2004;117(6): 420–8.
60. Kaushik RM, Kaushik R, Sharma A, et al. Tropical pyomyositis in a case of rheumatoid arthritis. Trans R Soc Trop Med Hyg 2006;100(9):895–8.
61. Jidpugdeebodin S, Punyagupta S. Salmonella crepitant pyomyositis in a patient with systemic lupus erythematosus. J Infect Dis Antimicrob Agents 2004;21(1): 11–5.
62. Aynaci O, Onder C, Kalaycioglu A. Anterior tibial compartment syndrome due to pyomyositis in a patient with rheumatoid arthritis. A case report. Joint Bone Spine 2003;70(1):77–9.
63. Wang TK, Wong SS, Woo PC. Two cases of pyomyositis caused by Klebsiella pneumoniae and review of the literature. Eur J Clin Microbiol Infect Dis 2001; 20(8):576–80.
64. Hsu CC, Chen WJ, Chen SY, et al. Fatal septicemia and pyomyositis caused by Salmonella typhi. Clin Infect Dis 2004;39(10):1547–8.
65. Schwartz DM, Morgan ER. Multimodality imaging of Candida tropicalis myositis. Pediatr Radiol 2008;38(4):473–6.
66. Gave AA, Torres R, Kaplan L. Cryptococcal myositis and vasculitis: an unusual necrotizing soft tissue infection. Surg Infect (Larchmt) 2004;5(3):309–13.
67. Bae YJ, Choi JS, Lee YA, et al. A case of pyomyositis due to Mycobacterium tuberculosis. Korean J Pediatr 2006;49(10):1116–9.
68. Batra S, Ab Naell M, Barwick C, et al. Tuberculous pyomyositis of the thigh masquerading as malignancy with concomitant tuberculous flexor tenosynovitis and dactylitis. Singapore Med J 2007;48(11):1042–6.
69. Lorenz U, Abele-Horn M, Bussen D, et al. Severe pyomyositis caused by Panton-Valentine leucocidin-positive methicillin-sensitive Staphylococcus aureus complicating a pilonidal cyst. Langenbecks Arch Surg 2007;392(6):761–5.

70. Zalavras CG, Rigopoulos N, Poultsides L, et al. Increased oxacillin resistance in thigh pyomyositis in diabetic patients. Clin Orthop Relat Res 2008;466(6): 1405–9.

71. Jahamy H, Ganga R, Al Raiy B, et al. *Staphylococcus aureus* skin/soft-tissue infections: the impact of SCCmec type and Panton-Valentine leukocidin. Scand J Infect Dis 2008;40(8):601–6.

72. Tlacuilo-Parra JA, Guevara-Gutierrez E, Gonzalez-Ojeda A, et al. Nontropical pyomyositis in an immunocompetent host. J Clin Rheumatol 2005;11(3): 160–3.

73. Tang WM, Wong JWK, Wong LLS, et al. Streptococcal necrotizing myositis: the role of magnetic resonance imaging. J Bone Joint Surg Am 2001;83(11):1723–6.

74. Sarui H, Maruyama T, Ito I, et al. Necrotising myositis in Behcet's disease: characteristic features on magnetic resonance imaging and a review of the literature. Ann Rheum Dis 2002;61(8):751–2.

75. Schalinski S, Tsokos M. Fatal pyomyositis: a report of 8 autopsy cases. Am J Forensic Med Pathol 2008;29(2):131–5.

76. Chiu SK, Lin JC, Wang NC, et al. Impact of underlying diseases on the clinical characteristics and outcome of primary pyomyositis. J Microbiol Immunol Infect 2008;41(4):286–93.

77. Johnson DW, Herzig KA. Isolated tuberculous pyomyositis in a renal transplant patient. Nephrol Dial Transplant 2000;15(5):743.

78. Baylan O, Demiralp B, Cicek EI, et al. A case of tuberculous pyomyositis that caused a recurrent soft tissue lesion localized at the forearm. Jpn J Infect Dis 2005;58(6):376–9.

79. Trikha V, Varshney MK, Rastogi S. Isolated tuberculosis of the vastus lateralis muscle: a case report. Scand J Infect Dis 2006;38(4):304–6.

80. Azevedo VF, Parchen C, Coelho SA, et al. Tuberculous myositis in a patient with ankylosing spondylitis treated with adalimumab. Rheumatol Int 2009; [epub ahead of print].

81. Wang JY, Lee LN, Hsueh PR, et al. Tuberculous myositis: a rare but existing clinical entity. Rheumatology 2003;42(7):836–40.

82. Schnall SB, Vu-Rose T, Holtom PD, et al. Tissue pressures in pyogenic flexor tenosynovitis of the finger. J Bone Joint Surg Br 1996;78(5):793–5.

83. Clark DC. Common acute hand infections. Am Fam Physician 2003;68(11): 2167–76.

84. Nourissat G, Fournier E, Werther JR, et al. Acute carpal tunnel syndrome secondary to pyogenic tenosynovitis. J Hand Surg [Br] 2006;31(6):687–8.

85. Small LN, Ross JJ. Suppurative tenosynovitis and septic bursitis. Infect Dis Clin North Am 2005;19(4):991–1005.

86. Rice PA. Gonococcal arthritis. Infect Dis Clin North Am 2005;19(4):853–61.

87. Faraj S, Stanley-Clarke D. Acute extensor hallucis longus tenosynovitis caused by gonococcal infection. N Z Med J 2003;116(1173):U421.

88. Craig JG, Van Holsbeeck M, Alva M. Gonococcal arthritis of the shoulder and septic extensor tenosynovitis of the wrist. J Ultrasound Med 2003;22(2):221–4.

89. Garcia Triana M, Fernandez Echevarria MA, Alvaro RL, et al. *Pasteurella multocida* tenosynovitis of the hand: sonographic findings. J Clin Ultrasound 2003; 31(3):159–62.

90. Hsu TC, Wang CL, Wang TG, et al. Ultrasonographic examination of the posterior tibial tendon. Foot Ankle Int 1997;18(1):34–8.

91. Aboudola S, Sienko A, Carey RB, et al. Tuberculous tenosynovitis. Hum Pathol 2004;35(8):1044–6.

92. Dhammi IK, Singh S, Jain AK, et al. Isolated tuberculous tenosynovitis of the flexor carpi ulnaris: a case report and review of the literature. Acta Orthop Belg 2006;72(6):779–82.
93. Higuchi S, Ishihara S, Kobayashi H, et al. A mass lesion of the wrist: a rare manifestation of tuberculosis. Intern Med 2008;47(4):313–6.
94. Rashid M, Sarwar SU, Haq EU, et al. Tuberculous tenosynovitis: a cause of carpal tunnel syndrome. J Pak Med Assoc 2006;56(3):116–8.
95. Uthman I, Bizri AR, Jajj AR, et al. Miliary tuberculosis presenting as tenosynovitis in a case of rheumatoid arthritis. J Infect 1998;37(2):196–8.
96. Le Meur A, Arvieux C, Geggenbuhl P, et al. Tenosynovitis of the wrist due to resistant *Mycobacterium tuberculosis* in a heart transplant patient. J Clin Microbiol 2005;43(2):988–90.
97. Oshima M, Fukui A, Takakura Y. A case of tuberculous tenosynovitis in a patient with systemic lupus erythematosus. Hand Surg 2004;9(1):109–13.
98. Varshney MK, Trikha V, Gupta V. Isolated tuberculosis of the Achilles tendon. Joint Bone Spine 2007;74(1):100–2.
99. Hooker MS, Schaefer RA, Fishbain JT, et al. Tuberculous tenosynovitis of the tibialis anterior tendon: a case report. Foot Ankle Int 2002;23(12):1131–4.
100. Ogut T, Gokce A, Kesmezacar H, et al. Isolated tuberculous tenosynovitis of the Achilles tendon: a report of two cases. Acta Orthop Traumatol Turc 2007;41(4): 314–20.
101. Titov AG, Vyshnevskaya EB, Mazurenko SI, et al. Use of polymerase chain reaction to diagnose tuberculous arthritis from joint tissues and synovial fluid. Arch Pathol Lab Med 2004;128(2):205–9.
102. Wongworawat MD, Holtom P, Learch TJ, et al. A prolonged case of *Mycobacterium marinum* flexor tenosynovitis: radiographic and histological correlation, and review of the literature. Skeletal Radiol 2003;32(9):542–5.
103. Pang HN, Lee JYL, Puhaindran ME, et al. *Mycobacterium marinum* as a cause of chronic granulomatous tenosynovitis in the hand. J Infect 2007;54(6): 584–8.
104. Gerster JC, Duvoisin B, Dudler J, et al. Tenosynovitis of the hands caused by *Mycobacterium kansasii* in a patient with scleroderma. J Rheumatol 2004; 31(12):2523–5.
105. Akahane T, Nakatsuchi Y, Tateiwa Y. Recurrent granulomatous tenosynovitis of the wrist and finger caused by *Mycobacterium* intracellulare: a case report. Diagn Microbiol Infect Dis 2006;56(1):99–101.
106. Carter TI, Frelinghuysen P, Daluiski A, et al. Flexor tenosynovitis caused by *Mycobacterium scrofulaceum*: a case report. J Hand Surg (Am) 2006;31(8): 1292–5.
107. Godreuil S, Marchandin H, Terru D, et al. *Mycobacterium* heckeshornense tenosynovitis. Scand J Infect Dis 2006;38(11–12):1098–101.
108. Eskesen AN, Skramm I, Steinbakk M. Infectious tenosynovitis and osteomyelitis caused by *Mycobacterium* nonchromogenicum. Scand J Infect Dis 2007;39(2): 179–80.
109. Thariat J, Leveque L, Tavernier C, et al. *Mycobacterium marinum* tenosynovitis in a patient with Still's disease. Rheumatology (Oxford) 2001;40(12): 1419–20.
110. Southern PM Jr. Tenosynovitis caused by *Mycobacterium kansasii* associated with a dog bite. Am J Med Sci 2004;327(5):258–61.
111. Anim-Appiah D, Bono B, Fleegler E, et al. *Mycobacterium avium* complex tenosynovitis of the wrist and hand. Arthritis Rheum 2004;51(1):140–2.

112. Hung GU, Lan JL, Yang KT, et al. Scintigraphic findings of *Mycobacterium avium* complex tenosynovitis of the index finger in a patient with systemic lupus erythematosus. Clin Nucl Med 2003;28(11):936–8.
113. Mateo L, Rufi G, Nolla JM, et al. *Mycobacterium chelonae* tenosynovitis of the hand. Semin Arthritis Rheum 2004;34(3):617–22.
114. Lidar M, Elkayam O, Goodwin D, et al. Protracted *Mycobacterium kansasii* carpal tunnel syndrome and tenosynovitis. Isr Med Assoc J 2003;5(6):453–4.
115. Aubry A, Chosidow O, Caumes E, et al. Sixty-three cases of *Mycobacterium marinum* infection: clinical features, treatment and antibiotic susceptibility of causative isolates. Arch Intern Med 2002;162(15):1746–52.
116. Noguchi M, Taniwaki Y, Tani T. Atypical Mycobacterium infections of the upper extremity. Arch Orthop Trauma Surg 2005;125(7):475–8.
117. Garrido G, Gomez-Reino JJ, Fernandez-Dapica P, et al. A review of peripheral tuberculous arthritis. Semin Arthritis Rheum 1988;18(2):142–9.
118. Roberts CC, Liu PT, Chew FS. Imaging evaluation of tendon sheath disease: self-assessment module. Am J Roentgenol 2007;188:S10–2.
119. Hsu CY, Lu HC, Shih TT. Tuberculous infection of the wrist: MRI features. Am J Roentgenol 2004;183(3):623–8.
120. Jaovisidha S, Chen C, Ryu KN, et al. Tuberculous tenosynovitis and bursitis: imaging findings in 21 cases. Radiology 1996;201(2):507–13.
121. Chau CLF, Griffith JF, Chan PT, et al. Rice-body formation in atypical mycobacterial tenosynovitis and bursitis: findings on sonography and MR imaging. Am J Roentgenol 2003;180(5):1455–9.
122. Cucurull E, Sarwar H, Williams CS IV, et al. Localized tenosynovitis caused by *Histoplasma capsulatum*: case report and review of the literature. Arthritis Rheum 2005;53(1):129–32.
123. Bruno KM, Farhoomand L, Libman BS, et al. Cryptococcal arthritis, tendinitis, tenosynovitis, and carpal tunnel syndrome: report of a case and review of the literature. Arthritis Care Res 2002;47(1):104–8.
124. Horcajada JP, Pena JL, Martinez-Taboada VM, et al. Invasive cryptococcosis and adalimumab treatment. Emerg Infect Dis 2007;13(6):953–5.
125. Gottlieb GS, Lesser CF, Holmes KK, et al. Disseminated sporotrichosis associated with treatment with immunosuppressants and tumor necrosis factor–α antagonists. Clin Infect Dis 2003;37(6):838–40.
126. Graffin B, Flin C, Fulpin J, et al. A case report of Blastomyces tenosynovitis, with a literature review on fungal tenosynovitis. Joint Bone Spine 2001;68(4):350–3.
127. Tucker JD, Montecino R, Winograd JM, et al. Pyogenic flexor tenosynovitis associated with *Cellulosimicrobium cellulans*. J Clin Microbiol 2008;46(12):4106–8.
128. Lee JS, Moon GH, Lee NY. Case report: protothecal tenosynovitis. Clin Orthop Relat Res 2008;466(12):3143–6.
129. Haroon N, Agarwal V, Aggarwal A, et al. Arthritis as presenting manifestation of pure neuritic leprosy – a rheumatologist's dilemma. Rheumatology 2007;46(4):653–6.
130. Landais C, Fenollar F, Constantin A, et al. Q fever osteoarticular infection: four new cases and a review of the literature. Eur J Clin Microbiol Infect Dis 2007;26(5):341–7.
131. Soderquist B, Hedstrom SA. Predisposing factors, bacteriology and antibiotic therapy in 35 cases of septic bursitis. Scand J Infect Dis 1986;18(4):405–11.
132. Hiemstra LA, MacDonald Froese W. Subacromial infection following corticosteroid injection. J Shoulder Elbow Surg 2003;12(1):91–3.

133. Khazzam M, Bansal M, Fealy S. Candida infection of the subacromial bursa. J Bone Joint Surg Am 2005;87(1):168–71.
134. Torres HA, Bodey GP, Tarrand JJ, et al. Protothecosis in patients with cancer: case series and literature review. Clin Microbiol Infect 2003;9(8):786–92.
135. Chartash EK, Good PK, Gould ES, et al. Septic subdeltoid bursitis. Semin Arthritis Rheum 1992;22(1):25–9.
136. Laupland KB, Davies HD. Olecranon septic bursitis managed in an ambulatory setting. Clin Invest Med 2001;24(4):171–8.
137. Llinas L, Olenginski TP, Bush D, et al. Osteomyelitis resulting from chronic filamentous fungus olecranon bursitis. J Clin Rheumatol 2005;11(5):280–2.
138. Wasserman AR, Melville LD, Birkhahn RH. Septic bursitis: a case report and primer for the emergency clinician. J Emerg Med 2007; [epub ahead of print].
139. Baskar S, Jassim IT, Al-Allaf AW. Symmetrical inflammatory polyarthritis of the hands concomitant to the diagnosis of Staphylococcus aureus olecranon bursitis. Scand J Rheumatol 2005;34(6):491–2.
140. Wessolossky M, Haran JP, Bagchi K. Paecilomyces lilacinus olecranon bursitis in an immunocompromised host: case report and review. Diagn Microbiol Infect Dis 2008;61(3):354–7.
141. Bossler AD, Richter SS, Chavez AJ, et al. Exophiala oligosperma causing olecranon bursitis. J Clin Microbiol 2003;41(10):4779–82.
142. Khoury JA, Dubberke ER, Devine SM. Fatal case of protothecosis in a hematopoietic stem cell transplant after infliximab. Blood 2004;104(10): 3414–5.
143. Jimenez-Palop M, Corteguera M, Ibanez R, et al. Olecranon bursitis due to Candida parapsilosis in an immunocompetent adult. Ann Rheum Dis 2002; 61(3):279–81.
144. Blankstein A, Ganel A, Givon U, et al. Ultrasonographic findings in patients with olecranon bursitis. Ultraschall Med 2006;27(6):568–71.
145. Sofka CM, Collins AJ, Adler RS. Use of ultrasonographic guidance in interventional musculoskeletal procedures: a review from a single institution. J Ultrasound Med 2001;20(1):21–6.
146. Floemer F, Morrison WB, Bongartz G, et al. MRI Characteristics of olecranon bursitis. Am J Roentgenol 2004;183(1):29–34.
147. Harwell JI, Fisher D. Pediatric septic bursitis: case report of retrocalcaneal infection and review of the literature. Clin Infect Dis 2001;32(6):E102–4.
148. Mysnyk MC, Wroble RR, Foster DT, et al. Prepatellar bursitis in wrestlers. Am J Sports Med 1986;14(1):46–54.
149. Coste N, Perceau G, Leone J, et al. Osteoarticular complications of erysipelas. J Am Acad Dermatol 2004;50(2):203–9.
150. Wang JP, Granlund KF, Bozzette S, et al. Bursal sporotrichosis: case report and review. Clin Infect Dis 2000;31(2):615–6.
151. Traboulsi R, Uthman I, Kanj SS. Prepatellar Brucella melitensis bursitis: case report and literature review. Clin Rheumatol 2007;26(11):1941–2.
152. Choi HR. Patellar osteomyelitis presenting as prepatellar bursitis. Knee 2007; 14(4):333–5.
153. Waters P, Kasser J. Infection of the infrapatellar bursa. J Bone Joint Surg Am 1990;72(7):1095–6.
154. Carr KC, Hanly S, Griffin J, et al. Sonography of the patellar tendon and adjacent structures in pediatric and adult patients. AJR Am J Roentgenol 2001;176(6): 1535–9.

155. Hill CL, Gale DR, Chaisson CE, et al. Periarticular lesions detected on magnetic resonance imaging: prevalence in knees with and without symptoms. Arthritis Rheum 2003;48(10):2836–44.

156. Taylor PW. Inflammation of the deep infrapatellar bursa of the knee. Arthritis Rheum 1989;32(10):1312–4.

157. Cornia PB, Raugi GJ, Miller RA. Phialophora richardsiae bursitis treated medically. Am J Med 2003;115(1):77–9.

158. Jeon IH, Choi CH, Seo JS, et al. Arthroscopic management of septic arthritis of the shoulder joint. J Bone Joint Surg Am 2006;88(8):1802–6.

159. Drezner JA, Sennett BJ. Subacromial/subdeltoid septic bursitis associated with isotretinoin therapy and corticosteroid injection. J Am Board Fam Pract 2004; 17(4):299–302.

160. Costantino TG, Roemer B, Leber EH. Septic arthritis and bursitis. Emergency ultrasound can facilitate diagnosis. J Emerg Med 2007;32(3):295–7.

161. Yuksel HY, Aksahin E, Celebi L, et al. Isolated tuberculosis of the greater trochanter: a case report. Joint Dis Rel Surg 2006;17(3):151–4.

162. Crespo M, Pigrau C, Flores X, et al. Tuberculous trochanteric bursitis: report of 5 cases and literature review. Scand J Infect Dis 2004;36(8):552–8.

163. Pookarnjanamorakot C, Sirikulchayanonta V. Tuberculous bursitis of the subacromial bursa. J Shoulder Elbow Surg 2004;13(1):105–7.

164. Kim RS, Lee JY, Jung SR, et al. Tuberculous subdeltoid bursitis with rice bodies. Yonsei Med J 2002;43(2):539–42.

165. Nishida J, Furumachi K, Ehara S, et al. Tuberculous bicipitoradial bursitis: a case report. Skeletal Radiol 2007;36(5):445–8.

166. Abdelwahab IF, Bianchi S, Martinoli C, et al. Atypical extraspinal musculoskeletal tuberculosis in immunocompetent patients: part II, tuberculous myositis, tuberculous bursitis, and tuberculous tenosynovites. Can Assoc Radiol J 2006;57(5):278–86.

167. Ihara K, Toyoda K, Ofuji A, et al. Tuberculous bursitis of the great trochanter. J Orthop Sci 1998;3(2):120–4.

168. Yamamoto T, Iwasaki Y, Kurosaka M. Tuberculosis of the greater trochanter bursa occurring 51 years after tuberculous nephritis. Clin Rheumatol 2002; 21(5):397–400.

169. Kawamura E, Kawabe J, Tsumoto C, et al. Gallium scintigraphy in a case of tuberculous trochanteric bursitis. Ann Nucl Med 2007;21(4):229–33.

170. Sastre S, Garcia S, Soriano A. Reactivation of ancient trochanteric tuberculosis 60 years after surgical drainage. Rheumatology 2003;42(10):1263–4.

171. Huang GS, Lee CH, Chen CY. Clinical images: Tuberculous rice bodies of the wrist. Arthritis Rheum 2005;52(6):1950.

172. Garrigues GE, Aldridge JM III, Toth AP, et al. Nontuberculous mycobacterial olecranon bursitis: case report and literature review. J Shoulder Elbow Surg; 2009;18(2):e1–5.

173. Mok MY, Wong SS, Chan TM, et al. Non-tuberculous mycobacterial infection in patients with systemic lupus erythematosus. Rheumatology (Oxford) 2007; 46(2):280–4.

174. Prasertsuntarasai T, Bello EF. Mycobacterium avium complex olecranon bursitis in a patient treated with alefacept. Mayo Clin Proc 2005;80(11):1530–3.

Gonococcal and Nongonococcal Arthritis

Ignacio García-De LaTorre, MD[a,b,*], Arnulfo Nava-Zavala, MD, MSc[a,c]

KEYWORDS

- Gonococcal arthritis • Nongonococcal arthritis
- Bacterial arthritis • Septic arthritis • Infectious arthritis
- Acute arthritis

Acute bacterial arthritis usually is caused by gonococcal or nongonococcal infection of the joints. This term usually refers to most bacterial arthritis caused by bacterial infection, including fungal and mycobacterial infection, and is also known as septic arthritis. This article reviews the risk factors, pathogenesis, clinical manifestations, diagnosis, and treatment of nongonococcal and gonococcal arthritis only. Prosthetic joint infections, fungal, and mycobacterial arthritis are not discussed here because of their unique clinical manifestations.

Nongonococcal and gonococcal arthritis are the most potentially dangerous and destructive forms of acute arthritis. These bacterial infections of the joints are usually curable with treatment, but morbidity and mortality are still significant in patients who have underlying rheumatoid arthritis, patients who have prosthetic joints, elderly patients, and patients who have severe and multiple comorbidities.[1]

RISK FACTORS

Experimental evidence suggests that normal joints are resistant to infections compared with diseased joints or prosthetic joints. Recognition of risk factors—systemic, local, and social—is important. Such factors act by increasing the risk for bacteremia or reducing the body's capacity to eliminate organisms from the joint.[2,3]

Systemic disorders that affect the host's response through an impaired immune system include diabetes mellitus, preexisting rheumatoid arthritis, liver disease, chronic renal failure, malignancies, intravenous drug abuse, hemodialysis, alcoholism, AIDS, hemophilia, organ transplantation, and hypogammaglobulinemia.[4–8]

[a] Department of Immunology and Rheumatology, Hospital General de Occidente, Secretaría de Salud, Justo Sierra 2821, Guadalajara, México, CP 44690
[b] Centro Universitario de Ciencias de la Salud, Universidad de Guadalajara, Guadalajara, Jalisco, México
[c] Unidad de Investigación en Epidemiología Clínica, UMAE, HE, CMO, IMSS, Jalisco, México
* Corresponding author. Department of Immunology and Rheumatology, Hospital General de Occidente, Secretaría de Salud, Justo Sierra 2821, Guadalajara, JAL, México, CP 44690.
E-mail address: igdlt@aol.com (I. García-De La Torre).

Rheum Dis Clin N Am 35 (2009) 63–73
doi:10.1016/j.rdc.2009.03.001   rheumatic.theclinics.com
0889-857X/09/$ – see front matter © 2009 Elsevier Inc. All rights reserved.

Local factors, such as damage of a specific joint, may be the result of earlier trauma, including acupuncture procedures or recent joint surgery or arthroscopy; also, the presence of arthritis, including osteoarthritis, or a prosthetic joint in the knee or the hip are important predisposing factors for septic arthritis. Age is also important, with newborns and elderly people, especially those older than 80 years of age, being particularly vulnerable.[9–14] Social factors include occupational exposure to animals with respect to brucellosis,[15] or patients who are inhabitants of regions where this zoonosis remains a public health issue.[16] The risk for tuberculosis is greatly increased in certain racial groups (eg, people from India).[17]

Over the past 25 years, however, we have seen a resurgence of tuberculosis in developed countries as a result of mass immigrations from endemic areas of the world; increasing numbers of immunocompromised individuals, including those who have AIDS; increased infection rates in association with drug abuse, homelessness, and therapeutic noncompliance; and the emergence of drug-resistant mycobacteria.[18] In some cases, these risk factors are compounded (eg, patients who have rheumatoid arthritis treated with immunosuppression or steroids are at higher risk for infections). It may also be difficult to distinguish infection from inflammatory synovitis, especially if the patient is receiving steroid therapy.

In a study from The Netherlands, risk factors for bacterial arthritis were identified. In nearly half of the Dutch patients, infections occurred in abnormal joints. More than one quarter of the infected joints in the Dutch study with available clinical information contained prosthetic or osteosynthetic material. All but one of 22 hip infections in Dutch adults involved a prosthesis. About 20% of the Dutch adults had rheumatoid arthritis and accounted for 5 of 16 polyarticular cases. The authors sought clinical factors that might be amenable to future prophylaxis; infected skin lesions, accounting for 38 of 60 adult cases with an identifiable infection source, were considered the most common reason for hematogenous bacterial arthritis in patients who had rheumatoid arthritis (16 of 22 cases). Invasive nonsterile medical interventions distant from the affected joints accounted for 7 cases, all but one in a native joint.[19,20]

A recent study from Italy[21] points out that the reported incidence of septic arthritis varies from 2 to 5 cases/100,000 person-years in the general population to 70 cases/100,000 person-years among patients who have rheumatoid arthritis. In fact, individuals who have rheumatoid arthritis are at particular risk for developing septic arthritis. This risk may be due to several reasons: joint disease predisposes to bacterial joint colonization and rheumatoid arthritis itself and its treatment with corticosteroids, disease-modifying antirheumatic drugs (DMARDs), and biologic therapies may decrease the immune function required for protection from pathogens. Steroids and DMARDs seem to affect the leukocyte synovial count; indeed, patients who have rheumatoid arthritis with septic arthritis have a leukocyte count in synovial fluid lower than patients who have septic arthritis without underlying rheumatic diseases. The diagnosis of septic arthritis in patients who have rheumatoid arthritis can be difficult because the development of a hot painful joint is often confused with a relapse of the underlying joint disease leading to delay in diagnosis. **Box 1** lists the most common risk factors that predispose to septic arthritis.

PATHOGENESIS

Septic arthritis is most often a consequence of occult bacteremia that spreads to the joint. Synovium is highly vascular, and contains no limiting basement membrane, making it vulnerable to bacteremic seeding.[22] Several microorganisms, such as staphylococci and streptococci, may gain initial access to the bloodstream from their initial

Box 1
Common risk factors in septic arthritis

Systemic disorders

Rheumatoid arthritis

Diabetes mellitus

Liver diseases

Alcoholism

Chronic renal failure

Malignancies

Intravenous drug use

Hemodialysis

AIDS

Hemophilia

Organ transplantation

Hypogammaglobulinemia

Immunosuppressive drugs and glucocorticosteroids

Biologic agents

Local factors

Direct joint trauma

Recent joint surgery

Open reduction of fractures

Arthroscopy

Acupuncture procedure

Rheumatoid arthritis in a specific joint

Osteoarthritis

Prosthetic joint in knee or hip

Age: elderly >80 years old or newborns

Social factors

Occupational exposure to animals (brucellosis)

Low social income: tuberculosis

Data from García-De La Torre I. Advances in the management of septic arthritis. Rheum Dis Clin North Am 2003;29(1):61–75.

innocuous location if the integrity of skin and mucosa natural barriers becomes disrupted. Gram-negative septic arthritis probably arises from bacteremia from the gastrointestinal or urinary tracts. Certain bacteria, such a *Neisseria gonorrhoeae*, are particularly likely to infect a joint during a bacteremic episode.[23] Occasionally septic arthritis results from penetrating trauma, such as bite wounds, stepping on nails, or illegal injection drug use. This trauma is the most common means of infection of the small joints of the hands and feet,[19] including also those related to plant thorns and wood slivers injuries.[24]

Rarely, arthroscopy or therapeutic joint injections with corticosteroids may be complicated by septic arthritis. Also, bacteria may be introduced during joint surgery. Orthopedic surgeons may encounter patients who have joint infections as a result of trauma or surgical procedures. Some examples include penetrating injury or foreign body accidentally introduced into a joint, arthroscopic surgery, open reduction of fractures that involve the joint, and arthroplasties, including total joint replacement.[25] Gram-positive organisms are responsible for most cases of septic arthritis. Enteric Gram-negative rods account for 43% of community-acquired bacteremias, but cause only 10% of septic arthritis.[26,27]

This finding likely relates to the superior ability of Gram-positive organisms to bind connective tissue and extracellular matrix proteins. Staphylococcus aureus, the most common cause of septic arthritis, produces several surface adhesions that bind extracellular matrix proteins, known as "microbial surface components recognizing adhesive matrix molecules." Staphylococcal strains defective in microbial surface components recognizing adhesive matrix molecules are less arthritogenic in animal models.[28]

Joint damage in septic arthritis results from bacterial invasion, host inflammation, and tissue ischemia. Bacterial enzymes and toxins are directly injurious to cartilage. Cartilage may suffer "innocent bystander" damage, as host neutrophils release active oxygen species and lysosomal proteases. Cytokines activate host matrix metalloproteinases, leading to autodigestion of cartilage. Ischemic injury also plays a role. Cartilage is avascular and highly dependent on diffusion of oxygen and nutrients from the synovium. As purulent exudates accumulate, joint pressure increases and synovial blood flow is tamponaded, resulting in cartilage anoxia.[29] Under these conditions, cartilage degradation accelerates and inhibition of cartilage synthesis and irreversible bone loss occur,[23] as evidenced in the specific case of hip joint septic arthritis in which delayed presentation beyond 3 weeks predicts higher joint damage, leading to a need for excision arthroplasty.[30]

CLINICAL FEATURES

Bacterial arthritis generally presents with characteristic signs and symptoms that can easily lead to a diagnosis of either gonococcal or nongonococcal arthritis. Acute infectious arthritis is most commonly monoarticular but it can overlap with other causes of polyarthritis and could also be the presentation form of any polyarticular disease. The differential diagnosis in patients who have monoarthritis should be made with two other main conditions, trauma and crystal-induced arthropaties.[31]

In a typical case nongonococcal arthritis presents in a patient who has a short history of high fever, leukocytosis, and with involvement of a single hot, swollen, and exquisitely painful joint, especially large joints, more than 50% affecting the knee.[32] Approximately 20% of nongonococcal arthritis is polyarticular and affects two to three large joints, although this is a characteristic presentation mainly in patients who have chronic degenerative diseases, such as rheumatoid arthritis and osteoarthritis.[22,31]

The clinical and laboratory diagnosis of a nongonococcal bacterial arthritis is often difficult, however. Some clinical manifestations, such as high-grade fever, are only present in 58% of the cases,[4] but low-grade fever may be present in approximately 90% of the patients; leukocytosis is found in only 50% of patients.[33] In patients who have rheumatoid arthritis or in those taking corticosteroids or immunosuppressive drugs the joint pain may be masked, a situation that may delay the diagnosis.

Gonococcal infection is by far the most common cause of monoarthritis in young sexually active adults, with a female/male ratio of 3:1. This difference might be because women usually have a more asymptomatic clinical picture and present more often with untreated genitourinary tract infections.[34–36] There is a characteristic triad of clinical components: migratory polyarthralgia, dermatologic lesions usually presenting as macules and papules, and tenosynovitis often affecting multiple joints simultaneously (particularly wrists, fingers, ankles, and toes), as well as systemic inflammatory symptoms.[37,38]

There are usually two forms of presentation of this form of infectious arthritis, one being the classic triad defined above and the other an asymmetric polyarticular or monoarticular disease, present in less than 50% of patients, with knees, ankles, and wrists being the most commonly affected joints. Tenosynovitis usually affects wrists, ankles, and other small joints and usually is painful. The dermatologic features usually exhibit nonpainful macules or papules in arms or legs, although there is no specific localization described.[37]

A recent exposure to sexual encounters should raise suspicion of this type of arthritis and even though a positive Gram stain of synovial fluid is present in less than 50% of these patients, simultaneous cultures of cervix, urethra, and rectus should be obtained to augment the positive result, especially searching for the presence of N gonorrhoea.[37] A summary of the distinguishing clinical characteristics between gonococcal and nongonococcal arthritis is shown in **Table 1**.

DIAGNOSIS

The diagnosis of bacterial arthritis has not changed substantially in the last decade. The mainstay of diagnosis continues to be culture and isolation of the pathogen itself, but it is of great importance to differentiate between the two major types of infectious arthritis. It is well recognized that gonococcal arthritis is an important cause of septic arthritis and its differentiation from nongonococcal arthritis is exceedingly important because of prognostic and disability factors.

To achieve an accurate diagnosis, a combination of clinical and laboratory data and radiologic imaging studies plays an important role. In this case clinical and laboratory data represent almost 100% of final diagnoses (**Box 2**).

A definite diagnosis of bacterial arthritis can be established only by visualizing bacteria on a Gram-stained smear or by culturing bacteria from the synovial fluid. Gram stain and culture of synovial fluid should be routinely obtained in any case of

Table 1		
Clinical characteristics of gonococcal and nongonococcal arthritis		
Characteristics	Gonococcal	Nongonococcal
Patient profile	Sexually active young adults, mainly women	Newborns or adults with chronic disease (diabetes, RA, OA)
Presentation	Migratory polyarthritis dermatitis, tenosynovitis	Single joint involvement
Pattern of joint involvement	Polyarticular ∼50%	Oligoarticular ∼90%
Culture positivity	Less than 50%	Nearly 90%
Prognosis	Good with adequate antibiotic therapy	Usually bad prognosis, requiring joint drainage in most cases

Abbreviations: OA, osteoarthritis; RA, rheumatoid arthritis.
Data from Goldberg DL. Septic arthritis. Lancet 1998;351:197–202.

Box 2
Clinical and laboratory data suggestive of infectious arthritis

Key clinical data

Recent onset of fever, general malaise

Arthralgia and synovitis (mono/polyarticular)

Risk factors for infectious arthritis

Joint fluid characteristics

More than 50,000 cells/mL

More than 90% polymorphonuclear cells

Positive Gram stain and culture

Low glucose and high lactate

Data from Shirtliff ME, Mader JT. Acute septic arthritis. Clin Microbiol Rev 2002;15:527–44.

---

undiagnosed arthritis. Gram staining of synovial fluid, however, lacks sensitivity for the diagnosis of septic arthritis. Gram stains are positive in 71% of Gram-positive septic arthritis,[4] 40% to 50% of cases of Gram-negative septic arthritis,[39] and less than 25% of cases of gonococcal septic arthritis.[23] Usually, synovial fluid cultures are positive in 70% to 90% of cases of nongonococcal bacterial arthritis.[23,40] Blood cultures are positive in 40% to 50% of cases of bacterial arthritis and are the only method of identifying the pathogen in about 10% of cases. Sometimes, an infection in an extra-articular site suggests a clue to the etiologic agent infecting the joint, as in the case of bacterial arthritis in association with pneumococcal pneumonia, or a urinary tract infection caused by *Escherichia coli*.

In cases of a gonococcal infection, the culture for *N gonorrhoeae* is almost always negative in skin lesions and is positive in less than 50% of synovial fluids and less than one third of blood cultures. This negativity may be the result of the difficulty in growing this organism in vitro. The tenosynovitis and dermatitis associated with disseminated gonococcal infection may not yield viable organisms; however, it can be easily recovered from the genitourinary tract. Patients who have the clinical features of gonococcal arthritis should have synovial, skin, urethral, or cervical cultures, and rectal cultures submitted on Thayer-Martin media. Approximately 50% of patients who have gonococcal arthritis have positive cultures from one of the last three mucosal sites.[41] If associated urethritis is simultaneously present, a Gram stain of the urethral exudate should be obtained and examined for the presence of the Gram-negative diplococci characteristic of *N gonorrhoeae* infection. Culture and Gram stain of specimens obtained from skin lesions or tendon sheaths are often negative. Polymerase chain reaction techniques can detect gonococcal DNA in the synovial fluid of some culture-negative cases of suspected gonococcal arthritis, but the technique is not standardized and is not widely available.[42,43]

The organisms causing nongonococcal septic arthritis in adults are 75% to 80% Gram-positive cocci and 15% to 20% Gram-negative bacilli.[4] *Staphylococcus aureus* is the most common organism in native and prosthetic joint infections. The next most common group of Gram-positive aerobes is the streptococci, including *Streptococcus pneumoniae*. *Streptococcus pyogenes* is followed by groups B, G, C, and F in frequency. Patients who have immunosuppression, diabetes mellitus, malignancy, and severe genitourinary or gastrointestinal infections usually present non–group A streptococcal disease.[44] Group B streptococcal arthritis in adults is rare; however, it can be a serious infection in patients who have diabetes and also in those who have prosthetic hip infections.[45] Infections with Gram-negative bacilli usually occur in patients who have a history of intravenous drug abuse, in immunocompromised patients, and in very old patients.[46] The most common Gram-negative organisms are E coli and Pseudomonas aeruginosa.

Infections caused by anaerobes occur in 5% to 7% of septic arthritis.[19,40] Common anaerobes include Bacteroides, Propionibacterium acnes, and various anaerobic Gram-positive cocci. Foul-smelling synovial fluid or air in the joint space should raise the suspicion of anaerobic infection, and appropriate cultures should be obtained and held for at least 2 weeks. This type of infection is most frequent in patients who have wound infections or joint arthroplasty and in immunocompromised hosts.

Polyarticular septic arthritis is much less common than monoarticular infection.[31] Many of the patients have one or more comorbidities, and some have been intravenous drug abusers. The occurrence of this type of arthritis in patients who have rheumatoid arthritis is high and averages 25% (range 18%–35%).[47] Although Staphylococcus aureus is the most common pathogen, group G streptococci, Haemophilus influenzae, Streptococcus pneumoniae, or mixed aerobic and anaerobic bacteria have been responsible for polyarticular infections.

Plain radiographs of the infected joint are usually normal at presentation but should be obtained in all patients because associated osteomyelitis or concurrent joint disease may rarely be present. In addition, a baseline radiograph is often useful for comparison purposes should the response to therapy be delayed or poor. Radiographs often show nonspecific changes of inflammatory arthritis, including periarticular osteopenia, joint effusion, soft tissue swelling, and joint space loss. Scintigraphy, ultrasound, CT, or MRI can detect effusions and inflammation in joints that are difficult to examine, especially in the hip and sacroiliac joints, and can provide useful images to delineate the extent of the infection.[48,49] MRI is highly sensitive in early detection of joint fluid and is superior to CT delineation of soft tissue structures. These images can show early bone erosion; reveal soft tissue extension; and facilitate arthrocentesis of joints, such as shoulders, hips, acromioclavicular, sternoclavicular, and sacroiliac joints.[50]

TREATMENT

Treatment of bacterial arthritis must begin immediately after the clinical evaluation is complete and appropriate cultures have been taken. The acuity with which a clinician decides to initiate treatment and the correct choice of antibiotic in a patient who has infectious arthritis determines a good prognosis. The mainstay of therapy in these patients is parenteral antibiotic in the acute phase of the disease and adequate joint drainage. Initial antibiotic therapy should always be broad spectrum until a definite pathogen is isolated and thus a specific antibiotic chosen.

Many proposals have been made on the use of antibiotics but this is something that always depends on local epidemiology, clinician experience, local hospital conditions, and availability of therapy, especially in developing countries. Gram stain and risk factors should guide therapeutic regimens. Most antibiotics show a good penetration into diseased joints and the duration of parenteral antibiotics should be approximately 15 to 21 days and afterward continue with oral antibiotics for a complete 4-week regimen.

The most frequently used regimens use third-generation cephalosporins with good effective outcomes, especially if there is a high suspicion for Staphylococcus aureus or

Table 2 Proposal for empiric antibiotic use in bacterial arthritis	
Gram Stain of Synovial Fluid	Antibiotic Therapy
Gram-positive cocci	Cefazolin 2 g IV q 8 h Cefotaxime 1 g IV q 8 h
Gram-negative cocci	Ceftriaxone 1 g IV q 24 h
Gram-negative rods	Cefepime 2 g IV q 8 h Piperacillin-tazobactam 4.5 g IV q 6 h
MRSA suspicion or risk factors	Vancomycin 1 g IV q 12 h

Abbreviations: IV, intravenous; MRSA, methicillin-resistant Staphylococcus aureus.
Data from Ross JJ. Septic arthritis. Infect Dis Clin N Am 2005;19:799–817.

streptococci.[51] The use of B-lactam and aminoglycosides or quinolones for Gram-negative rods is usually a good choice, but recently the use of quinolones has shown an increased resistance from N gonorrhoeae and this has made the Centers for Disease Control discard its use as a viable therapy.[52,53]

The use of oral cefixime should continue after a course of intravenous antibiotic with other cephalosporins for the suggested time, always ensuring that Chlamydia is not the offending pathogen because of the lack of effectiveness against it.[41] In all cases, osteomyelitis is a feared outcome, especially in those patients who have involvement of a cartilaginous joint (sternoclavicular and sacroiliac), so therapy in those cases might need to have a duration of up to 6 weeks.[54] **Table 2** summarizes empiric antibiotic regimens.

Joint drainage has shown good results when combined with antibiotics, especially because it has the advantage of improving vascularization in the joint; it decompresses the joint, and it removes the organism and its offending cascade of inflammatory reactions. Whether to use arthrocentesis or open surgery is still debatable, but available data suggest that arthrocentesis is more effective than open drainage; patient selection might be biased and critically ill patients are not good candidates for surgical procedures, having worse mortality outcomes than arthrocentesis.[32,55] There is no consensus about joint immobilization in patients who have bacterial arthritis but it is generally suggested by several authors that early rehabilitation and joint mobilization provide better outcomes than immobilization, especially in the prevention of muscle atrophy and joint contractures.[56]

PROGNOSIS

The ability to diagnose and treat an infected joint as soon as possible is the key for a good prognosis. Mortality occurs in approximately 10% of patients and permanent joint damage affects almost half of the patients affected with infectious arthritis. Outcome is closely related to multiple factors, especially comorbid conditions (eg, immunocompromised state, presence of underlying osteoarthritis and rheumatoid arthritis, and previous joint damage and pathogen virulence factors). All clinicians should be aware of the presence of an infectious process as a potential cause of acute arthritis to do an adequate screening to diagnose and treat it promptly.

ACKNOWLEDGMENTS

We thank Ignacio García-Valladares for his help in the preparation of this article.

REFERENCES

1. Atkins BL, Bowler IC. The diagnosis of large joint sepsis. J Hosp Infect 1998;40: 263–74.
2. Goldenberg DL, Chisholm PL, Rice PA. Experimental models of bacterial arthritis: a microbiologic and histopathologic characterization of the arthritis after the intra-articular injections of *Neisseria gonorrhoeae*, *Staphylococcus aureus*, group A streptococci, and *Escherichia coli*. J Rheumatol 1983;10:5–11.
3. Schurman DJ, Mirra J, Ding A, et al. Experimental *E. coli* arthritis in the rabbit. A model of infectious and post-infectious inflammatory synovitis. J Rheumatol 1977; 4:118–28.
4. Goldenberg DL, Cohen AS. Acute infectious arthritis. A review of patients with a non-gonococcal joint infection. Am J Med 1976;60:369–77.
5. Roca RP, Yoshikawa TT. Primary skeletal infections in heroin users: a chemical characterization, diagnosis and therapy. Clin Orthop 1979;144:238–48.
6. Mitchell WS, Brooks PM, Stevenson RD, et al. Septic arthritis in patients with rheumatoid disease: a still under-diagnosed complication. J Rheumatol 1976;3: 124–33.
7. Douglas GW, Levin RU, Sokololf L. Infectious arthritis complicating neoplastic disease. N Engl J Med 1964;270:299–302.
8. Franz A, Webster AD, Furr PM, et al. Mycoplasmal arthritis in patients with primary immunoglobulin deficiency: clinical features and outcome in 18 patients. Br J Rheumatol 1997;36:661–8.
9. Cooper C, Cawley MID. Bacterial arthritis in an English health district: a 10 year review. Ann Rheum Dis 1986;45:458–63.
10. Woo PC, Lau SK, Yuen KY. First report of methicillin-resistant *Staphylococcus aureus* septic arthritis complicating acupuncture: simple procedure resulting in most devastating outcome. Diagn Microbiol Infect Dis 2009;63:92–5.
11. Armstrong RW, Bolding F, Joseph R. Septic arthritis following arthroscopy: clinical syndromes and analysis of risk factors. Arthroscopy 1992;8:213–23.
12. Klein DM, Barbera C, Gray ST, et al. Sensitivity of objective parameters in the diagnosis of pediatric septic hips. Clin Orthop 1997;338:153–9.
13. Kallio MJ, Unkila-Kallio L, Aalto K, et al. Serum C-reactive protein, erythrocyte sedimentation rate and white blood cell count in septic arthritis of children. Pediatr Infect Dis J 1997;16:411–3.
14. Wilkins RF, Healy RA, Decker JL. Acute infectious arthritis in the aged and chronically ill. Arch Intern Med 1996;106:354–67.
15. Brucellosis in Britain [editorial]. BMJ 1984;289:817.
16. Trujillo IZ, Zavala AN, Caceres JG, et al. Brucellosis. Infect Dis Clin North Am 1994;8:225–41.
17. Hasley JP, Reebak JS, Barnes CG. A decade of skeletal tuberculosis. Ann Rheum Dis 1982;41:7–10.
18. Niall DM, Murphy PG, Fogarty EE, et al. Puncture wound related pseudomonas infections of the foot in children. Ir J Med Sci 1997;166:98–101.
19. Kaandorp CJ, Dinant HJ, van de Laar MA, et al. Incidence and sources of native and prosthetic joint infection: a community based prospective survey. Ann Rheum Dis 1997;56:470–5.
20. Kaandorp CJ, Krijnen P, Moens HJ, et al. The outcome of bacterial arthritis: a prospective community-based study. Arthritis Rheum 1997;40:884–92.
21. Favero M, Schiavon F, Riato L, et al. Rheumatoid arthritis is the major risk factor for septic arthritis in rheumatological settings. Autoimmun Rev 2008;8:59–61.

22. Goldenberg DL, Reed JI. Bacterial arthritis. N Engl J Med 1985;312:764–71.
23. Goldenberg DL. Septic arthritis. Lancet 1998;351:197–202.
24. De Champs C, Le Seaux S, Dubost JJ, et al. Isolation of *Pantoea agglomerans* in two cases of septic monoarthritis after plant thorn and wood sliver injuries. J Clin Microbiol 2000;38:460–1.
25. Tong DC, Rothwell BR. Antibiotic prophylaxis in dentistry: a review and practice recommendations. J Am Dent Assoc 2000;131:366–74.
26. Haug JB, Harthug S, Kalager T, et al. Bloodstream infections at a Norwegian university hospital, 1974–1979 and 1988–1989: changing etiology, clinical features, and outcome. Clin Infect Dis 1994;19:246–56.
27. Ross JJ, Saltzman CL, Carling P, et al. Pneumococcal septic arthritis: review of 190 cases. Clin Infect Dis 2003;36:319–27.
28. Patti JM, Bremell T, Krajewska-Pietrasik D, et al. The *Staphylococcus aureus* collagen adhesin is a virulence determinant in experimental septic arthritis. Infect Immun 1994;62:152–61.
29. Stevens CR, Williams RB, Farrell AJ, et al. Hypoxia and inflammatory synovitis: observations and speculation. Ann Rheum Dis 1991;50:124–32.
30. Matthews PC, Dean BJ, Medagoda K, et al. Native hip joint septic arthritis in 20 adults: delayed presentation beyond three weeks predicts need for excision arthroplasty. J Infect 2008;57:185–90.
31. Dubost J, Fis I, Denis P, et al. Polyarticular septic arthritis. Medicine 1993;72:296–310.
32. Weston VC, Jones AC, Bradbury N, et al. Clinical features and outcome of septic arthritis in a single UK Health District 1982–1991. Ann Rheum Dis 1999;58:214–9.
33. Edwards SA, Cranfield T, Clarke HJ. Atypical presentation of septic arthritis in the immunosuppressed patient. Orthopedics 2002;25:1089–90.
34. Brown TJ, Yen-Moore A, Tyring SK. An overview of sexually transmitted diseases, Part I. J Am Acad Dermatol 1999;41:511–32.
35. Cucurull E, Espinoza LR. Gonococcal arthritis. Rheum Dis Clin North Am 1998;24:305–22.
36. Al-Suleiman SA, Grimes EM, Jonas HS. Disseminated gonococcal infections. Obstet Gynecol 1983;61:48–51.
37. O'Brien JP, Goldenberg DL, Rice PA. Disseminated gonococcal infection: a prospective analysis of 49 patients and a review of pathophysiology and immune mechanisms. Medicine (Baltimore) 1983;62:395–406.
38. Wise CM, Morris CR, Wasilauskas BL, et al. Gonococcal arthritis in an era of increasing penicillin resistance: presentations and outcomes in 41 recent cases (1985–1991). Arch Intern Med 1994;154:2690–5.
39. Newman ED, Davis DE, Harrington TM. Septic arthritis due to Gram negative bacilli: older patients with good outcome. J Rheumatol 1988;15:659–62.
40. Pioro MH, Mandell BF. Septic arthritis. Rheum Dis Clin North Am 1997;23:239–58.
41. Rice PA. Gonococcal arthritis (disseminated gonococcal infection). Infect Dis Clin North Am 2005;19:853–61.
42. Liebling MR, Arkfeld DG, Michelini GA, et al. Identification of Neisseria gonorrhoeae in synovial fluid using the polymerase chain reaction. Arthritis Rheum 1994;37:702–9.
43. Muralidhar B, Rumore PM, Steinman CR. Use of the polymerase chain reaction to study arthritis due to *Neisseria gonorrhoeae*. Arthritis Rheum 1994;37:710–7.
44. Schattner A, Vosti KL. Bacterial arthritis due to beta-hemolytic streptococci of serogroups A, B, C, F, and G: analysis of 23 cases and review of the literature. Medicine 1998;77:122–39.

45. Dugan JM, Geogiades G, VanGorp C, et al. Group B streptococcal prosthetic joint infections. J South Orthop Assoc 2001;10:209–14.
46. Goldenberg DL, Brandt K, Cathcart E, et al. Acute arthritis caused by gram-negative bacilli: a clinical characterization. Medicine 1974;53:197–208.
47. Ho G Jr. Bacterial arthritis. In: McCarty DJ, Koopman WJ, editors. Arthritis and allied conditions. 12th edition. Philadelphia: Lea and Febiger; 1993. p. 2003–23.
48. Zimmermann B 3rd, Mikolich DJ, Lally EV. Septic sacroiliitis. Semin Arthritis Rheum 1996;26:592–604.
49. Sanchez RB, Quinn SF. MRI of inflammatory synovial processes. Magn Reson Imaging 1989;7:529–40.
50. Widman DS, Craig JG, Van Holsbeeck MT. Sonographic detection, evaluation and aspiration of infected acromioclavicular joints. Skeletal Radiol 2001;30: 388–92.
51. Hamed KA, Tam JY, Prober CG. Pharmacokinetic optimisation of the treatment of septic arthritis. Clin Pharmacokinet 1996;21:156–63.
52. Le Dantec L, Mabry F, Flipo RM, et al. Peripheral pyogenic arthritis. A study of one hundred seventy-nine cases. Rev Rhum Engl Ed 1996;63:103–10.
53. Centers for Disease Control and Prevention. Update to CDC's sexually trans-mitted diseases treatment guidelines, 2006: fluoroquinolones no longer recom-mended for treatment of gonococcal infections. Morb Mortal Wkly Rep 2007; 56:332–6.
54. Ross JJ, Shamsuddin H. Sternoclavicular septic arthritis: review of 180 cases. Medicine (Baltimore) 2004;83:139–48.
55. Broy SB, Schmid FR. A comparison of medical drainage (needle aspiration) and surgical drainage (arthrotomy or arthroscopy) in the initial treatment of infected joints. Clin Rheum Dis 1986;12:501–22.
56. Tarkowski A. Infectious arthritis. Best Pract Res Clin Rheumatol 2006;20:1029–44.

Pathophysiology and Clinical Spectrum of Infections in Systemic Lupus Erythematosus

Raquel Cuchacovich, MD[a],*, Abraham Gedalia, MD[b]

KEYWORDS

- Systemic lupus erythmatosus • Infections • Pathogenesis
- Immunosuppression • Immunodeficiencies

Systemic lupus erythematosus (SLE) is an inflammatory and multisystemic autoimmune disorder characterized by an uncontrolled autoreactivity of B and T lymphocytes leading to the production of autoantibodies (auto-Abs) against self-directed antigens and tissue destruction. The breakdown of tolerance, which is poorly understood, is the main feature of the disease. It involves intrinsic and extrinsic mechanisms, such as genes, deficiency of regulatory T/B cells, and hormonal and environmental factors (**Box 1**).[1–23]

Several lines of evidence suggest that there is familial aggregation; a sibling of an SLE patient is approximately 20 times more likely to develop disease. In a prospectively followed cohort from South Sweden, 15% of the patients who had SLE had a first-degree relative who had SLE. Twin studies support a concordance rate of 2% in dizygotic compared with 24% in monozygotic twins. Deficiencies in C1q (>90% develop the disease), C_2, C_4, and CR1 receptor, and polymorphic variants of the mannose binding lectin (MBL)–2 gene, and certain human leukocyte antigen (HLA) class II haplotypes, such as DR2-DQ6, the extended haplotype HLA A1-B8-DR3-DQ2-C4AQ0, and tumor necrosis factor (TNF) gene variants are associated. Other polymorphic genes implicated are Fc-receptor genes IIa and IIIa, C-reactive protein, programmed cell death-1 (PDCD-1), IL-1 receptor antagonist (Ra), chemokines (CCL2), and genes being part of interferon (IFN) pathways.[13,24–36]

Environmental factors, such as infections, which are an important cause of morbidity and mortality, hormones, smoking, alcohol intake, exposure to aromatic amines, pesticides, silica, organic solvents, heavy metals, ultraviolet light, dietary

[a] Section of Rheumatology, Department of Internal Medicine, Louisiana State University Health Sciences Center, 1542 Tulane Avenue, New Orleans, LA 70112, USA
[b] Department of Pediatrics, Louisiana State University Health Sciences Center, 1542 Tulane Avenue, New Orleans, LA 70112, USA
* Corresponding author.
E-mail address: rcucha@lsuhsc.edu (R. Cuchacovich).

Rheum Dis Clin N Am 35 (2009) 75–93
doi:10.1016/j.rdc.2009.03.003   rheumatic.theclinics.com
0889-857X/09/$ – see front matter © 2009 Elsevier Inc. All rights reserved.

Box 1

Impaired immune functions in systemic lupus erythematosus that may predispose to infection

Breakdown in the mechanisms that maintain T- and B-cell tolerance

Production of autoantibodies, which react with nuclear, cytoplasmic, cell membrane, and extracellular matrix components; these immune complexes (IC) initiate inflammation and tissue damage

Failure to remove autoreactive B cells: FcγRIIb induce cell death, inhibit migration, and control plasma cell survival, which contribute to autoimmunity and infection

Posttranslational modifications of nuclear autoantigens, such as ubiquitination, citrullination, phosphorylation, and methylation, result in the presentation of cryptic self-antigens

Significant lower level of CD24+CD25+ T reg cells

Decreased phagocytosis, clearance of apoptotic blebs, impaired nitroblue tetrazolium reduction, and reduced production of interleukin (IL)-8 and IL-12 by polymorph nuclear cells

Inappropriate activation of toll-like receptor (TLR) for self-antigens, TLR3 (ds) RNA, TLR7 (ss) RNA, and TLR9 (unmethylated CpG motifs within ssDNA)

TLR9 is expressed in B cells, dendritic cells (DCs), and macrophages, recognizes bacterial DNA with multiple CpG nucleotides; and co-ligation of the B cell receptor and TLRs induces proliferation and differentiation of plasmacytoid DC (pDC)

Internalization of mammalian DNA-containing IC in DCs is mediated by FcγRIIa, delivering the antigen into lysosomes containing TLR9, which subsequently initiates DC activation and the production of Type I IFNs

Clearance of IgG-coated erythrocytes and soluble IC is delayed because of reduced complement- and Fc-mediated uptake

Mannose-binding lectin deficiency may be a susceptibility for SLE and high frequency of infections, particularly bacterial and mainly pulmonary

---

factors, such as alfalfa sprouts and saturated fats, and the drugs hydralazine, procainamide, estrogens, TNF-inhibitors, antiepileptics, sulfasalazine (SSZ), statins, and type I IFN are potential triggers of the disease.[37,38]

BACTERIAL INFECTION

About 80% of SLE infections are caused by bacteria. The most frequent sites of infection are skin, respiratory tract, and urinary tract, accounting for more than two thirds of the infections seen in SLE (**Box 2**).[39–42]

Depressed IL-12 production by polymorph nuclear cells (PMNs) in patients who have SLE could be of significance in acute infections, such as bacterial pneumonia, candidiasis, and urinary tract infection.[43] Several risk factors predispose patients who have lupus to infections, such as active disease, lymphopenia,[44] presence of renal involvement, immunosuppressive therapy, and central nervous system (CNS) damage.[45–48] Antigranulocyte antibodies, found in approximately 50% of patients who have SLE, can cause neutropenia through direct cytotoxicity and opsonization. Bosch and colleagues[49] studied the incidence and characteristics of infection in SLE, as well as the risks factors. A total of 110 patients who had SLE and 220 controls were prospectively followed up over 3 years and all the infectious episodes were recorded. Thirty-nine patients who had SLE experienced at least one infection (36%) versus 53 controls (22%), (P<.05). The incidence of urinary infections, pneumonia, and bacteremia without known focus was significantly greater in SLE. *Escherichia coli* was the most common microorganism (21.3%). In the univariate analysis,

Box 2
Most frequent microorganisms found in patients who have systemic lupus erythematosus
Bacteria
Staphylococcus aureus
Nontyphoidal *Salmonella*
Escherichia coli
Streptococcus pneumoniae
Haemophilus influenzae
Klebsiella spp
Acinetobacter spp
Pseudomonas spp
Mycoplasma spp
Virus
Parvovirus B19
Cytomegalovirus
Epstein-Barr virus
Herpes simplex/varicella zoster
Human papillomavirus
Hepatitis A
Fungus
Candida spp
Aspergillus spp
Cryptococcus neoformans
Nocardia spp
Mycobacterium
Nontuberculous mycobacterium
Mycobacterium chelonae
M avium complex (MAC)
M haemophilum
M fortuitum
M marinum
M tuberculosis

nephritis, SLE activity, leukopenia, anti-dsDNA Abs, low CH50, and ever use of steroids or cyclophosphamide were significantly associated with infection. In the multivariate analysis, total serum complement levels and a daily dose of prednisone greater than 20 mg during at least 1 month plus use of cyclophosphamide were found to be significant ($P<.0001$). Hypocomplementemia seems to be an independent predictive factor for infection (**Box 3**). Hsieh and colleagues[50] demonstrated that anti-SSB/La antibodies cause increased neutrophil apoptosis, IL-8 production, and decreased phagocytosis. Biswas and colleagues[51] assessed the phagocytic efficiency of PMNs in patients who had SLE with and without history of infections and

Box 3
Systemic lupus erythematosus risk factors that predispose to infections

Active disease

Long-term disease damage

Cytopenias (neutropenia/lymphopenia)

Hypocomplementemia

Renal involvement

CNS involvement

Immunosuppressive therapy

correlated it with disease activity, duration, and presence of anti-SSB/La antibodies. They also analyzed the ability of PMNs from patients who had SLE to produce IL-12 in response to LPS with or without IFN-γ. Findings showed that PMNs from patients who have SLE have impaired phagocytic efficiency and decreased production of IL-12, which is more pronounced in patients who have a history of infections, and the phagocytic efficiency is significantly lower in patients who are anti-SSB/La positive.[52]

A study on adult patients who had SLE in Hong Kong revealed that infections accounted for 60% of mortality, followed by cardiovascular (12%) and cerebrovascular (16%) diseases. Bacteremia is common in patients who have SLE and bacteremia-related mortality is higher than mortality caused by other infections. The prevalence of bacteremia in patients who have SLE fluctuates between 16% and 47% and is mainly caused by opportunistic pathogens and microorganisms that are responsible for common infections in the general population. Mok and colleagues[53,54] indicated that age is an important factor that affects the clinical manifestations and prognosis of SLE and that infection is a major cause of mortality in late-onset SLE.

Multiple studies have identified that active lupus is one of the risk factors for infection; in the Toronto study, patients who had SLE who developed infections required longer hospitalization (28.5 versus 11.2 days, P<.001) and had higher SLE Disease Activity Index (SLEDAI) scores (11.6 versus 7.1). A prospective study in the Hopkins Lupus Cohort[55] also demonstrated that SLE activity (SLEDAI) was a predictive factor for hospitalization because of infection. Gram-negative bacilli are the most common microorganisms responsible for bacteremia in Asian patients who have SLE, but Gram-positive coccid are more often encountered in Western patients who have bacteremic SLE. Nontyphoidal salmonella is the main cause of Gram-negative bacteremia in patients who have SLE.[56–59] In immunocompromised patients, the overall mortality of salmonella bacteremia has been reported as 26%. Chen and colleagues[56] described the nature of bacteremia in patients who have SLE and determined the short-term survival and long-term outcome of these patients. They analyzed medical records of 1442 patients who had SLE who were regularly followed up in a tertiary teaching medical center for a 6-year observation period. Among 1442 patients who had SLE, 240 patients (17%) developed at least one episode of bacteremia, corresponding to an incidence of 92.7 cases/1000 hospital admissions. Since SLE diagnosis, the overall survival of their patients was 92% at 5 years, 86% at 10 years and 79% at 15 years. After one episode of bacteremia, however, the survival decreased to 76% at 30 days and 67% at 360 days. Of the 336 episodes of bacteremia, 167 were community acquired (49.7%) and 169 were nosocomial (50.3%). Staphylococcus aureus was the leading cause of Gram-positive bacteremia. Among Gram-negative bacteria, nontyphoidal salmonella and E coli were the most common species.

Community-acquired salmonella and streptococcus bacteremia were more common than nosocomial infections. *Klebsiella* and *Acinetobacter* spp were significantly more responsible for nosocomial than community-acquired bacteremia. Patients infected with *Acinetobacter*, *Klebsiella*, or *Pseudomonas* had lower probabilities of 14-day survival (71.4%, 55.6%, and 42.9%, respectively). There was a significant difference in the SLEDAI scores between patients who developed bacteremia infection and those who did not. Use of oral corticosteroids was more common in patients who developed bacteremia. There were no significant differences between the two groups in the use of other immunosuppressants (methylprednisolone pulse therapy, azathioprine [AZA], or cyclophosphamide).[60]

Risk factors for long-term disease damage in juvenile-onset SLE are disease duration, cumulative disease activity, neuropsychiatric lupus, acute thrombocytopenia, hypertension, seropositivity for antiphospholipid antibody, corticosteroid and cyclophosphamide therapy, renal involvement, duration of AZA, and recurrent infections. In a retrospective study Lee and colleagues[61] analyzed the pattern of infections and disease damage that occurred in a cohort of patients who had juvenile-onset SLE; the second endpoint was whether cumulative disease damage was associated with recurrent infections in these patients. Thirty-two (68.1%) patients had lupus nephropathy and 16 patients (34%) had neuropsychiatric lupus. Sixty-one episodes of major infections, defined as infections requiring more than 1 week of antimicrobial agents, occurred in 27 patients (57.4%), and 18 patients (31.4%) had recurrent major infections (two episodes). Organ damage using the Systemic Lupus International Collaborating Clinics/American College of Rheumatology Damage Index (SDI) was documented in 21 subjects (44.7%). The occurrence of major infections (*P*<.001) was the only significant risk factor for disease damage. There was a positive correlation between SDI score with the number of recurrent major infections (*P*<.001). This study showed that long-term disease damage and recurrent infections were a significant burden to patients who had juvenile-onset SLE despite good overall survival. Lupus nephritis, duration of use of AZA, and the occurrence of major infections were significantly more common in patients who had long-term damage.[62] Rojas-Serrano and colleagues[63] assessed the prevalence of infections in patients who had SLE with pulmonary hemorrhage. Fourteen events in 13 patients were evaluated. In eight (57%), infection was demonstrated; the most common pathogenic agents were *Pseudomonas* spp and *Aspergillus fumigatus*. Four patients died, 3 of them of pulmonary infection and 1 of a cerebral hemorrhage secondary to severe hypertension.

VIRAL INFECTIONS IN SYSTEMIC LUPUS ERYTHEMATOSUS

Acute viral infections in children and adults induce transient autoimmune responses, including generation of autoantibodies in low titers with a transient course, but the progression into an established autoimmune disease is rare.[64,65] The most common viral infections in patients who have SLE are parvovirus B19 (there are more than 30 reports of primary B19 infection reported as lupus-like syndrome)[66–70] and cytomegalovirus (CMV, predominantly presenting in severely immunosuppressed patients). CMV infection may mimic a lupus flare or present with specific organ involvement, such as gastrointestinal bleeding or pulmonary infiltrates. Ramos-Casals and colleagues[71] studied the cause and clinical features of acute viral infections in 88 (23 from their clinics and 65 from the literature review) patients who had SLE and their influence on the diagnosis, prognosis, and treatment. Twenty-five patients were diagnosed with new-onset SLE associated with infection by human parvovirus B19 (n = 15), CMV (n = 6), Epstein-Barr virus (EBV; n = 3), and hepatitis A virus (n = 1). The remaining 63 cases of acute viral infections arose in patients already diagnosed with SLE. In 18 patients symptoms related to infection mimicked a lupus flare; 36 patients, including 1 patient from the former group who presented with both conditions, presented organ-specific viral infections (mainly pneumonitis, colitis, retinitis, and hepatitis). Ten patients had a severe multiorgan process similar to that described in catastrophic antiphospholipid syndrome; the final diagnosis was hemophagocytic syndrome in 5 cases and disseminated viral infection in 5 cases. Twelve patients died of infection caused by CMV (n = 5), herpes simplex virus (n = 4), EBV (n = 2), and varicella-zoster virus (VZV; n = 1). Autopsies were performed in 9 patients and disclosed disseminated herpetic infection in 6 patients (caused by herpes simplex in 4 cases, varicella in 1, and CMV in 1) and hemophagocytic syndrome in 3. A higher frequency of renal failure (54% versus 19%, P = .024), antiphospholipid syndrome (33% versus 6%, P = .023), treatment with cyclophosphamide (82% versus 37%, P = .008), and multisystemic involvement at presentation (58% versus 8%, P<.001), and a lower frequency of antiviral therapy (18% versus 76%, P<.001) were found in patients who died, compared with survivors.[72]

Some viral infections, especially CMV and B19 but also EBV, varicella, hepatitis A virus, norovirus, measles, and mumps, can mimic lupus flares in patients who have SLE. Fever, arthralgia, malaise, cutaneous rash, lymphadenopathy, and cytopenia and could be easily confused with a lupus flare. In patients who have SLE with a suspected flare who do not respond to SLE-specific therapy, careful evaluation of virus-specific features (elevated transaminases for hepatitis A virus, acute onset of diarrhea and vomiting for norovirus, cutaneous vesicular rash for varicella, and parotid enlargement for mumps), together with investigations for the most frequent viruses involved (herpesviruses and B19), should be performed.[67,73,74]

Patients who have SLE with acute viral infections often present comorbid processes that may complicate the diagnosis and outcome, such as severe cytopenias, thrombocytopenia, leukopenia, hemolytic anemia, pure red cell aplasia, and hemophagocytic syndrome.[75–82] Disseminated viral infections (associated with hemophagocytic syndrome or not) should be included in the differential diagnosis of life-threatening situations (of which catastrophic antiphospholipid syndrome [APS] is the main differential diagnosis) in patients who have SLE. Parvovirus B19 mainly affects patients who are not immunosuppressed and mimics SLE, whereas CMV preferentially affects immunosuppressed patients.

Epstein-Barr Virus

EBV is a member of the herpesvirus family, causes acute infectious mononucleosis and lymphoproliferative diseases, and triggers the development of autoimmune diseases. In 1971 Evans[83] described a high prevalence of the virus in the sera of patients who had SLE, and in 1997 EBV was proposed as an etiologic cause for SLE, rather than an incidental finding. The pathogenesis is molecular mimicry, between EBV antigen 1 and lupus-specific antigens, such as Ro, La, or dsDNA, through induction of TLR hypersensitivity by EBV latent membrane protein 2A or by creating immortal B and T cells by loss of apoptosis. Pender and colleagues[84] state that during primary infection, autoreactive B cells are infected by EBV, proliferate, and become latently infected memory B cells, which are resistant to apoptosis as a consequence of expression of virus-encoded antiapoptotic molecules. Then autoreactive T cells, which were activated by the impaired B cells, also fail to undergo apoptosis because they receive a costimulatory survival signal from the infected B cells. The autoreactive T cells proliferate and produce cytokines, which recruit other inflammatory cells, with resultant target-organ damage and chronic autoimmune disease.[85–93]

Cytomegalovirus

CMV, a member of the herpesvirus family, has a potential role in the development and progression of SLE. There seems to be a higher prevalence of CMV IgG and IgM antibodies in patients who have SLE, antiphospholipid syndrome, primary biliary cirrhosis, systemic sclerosis, polymyositis, Sjögren syndrome, and vasculitis. CMV may produce a systemic infection mimicking SLE, either superimposed upon a flare or presenting with isolated organ involvement that may not be immediately attributable to infection (gastrointestinal bleeding from colitis or pulmonary infiltrates from pneumonitis).[94–99]

Varicella–Zoster Virus

Following primary infection, VZV is latent in the cranial nerve ganglia or the dorsal root ganglia throughout its lifetime. VZV infection is common among patients who have SLE, but disseminated or aggressive episodes are rare. In Kahl's study,[100] disseminated infections accounted for 11% of episodes, but this experience is not confirmed by other authors. Moga and colleagues[101] followed 145 patients who had SLE for a mean period of 7.6 years. They detected 20 VZV infections in 19 patients (13.1%) with no disseminated episode among them. Higher incidence was in patients under immunosuppressive therapy or corticosteroids. There was no evidence of a deleterious effect of VZV infection on SLE evolution and patients responded to established therapy. In a retrospective study Hellman and colleagues[102] reviewed the charts of 44 patients who had SLE who died during the hospital admission. A total of 24 of 44 (55%) of the patients had an infection and in 13 of those 24 (50%) infection was the cause of death, but only 1 patient presented with disseminated herpes zoster. Corticosteroids are a risk factor for VZV infections; most infections appear in patients who take daily doses of prednisone less than 20 mg or in patients not taking any prednisone.

Human Papillomavirus

Women who have SLE are at enhanced risk for acquiring HPV-16 infections and developing cervical premalignancies.[103,104] Women in the United Kingdom who had a recent SLE diagnosis had elevated levels of HPV infections (European HPV-16 variants at a high viral load), abnormal cervical cytology, and squamous intraepithelial lesions (SIL). Previous studies of HPV infections among patients who had SLE have demonstrated that wart-virus antibodies are less frequent among patients than controls, suggesting an inability to produce an effective immune response to HPV, and that 11% of patients had high-risk HPV infections, which are not associated with therapy.[105,106] Nath and colleagues[107] studied the rates of HPV infections, abnormal cervical smears, and SIL in 30 women in the United Kingdom who had SLE and compared them with 67 abnormal smears from colposcopy clinics, and 15 community subjects who had normal smears. SLE and colposcopy patients were more likely ($P<.05$) to be HPV positive (15 [54%] and 37 [67%] patients, respectively) and HPV-16 DNA positive (16 [57%] and 17 [31%] patients, respectively) than community subjects (0% HPV DNA positive and 1 [6%] HPV-16 DNA positive). SLE patients were also more likely to be HPV-16 DNA positive than colposcopy patients ($P<.05$). Patients who had SLE with a high HPV-16 viral load more frequently had SIL (n = 6) than those who had a low HPV-16 viral load (n = 1; $P<.05$). HPV and HPV-16 DNA positivity were not associated with previous or current drug therapy for patients who had SLE. Eighteen (60%) patients who had SLE had a previous or current cervical abnormality. At the time of study, 5 (17%) patients who had SLE had an abnormal cervical smear and 8 (27%) had SIL. For those diagnosed with SLE for greater than 10 years, the rate of SIL was 44% lower than those who had SLE for less than 5 years (odds ratio 0.56, 95% confidence interval 0.1–3.5). The results demonstrated that patients who have SLE are at significantly heightened risk for HPV-16 infections and for developing cervical abnormalities, particularly SIL.

OPPORTUNISTIC MICROORGANISMS
Fungal Infections

Cases of SLE with fungemia or invasive fungal infection have seldom been described. During the past 35 years, only case reports (the largest consisting of three cases) have described fungal infections in patients who had SLE. Sieving and colleagues[108] reported three SLE cases who had deep fungal infections and reviewed 30 cases in the literature; most patients were young females. Among these 30 patients, the most common infection was Candida spp (n = 13), C neoformans in 10 and Aspergillus spp in 4. Candida infection was identified as the most common fungal infection.[109] In contrast, cryptococcal infection was the most common pathogen in this study. Nocardial infections are common fungal infections in steroid-treated patients who have SLE, particularly for lung lesions.[110–114] Severe candida infection is the most frequently identified opportunistic fungal infection in several SLE series, associated with steroid and cytotoxic drug therapy. Patients who had fungal infections had active SLE (SLE-DAI > 7), indicating that SLEDAI greater than 7 may be a predisposing factor for fungal infection. In this study, survival was 80% at 1 year (SLE diagnosis to death) for patients who had SLE who were suffering fungal infections, 73.3% at 2 years, 66.7% at 5 years and 60% at 10 years. Patients who had SLE with fungal infections in this study had poorer prognosis than the general SLE population. Currently there is no consensus as to whether different corticosteroid doses predispose patients to fungal infection regardless of earlier lupus involvement (such as hemolytic anemia or positive anticardiolipin antibody) in patients who have SLE.

Chen and colleagues[115] studied invasive fungal infections in 15 Taiwanese patients who had SLE and compared the characteristics of their infections with those reported in the literature. Cryptococcus neoformans was the most commonly identified fungus in this Taiwanese series. The prevalence of autoimmune hemolytic anemia and positive results for the anticardiolipin antibody in this study were significantly higher than those in patients who had SLE in general (P<.0001 and P<.0001, respectively). Fungal infection contributed to cause of death in 7 of 15 (46.7%) patients; C neoformans accounted for 6 of these infections. Low-dose prednisolone (<1 or <0.5 mg/kg/d based on arbitrary division) before fungal infection tended to correlate with 1-year mortality after diagnosis of SLE (P = .077 or P = .080). Following fungal infection, however, patients who died of infection itself had been prescribed with higher prednisolone dose or equivalent than surviving patients (P = .016). All patients who had SLE who had fungal infections had active SLE (SLEDAI > 7). C neoformans infection accounted for most fatalities in patients who had SLE with fungal infections in this series. Active lupus disease is probably a risk factor for fungal infection in patients who have SLE. Notably, low prednisolone doses before fungal infection or high prednisolone doses following fungal infection tended to associate with or correlated to fatality, respectively.

MYCOBACTERIAL INFECTIONS

Nontuberculous mycobacterium (NTM) infections have been described in patients who have autoimmune diseases in isolated case reports, especially in those who have SLE.[116–119] Mok and colleagues[120] examined the clinical manifestations of NTM infections with those of *M tuberculosis* (MTB) infections in 725 patients who had SLE. Eleven cases were identified (prevalence 1.5%). The mean ± SD age at the time of infection was 42.8 ± 13.9 years, 9.3 ± 5.8 years after the onset of SLE. The mean ± SD time taken from onset of symptoms to the diagnosis of NTM infection was 5.7 ± 7.2 months. Sites of involvement included skin and soft tissue (n = 8), chest (n = 2), and disseminated infection (n = 1). NTM infections were more likely to involve extrapulmonary sites (soft tissue and skin) (*P* = .006), presented in patients with longer lupus disease duration (*P*<.001), and occurred in older patients (*P*<.001) and in those who had a higher cumulative dose of prednisolone (*P* = .01) than MTB infections. Disease duration was found to be the only independent predictive factor (*P* = .005) for NTM infections. Ten (25.6%) patients who had MTB infections but none of the patients who had NTM infections presented concomitantly at the onset of SLE (*P* = .09). MTB occurred in 33.3% of our cohort and may manifest as synovitis, skin ulcer, and lymphadenitis. There were no differences in the recurrence rate (*P* = .64) and frequency of disseminated infections (*P* = .40) between NTM and MTB infections.

NTM infections tended to develop in patients who had SLE later in their disease course than MTB infections. Local implantation of the organism from skin abrasion is likely to be the route of transmission, because most NTM are found in water and soil. *M chelonae* viz *M avium complex* (MAC) and *M haemophilum* cause cutaneous infections in SLE.[121] In acute synovitis, mainly monoarticular involvement and periarticular tissue, *M fortuitum*, MAC, and *M marinum* have been found.[122–126]

MTB infection occurs earlier in the clinical course of SLE than NTM infection. Most NTM that causes disease involve the lungs, skin, soft tissue, lymph node, and bone, and rarely disseminate. NTM presentation may be insidious in onset, have different sites of involvement, and present as multifocal lesions. Tissue culture is often required for a definitive diagnosis because the clinical manifestations of NTM infections are not pathognomonic and may mimic other infective or noninfective conditions. NTM infections tend to occur in the chronically and more heavily immunosuppressed patients who have SLE as compared with tuberculosis.[127]

IS THERE ANY ASSOCIATION BETWEEN IMMUNOSUPPRESSIVE THERAPY AND INCREASED MORBIDITY AND MORTALITY DUE TO INFECTIONS IN SYSTEMIC LUPUS ERYTHEMATOSUS?

The use of immunosuppressive therapies in SLE carries a significantly increased risk for developing infections, especially in patients treated with high-dose corticosteroids and cyclophosphamide. Infections in immunosuppressed patients are usually caused by bacteria, but patients may also develop severe viral infections. Patients who had viral infections who had received cyclophosphamide had a poorer survival. Staples and colleagues[128–130] suggested that the incidence of infection among patients who had SLE increased when steroid dose increased, whereas disseminated or deep tissue infections occurred more frequently in patients who had azotemia receiving high doses of steroids. In a study by Petri and Genovese,[55] hospitalized patients who had SLE received a mean prednisone dose of more than 10 mg significantly more commonly compared with nonhospitalized patients. The mean prednisone dose was not found to be significantly different between patients who had SLE who developed infections and those who did not in two other studies. In another study, the median prednisolone dose was not found to be significantly different between patients who had SLE who developed three or more bacterial infections other than urinary tract infections and those who did not have SLE. Recent administration of methylprednisolone pulse was outlined as a risk factor for infection in another study. Prolonged treatment with corticosteroids was found to be more common among patients who had SLE who had more than two bacterial infections (other than urinary) compared with those who did not have such infections in another study. Rosner and colleagues[131] reported that deaths attributable to infections were statistically significant related only to the peak of steroid dose without any correlation with other immunosuppressants used. Petri and Genovese[55] reported that even though patients who had infections were treated with higher doses of prednisone, this relation was not statistically significant.

IMMUNODEFICIENCIES IN SYSTEMIC LUPUS ERYTHEMATOSUS
Common Variable Immunodeficiency

Hypogammaglobulinemia in SLE may occur as part of common variable immunodeficiency (CVID).[132–136] Patients who have CVID develop recurrent respiratory and sinus infections; a subset of these patients can also develop features suggestive of immune dysregulation, including autoimmunity (usually cytopenias and SLE); granulomatous inflammation, which can affect liver, spleen, and lungs; and bowel disease. Transition from one state to the other is clearly unusual.[137,138] Whether these two entities just coexist or CVID is a complication of SLE or is caused by the immunosuppressive treatment given for controlling the autoimmune disease is an open question.

CVID has been described in patients after the diagnosis of SLE; immunosuppressive agents, such as cyclophosphamide, AZA, mycophenolate mofetil, SSZ, long-term low-dose corticosteroids, and repeated courses of rituximab, had been used for treatment of SLE before detection of hypogammaglobulinemia. Drug-induced hypogammaglobulinemia is potentially reversible with cessation of therapy, unlike CVID, although the duration of post-cessation hypogammaglobulinemia can be prolonged. Fernández-Castro and colleagues[139] reviewed 18 SLE-associated CVID cases and identified clinical characteristics and laboratory features in these patients. In 50% of patients CVID developed within the first 5 years after the diagnosis of SLE. All patients had been treated with corticosteroids and 72% had also received immunosuppressive therapy. Sinopulmonary infections were the most frequent symptom. SLE disease activity decreased after the development of CVID in 67% of patients. Most patients (89%) were treated with gamma globulin therapy. In 60% of the patients there was a reduced number or percentage of B cells.

CVID should be suspected in any patient who has SLE with recurrent sinopulmonary infections in the absence of SLE activity or immunosuppressive treatment. Although SLE-associated CVID is uncommon, because of its potentially fatal outcome it should be considered in any patient who has SLE with hypogammaglobulinemia (at least 2 standard deviations below the mean for age in serum concentration of IgG and IgA), poor or absent response to immunization (twofold or less increase in antibody titer), and acute, chronic, or recurrent infections, specifically, pneumonia, bronchitis, sinusitis, conjunctivitis, and otitis. The clinical and bacteriologic spectrums of infections in patients who have SLE who develop CVID do not seem to be significantly different from those of patients who have SLE in the absence of CVID. The deficiency in IgG production leads to recurrent infections with encapsulated organisms, including *Streptococcus pneumoniae* and *Haemophilus influenzae*; there is also an unusual susceptibility to mycoplasma infections. Chronic or recurrent conjunctivitis is mainly due to nonencapsulated *H influenzae*. Bacterial meningitis and sepsis are also common. Unusual or opportunistic infections with viral and fungal pathogens have been reported. Patients may have an increased susceptibility to enterovirus infection, either presenting with classical meningoencephalitic symptoms or more rarely with cognitive impairment that may be misdiagnosed. Arthritis may be a prominent feature in adults who have CVID. Mycoplasma species, such as *M pneumoniae*, *M salivarium*, and *M hominis*, and *Ureaplasma urealyticum* are the most common causes of septic arthritis. The more characteristic, aseptic form of arthritis developing in individuals who have CVID is symmetric, nonerosive polyarthritis of the large joints. Chronic lung disease, specifically the development of bronchiectasis, liver dysfunction with hepatitis B and C virus infection, primary biliary cirrhosis, and granulomatous disease, have also been reported.

IgA Deficiency

Rankin and colleagues[140] investigated the occurrence of IgA deficiency in SLE and reported a prevalence of 5% in 96 patients who had SLE. Cassidy and colleagues[141] estimated the prevalence of IgA deficiency at 2.6% in adults (n = 152) and 5.2% in children (n = 77) who had SLE. These patients have a similar clinical course compared with patients who have SLE without IgA deficiency.

IgM Deficiency

Selective IgM deficiency has been described in patients who have SLE and there is a suggestion that it correlates with more severe or long-standing SLE.[142–146] They have recurrent sinopulmonary infections that respond to conventional courses of antibiotics without the need for prolonged antibiotic course or intravenous immunoglobulin (Ig) therapy. Other unrelated causes of hypogammaglobulinemia in patients who have SLE are lymphoproliferative disorders, including myeloma, chronic lymphocytic leukemia, and lymphoma.

IMMUNIZATIONS

SLE exacerbation and onset with pneumococcal vaccination, tetanus toxoid, *H influenza* B vaccines, and vaccinations for hepatitis B and influenza have been described.[147–149] Autoimmune phenomena have been observed in response to measles, mumps, and rubella, and bacille Calmette-Guérin vaccinations. In the Carolina Lupus Study, there seemed to be no association between hepatitis B vaccination and SLE. Whether there is truly an association between immunizations and incident SLE is not well known, however. Possible mechanisms are molecular mimicry and the host type I IFN response (initiation and flares).[150]

REFERENCES

1. Uccellini MB, Busconi L, Green NM, et al. Autoreactive B cells discriminate CpG-rich and CpG-poor DNA and this response is modulated by IFN-alpha. J Immunol 2008;181(9):5875–84.
2. Nakou M, Knowlton N, Frank MB, et al. Gene expression in systemic lupus erythematosus: bone marrow analysis differentiates active from inactive disease and reveals apoptosis and granulopoiesis signatures. Arthritis Rheum 2008;58(11): 3541–9 IFN.
3. Cooper GS, Gilbert KM, Greidinger EL, et al. Recent advances and opportunities in research on lupus: environmental influences and mechanisms of disease. Environ Health Perspect 2008;116(6):695–702.

4. Wu P, Wu J, Liu S, et al. TLR9/TLR7-triggered downregulation of BDCA2 expression on human plasmacytoid dendritic cells from healthy individuals and lupus patients. Clin Immunol 2008;129(1):40–8.

5. He B, Qiao X, Cerutti A. CpG DNA induces IgG class switch DNA recombination by activating human B cells through an innate pathway that requires TLR9 and cooperates with IL-10. J Immunol 2004;173(7):4479–91.

6. Mozaffarian N, Wiedeman AE, Stevens AM. Active systemic lupus erythematosus is associated with failure of antigen-presenting cells to express programmed death ligand-1. Rheumatology 2008;47(9):1335–41.

7. Takeuchi T, Tsuzaka K, Abe T, et al. T cell abnormalities in systemic lupus erythematosus. Autoimmunity 2005;38(5):339–46.

8. Know SK, Lee JY, Park SH, et al. Dysfunctional interferon alpha production by peripheral plasmacytoid dendritic cells upon Toll-like receptor 9 stimulation in patients with lupus erythematosus. Arthritis Res Ther 2008;10(2):R29.

9. Sawalha AH, Jeffries M, Webb R, et al. Defective T-cell ERK signaling induces interferon-regulated gene expression and overexpression of methylation-sensitive genes similar to lupus patients. Genes Immun 2008;9(4):368–78.

10. Lee HY, Hong YK, Yun HJ, et al. Altered frequency and migration capacity of CD4+CD25+ regulatory T cells in systemic lupus erythematosus. Rheumatology 2008;47(6):789–94.

11. Munoz LE, van Bavel C, Franz S, et al. Apoptosis in the pathogenesis of systemic lupus erythematosus. Lupus 2008;17(5):371–5.

12. Komatsuda A, Wakui, Iwamoto K, et al. Up-regulated expression of Toll-like receptors mRNAs in peripheral blood mononuclear cells from patients with systemic lupus erythematosus. Clin Exp Immunol 2008;152(3):482–7.

13. Pan F, Tang X, Zhang K, et al. Genetic susceptibility and haplotype analysis between Fcγ receptor IIB and IIIA gene with systemic lupus erythematosus in Chinese population. Lupus 2008;17(8):733–8.

14. Anolik JH. B cell biology and dysfunction in SLE. Bull NYU Hosp Jt Dis 2007; 65(3):182–6.

15. Parietti V, Chifflot H, Muller S, et al. Regulatory T cells and systemic lupus erythematosus. Ann N Y Acad Sci 2007;1108:64–75.

16. Pickering MC, Macor P, Fish J, et al. Complement C1q and C8β deficiency in an individual with recurrent bacterial meningitis and adult-onset systemic lupus erythematosus-like illness. Rheumatology 2008;47(10):1588–9.

17. Wenger ME, Bole GG. Nitroblue tetrazolium dye reduction by peripheral leukocytes from patients with rheumatoid arthritis and systemic lupus erythematosus measured by a histochemical and spectrophotometric method. J Lab Clin Med 1973;82:513–21.

18. Su K, Yang H, Li X, et al. Expression profile of FcγRIIb on leukocytes and its dysregulation in systemic lupus erythematosus. J Immunol 2007;178:3272–80.

19. Clatworthy MR, Willcocks L, Urban J, et al. Systemic lupus erythematosus associated defects in the inhibitory receptor Fc γR IIb reduce susceptibility to malaria. Proc Natl Acad Sci U S A 2007;104:7169–74.

20. Mok MY, Ip WK, Lau CS, et al. Mannose-binding lectin and susceptibility to infection in Chinese patients with systemic lupus erythematosus. J Rheumatol 2007;34(6):1270–6.

21. Truedsson L, Bengtsson AA, Sturfelt G. Complement deficiencies and systemic lupus erythematosus. Autoimmunity 2007;40(8):560–6.

22. Alvarado-Sanchez B, Hernandez-Castro B, Portales-Perez D, et al. Regulatory T cells in patients with systemic lupus erythematosus. J Autoimmun 2007;27:110–8.

23. Monticielo OA, Mucenic T, Xavier RM, et al. The role of mannose-binding lectin in systemic lupus erythematosus. Clin Rheumatol 2008;27(4):413–9.

24. Rhodes B, Vyse TJ. The genetics of SLE: an update in the light of genome-wide association studies. Rheumatology 2008;47(11):1603–11.

25. Pickering MC, Botto M, Taylor PR, et al. Systemic lupus erythematosus, complement deficiency, and apoptosis. Adv Immunol 2000;76:227–324.

26. Tsutsumi A, Takahashi R, Sumida T. Mannose binding lectin: genetics and autoimmune disease. Autoimmun Rev 2005;4(6):364–72.

27. Mamtani M, Rovin B, Brey R, et al. CCL3L1 gene-containing segmental duplications and polymorphisms in CCR5 affect risk of systemic lupus erythaematosus. Ann Rheum Dis 2008;67(8):1076–83.

28. Jonsen A, Bengtsson AA, Nived O, et al. Gene-environment interactions in the aetiology of systemic lupus erythematosus. Autoimmunity 2007;40(8):613–7.

29. Namjou B, Kilpatrick J, Harley JB. Genetics of clinical expression in SLE. Autoimmunity 2007;40(8):602–12.

30. Brown EE, Edberg JC, Kimberly RP. Fc receptor genes and the systemic lupus erythematosus diathesis. Autoimmunity 2007;40(8):567–81.

31. Gergely P Jr, Isaak A, Szekeres Z, et al. Altered expression of Fcγ and complement receptors on B cells in systemic lupus erythematosus. Ann N Y Acad Sci 2007;1108:183–92.

32. Sestak AL, Nath SK, Sawalha AH, et al. Current status of lupus genetics. Arthritis Res Ther 2007;9(3):210.

33. Kyogoku C, Tsuchiya N. A compass that points to lupus: genetic studies on type I interferon pathway. Genes Immun 2007;8(6):445–55.

34. Brownlie RJ, Lawlor KE, Heather A, et al. Distinct cell-specific control of autoimmunity and infection by FcγRIIb. J Exp Med 2008;205(4):883–95.

35. Crocker JA, Kimberly RP. Genetics of susceptibility and severity in systemic lupus erythematosus. Curr Opin Rheumatol 2005;17(5):529–37.

36. Garred P, Madsen HO, Halberg P, et al. Mannose-binding lectin polymorphisms and susceptibility to infection in systemic lupus erythematosus. Arthritis Rheum 1999;42:2145–52.

37. Tsay GJ, Zouali M. Toxicogenomics – a novel opportunity to probe lupus susceptibility and pathogenesis. Int Immunopharmacol 2008;8(10):1330–7.

38. Kelly JA, Kelley JM, Kaufman KM, et al. Interferon regulatory factor-5 is genetically associated with systemic lupus erythematosus in African Americans. Genes Immun 2008;9(3):187–94.

39. Atzeni F, Bendtzen K, Bobbio-Pallavicini F, et al. Infections and treatment of patients with rheumatic diseases. Clin Exp Rheumatol 2008;26(1 Suppl 48): S67–73.

40. Amital H, Govoni M, Maya R, et al. Role of infectious agents in systemic rheumatic diseases. Clin Exp Rheumatol 2008;26(1 Suppl 48):S27–32.

41. Wucherpfennig KW. Structural basis of molecular mimicry. J Autoimmun 2001; 16:293–302.

42. Lehmann PV, Forsthuber T, Miller A, et al. Spreading of T-cell autoimmunity to cryptic determinants of an autoantigen. Nature 1992;358:155–7.

43. Tsai CY, Wu TH, Yu CL, et al. Decreased IL-12 production by polymorphonuclear leukocytes in patients with active systemic lupus erythematosus. Immunol Invest 2002;31:177–89.

44. Ng WL, Chu CM, Wu AK, et al. Lymphopenia at presentation is associated with increased risk of infections in patients with systemic lupus erythematosus. QJM 2006;99(1):37–47.

45. Zandman-Goddard G, Berkun Y, Barzilai O, et al. Neuropsychiatric lupus and infectious triggers. Lupus 2008;17(5):380–4.
46. Duffy KN, Duffy CM, Gladman DD. Infection and disease activity in systemic lupus erythematosus: a review of hospitalized patients. J Rheumatol 1991;18: 1180–4.
47. Noel V, Lortholary O, Casassus P, et al. Risk factors and prognostic influence of infection in a single cohort of 87 adults with systemic lupus erythematosus. Ann Rheum Dis 2001;60:1141–4.
48. Fessler BJ. Infectious diseases in systemic lupus erythematosus: risk factors, management and prophylaxis. Best Pract Res Clin Rheumatol 2002;16:281–91.
49. Bosch X, Guilabert A, Pallares L, et al. Infections in systemic lupus erythematosus: a prospective and controlled study of 110 patients. Lupus 2006;15(9):584–9.
50. Hsieh S-C, Yu H-S, Lin W-W, et al. Anti-SSB/La is one of the antineutrophil auto-antibodies responsible for neutropenia and functional impairment of polymor-phonuclear neutrophils in patients with systemic lupus erythematosus. Clin Exp Immunol 2003;131:506–16, 1999.
51. Biswas D, Mathias A, Dayal R, et al. Presence of antibodies to SSB/La is asso-ciated with decreased phagocytic efficiency of neutrophils in patients with systemic lupus erythematosus. Clin Rheumatol 2008;27(6):717–22.
52. Strandberg L, Ambrosi A, Espinosa A, et al. Interferon-alpha induces up-regula-tion and nuclear translocation of the Ro52 autoantigen as detected by a panel of novel Ro52-specific monoclonal antibodies. J Clin Immunol 2008;28(3):220–31.
53. Mok CC, Mak A, Chu WP, et al. Long-term survival in Southern Chinese patients with systemic lupus erythematosus: a prospective study of all age-groups. Medi-cine 2005;84:218–24.
54. Mok CC, Lee KW, Ho CTK, et al. A prospective study of survival and prognostic indicators of systemic lupus erythematosus in a southern Chinese population. Rheumatology 2000;39:399–406.
55. Petri M, Genovese M. Incidence of and risk factors for hospitalizations in systemic lupus erythematosus: a prospective study of the Hopkins lupus cohort. J Rheumatol 1992;19:1559–65.
56. Chen MJ, Tseng HM, Huang YL, et al. Long-term outcome and short-term survival of patients with systemic lupus erythematosus after bacteraemia episodes: 6-yr follow-up. Rheumatology 2008;47(9):1352–7.
57. Chiu KM, Lin TY, Chen JS, et al. Rupture of renal artery aneurysm due to Salmo-nella infection in a patient with systemic lupus erythematosus. Lupus 2008;17(2): 135–8.
58. Huang JL, Hung JJ, Wu KC, et al. Septic arthritis in patients with systemic lupus erythematosus: salmonella and nonsalmonella infections compared. Semin Arthritis Rheum 2006;36(1):61–7.
59. van de Vosse E, Hoeve MA, Ottenhoff TH. Human genetics of intracellular infec-tious diseases: molecular and cellular immunity against mycobacteria and salmonellae. Lancet Infect Dis 2004;4:739–49.
60. Tsao CH, Chen CY, Ou LS, et al. Risk factors of mortality for salmonella infection in systemic lupus erythematosus. J Rheumatol 2002;29:1214–8.
61. Lee PP, Lee TL, Ho MH, et al. Recurrent major infections in juvenile-onset systemic lupus erythematosus—a close link with long-term disease damage. Rheumatology 2007;46(8):1290–6.
62. Chen YS, Yang YH, Lin YT, et al. Risk of infection in hospitalized children with systemic lupus erythematosus: a 10-year follow-up. Clin Rheumatol 2004;23: 235–8.

63. Rojas-Serrano J, Pedroza J, Regalado J, et al. High prevalence of infections in patients with systemic lupus erythematosus and pulmonary haemorrhage. Lupus 2008;17(4):295–9.
64. Barzilai O, Ram M, Shoenfeld Y. Viral infection can induce the production of autoantibodies. Curr Opin Rheumatol 2007;19(6):636–43.
65. Su BY, Su CY, Yu SF, et al. Incidental discovery of high systemic lupus erythematosus disease activity associated with cytomegalovirus viral activity. Med Microbiol Immunol 2007;196(3):165–70.
66. Aslanidis S, Pyrpasopoulou A, Kontotasios K, et al. Parvovirus B19 infection and systemic lupus erythematosus: activation of an aberrant pathway? Eur J Intern Med 2008;19(5):314–8.
67. Sugimoto T, Tsuda A, Uzu T, et al. Emerging lupus-like manifestations in acute parvovirus B19 infection. Clin Rheumatol 2008;27(1):119–20.
68. Pugliese A, Beltramo T, Torre D, et al. Parvovirus B19 and immune disorders. Cell Biochem Funct 2007;25(6):639–41.
69. Seve P, Ferry T, Koenig M, et al. Lupus-like presentation of parvovirus B19 infection. Semin Arthritis Rheum 2005;34(4):642–8.
70. Narvaez Garcia F, Domingo-Domenech E, Castro-Bohorquez F, et al. Lupus-like presentation of parvovirus B19 infection. Am J Med 2001;111:573–5.
71. Ramos-Casals M, Cuadrado MJ, Alba P, et al. Acute viral infections in patients with systemic lupus erythematosus: description of 23 cases and review of the literature. Medicine 2008;87(6):311–8.
72. Chung A, Fas N. Successful acyclovir treatment of herpes simplex type 2 hepatitis in a patient with systemic lupus erythematosus: a case report and meta analysis. Am J Med Sci 1998;316:404–7.
73. Suzuki T, Saito S, Hirabayashi Y, et al. Human parvovirus B19 infection during the inactive stage of systemic lupus erythematosus. Intern Med 2003;42:538–40.
74. Barzilai O, Sherer Y, Ram M, et al. EBV and CMV in autoimmune diseases. Are they truly notorious? A preliminary report. Ann N Y Acad Sci 2007;1108:567–77.
75. Fish P, Handgretinger R, Schaefer H. Pure red cell aplasia. Br J Haematol 2000; 111:1010–22.
76. Ideguchi H, Ohno S, Ishigatsubo Y. A case of pure red cell aplasia and systemic lupus erythematosus caused by human parvovirus B19 infection. Rheumatol Int 2007;27:411–4.
77. Isome M, Suzuki J, Takahashi A, et al. Epstein-Barr virus-associated hemophagocytic syndrome in a patient with lupus nephritis. Pediatr Nephrol 2005;20(2): 226–8.
78. Kawashiri S, Nakamura H, Kawakami A, et al. Emergence of Epstein-Barr virus-associated haemophagocytic syndrome upon treatment of systemic lupus erythematosus. Lupus 2006;15:51–3.
79. Kwon C, Jung Y, Yun D, et al. A case of acute pericarditis with hemophagocytic syndrome, cytomegalovirus infection and systemic lupus erythematosus. Rheumatol Int 2008;28:271–3.
80. Lee S, Sugiyama M, Hishikawa T, et al. Thrombocytopenia in systemic lupus erythematosus associated with cytomegalovirus infection. Scand J Rheumatol 1997;26:69.
81. Rouphael N, Talati N, Vaughan C, et al. Infections associated with haemophagocytic syndrome. Lancet Infect Dis 2007;7:814–22.
82. Sakamoto O, Ando M, Yoshimatsu S, et al. Systemic lupus erythematosus complicated by cytomegalovirus-induced hemophagocytic syndrome and colitis. Intern Med 2002;41:151–5.

83. Evans AS. E.B. virus antibody in systemic lupus erythematosus. Lancet 1971;1: 1023–4.
84. Pender MP. Infection of autoreactive B lymphocytes with EBV, causing chronic autoimmune diseases. Trends Immunol 2003;24:584–8.
85. Niller HH, Wolf H, Minarovits J. Regulation and dysregulation of Epstein-Barr virus latency: implications for the development of autoimmune diseases. Autoimmunity 2008;41(4):298–328.
86. Lu JJ, Chen DY, Hsieh CW, et al. Association of Epstein-Barr virus infection with systemic lupus erythematosus in Taiwan. Lupus 2007;16(3):168–75.
87. Harley JB, James JA. Epstein-Barr virus infection induces lupus autoimmunity. Bull NYU Hosp Jt Dis 2006;64(1–2):45–50.
88. Harley JB, Harley IT, Guthridge JM, et al. The curiously suspicious: a role for Epstein-Barr virus in lupus. Lupus 2006;15(11):768–77.
89. Gross AJ, Hochberg D, Rand WM, et al. EBV and systemic lupus erythematosus: a new perspective. J Immunol 2005;174(11):6599–607.
90. Sundar K, Jacques S, Gottlieb P, et al. Expression of the Epstein-Barr virus nuclear antigen-1 (EBNA-1) in the mouse can elicit the production of anti-dsDNA and anti-Sm antibodies. J Autoimmun 2004;23:127–40.
91. Poole BD, Scofield RH, Harley JB, et al. Epstein-Barr virus and molecular mimicry in systemic lupus erythematosus. Autoimmunity 2006;39:63–70.
92. Swanson-Mungerson M, Longnecker R. Epstein-Barr virus latent membrane protein 2A and autoimmunity. Trends Immunol 2007;28:213–8.
93. Wang H, Nicholas MW, Conway KL, et al. EBV latent membrane protein 2A induces autoreactive B cell activation and TLR hypersensitivity. J Immunol 2006;177:2793–802.
94. Finger E, Romaldini H, Lewi DS, et al. Ganciclovir-resistant, cytomegalic interstitial lung disease in a patient with systemic lupus erythematosus. Clin Rheumatol 2007;26(10):1753–5.
95. Takei M, Yamakami K, Mitamura K, et al. A case of systemic lupus erythematosus complicated by alveolar hemorrhage and cytomegalovirus colitis. Clin Rheumatol 2007;26(2):274–7.
96. Diaz F, Urkijo JC, Mendoza F, et al. Systemic lupus erythematosus associated with acute cytomegalovirus infection. J Clin Rheumatol 2006;12(5):263–4.
97. Lee JJ, Teoh SC, Chua JL, et al. Occurrence and reactivation of cytomegalovirus retinitis in systemic lupus erythematosus with normal CD4(+) counts. Eye 2006; 20(5):618–21.
98. Hrycek A, Kusmierz D, Mazurek U, et al. Human cytomegalovirus in patients with systemic lupus erythematosus. Autoimmunity 2005;38(7):487–91.
99. Ikura Y, Matsuo T, Ogami M, et al. Cytomegalovirus associated pancreatitis in a patient with systemic lupus erythematosus. J Rheumatol 2000;27:2715–7.
100. Kahl LE. Herpes-zoster infections in systemic lupus erythematosus: risk factors and outcome. J Rheumatol 1994;21:84.
101. Moga I, Formiga F, Canet R, et al. Herpes-zoster virus infection in patients with systemic lupus erythematosus. Rev Clin Esp 1995;195:530.
102. Hellman DB, Petri M, Whiting-O'Keefe Q. Fatal infections in systemic lupus erythematosus: the role of opportunistic organisms. Medicine 1987;66:341–8.
103. Dhar JP, Kmak D, Bhan R, et al. Abnormal cervicovaginal cytology in women with lupus: a retrospective cohort study. Gynecol Oncol 2001;82:4–6.
104. Tam LS, Chan AY, Chang AR, et al. Increased prevalence of squamous intraepithelial lesions in systemic lupus erythematosus: association with papilloma virus infection. Arthritis Rheum 2004;501(11):3619–25.

105. Bernatsky S, Ramsey-Goldman R, Gordon C, et al. Factors associated with abnormal Pap results in systemic lupus erythematosus. Rheumatology 2004; 43:1386–9.

106. Bateman H, Yazici Y, Leff L, et al. Increased cervical dysplasia in intravenous cyclophosphamide-treated patients with SLE: a preliminary study. Lupus 2000;9:542–4.

107. Nath R, Mant C, Luxton J, et al. High risk of human papillomavirus type 16 infections and of development of cervical squamous intraepithelial lesions in systemic lupus erythematosus patients. Arthritis Rheum 2007;57(4):619–25.

108. Sieving RR, Kauffman CA, Watanakukorn C. Deep fungal infection in systemic lupus erythematosus. Three cases reported, literature reviewed. J Rheumatol 1975;2:61–72.

109. Choi SJ, Rho YH, Lee YH, et al. Disseminated candidiasis in systemic lupus erythematosus. Clin Exp Rheumatol 2007;25(3):503.

110. Cassar CL. Nocardia sepsis in a multigravida with systemic lupus erythematosus and autoimmune hepatitis. Anaesth Intensive Care 2007;35(4):601–4.

111. Justiniano M, Glorioso S, Dold S, et al. Nocardia brain abscesses in a male patient with SLE: successful outcome despite delay in diagnosis. Clin Rheumatol 2007;26(6):1020–2.

112. Kilincer C, Hamamcioglu MK, Simsek O, et al. Nocardial brain abscess: review of clinical management. J Clin Neurosci 2006;13(4):481–5.

113. Cheng HM, Huang DF, Leu HB. Disseminated nocardiosis with initial manifestation mimicking disease flare-up of systemic lupus erythematosus in an SLE patient. Am J Med 2005;118(11):1297–8.

114. Santen RJ, Wright IS. Systemic lupus erythematosus associated with pulmonary nocardiosis. Arch Intern Med 1967;119:202–5.

115. Chen HS, Tsai WP, Leu HS, et al. Invasive fungal infection in systemic lupus erythematosus: an analysis of 15 cases and a literature review. Rheumatology 2007;46(3):539–44.

116. Zumla A, Grange J. Infection and disease caused by environmental mycobacteria. Curr Opin Pulm Med 2002;8:166–72.

117. Hsu PY, Yang YH, Hsiao CH, et al. Mycobacterium kansasii infection presenting as cellulitis in a patient with systemic lupus erythematosus. J Formos Med Assoc 2002;101:581–4.

118. Gordon MM, Wilson HE, Duthie FR, et al. When typical is atypical: mycobacterial infection mimicking cutaneous vasculitis. Rheumatology 2002;41:685–90.

119. Laborde H, Rodrigue S, Cattoglio PM. Mycobacterium fortuitum in systemic lupus erythematosus. Clin Exp Rheumatol 1989;7:291–3.

120. Mok MY, Wong SS, Chan TM, et al. Non-tuberculous mycobacterial infection in patients with systemic lupus erythematosus. Rheumatology 2007;46(2):280–4.

121. Enzenauer RJ, McKoy J, Vincent D, et al. Disseminated cutaneous and synovial Mycobacterium marinum infection in patient with systemic lupus erythematosus. South Med J 1990;83:471–4.

122. Rutten MJ, van den Berg JC, van den Hoogen FH, et al. Nontuberculous mycobacterial bursitis and arthritis of the shoulder. Skeletal Radiol 1998;27:33–5.

123. Telgt DS, van den Hoogen FH, Meis JF, et al. Arthritis and spondylodiscitis caused by Mycobacterium xenopi in a patient with systemic lupus erythematosus. Br J Rheumatol 1996;35:1008–10.

124. Nakamura T, Yamamura Y, Tsuruta T, et al. Mycobacterium kansasii arthritis of the foot in a patient with systemic lupus erythematosus. Intern Med 2001;40: 1045–9.

125. Hoffman GS, Myers RL, Stark FR, et al. Septic arthritis associated with Mycobacterium avium: a case report and literature review. J Rheumatol 1978;5: 199–209.
126. Zventina JR, Demos TC, Rubinstein H. Mycobacterium intracellulare infection of the shoulder and spine in a patient with steroid-treated systemic lupus erythematosus. Skeletal Radiol 1982;8:111–3.
127. Huang HC, Yu WL, Shieh CC, et al. Unusual mixed infection of thoracic empyema caused by Mycobacteria tuberculosis, nontuberculosis mycobacteria and Nocardia asteroides in a woman with systemic lupus erythematosus. J Infect 2007;54(1):e25–8.
128. Staples PJ, Gerding DN, Decker JL, et al. Incidence of infection in systemic lupus erythematosus. Arthritis Rheumatology 1974;17:1–10.
129. Kang I, Park SH. Infectious complications in SLE after immunosuppressive therapies. Curr Opin Rheumatol 2003;15:528–34.
130. Pillay VKG, Wilson DM, Ing TS, et al. Fungus infection in steroid-treated systemic lupus erythematosus. JAMA 1968;205:261–5.
131. Rosner S, Ginzler EM, Diamond HS, et al. A multicenter study of outcome in systemic lupus erythematosus. II. Causes of death. Arthritis Rheum 1982;25: 612–7.
132. Ashman RF, White RH, Wiesenhutter C, et al. Panhypogammaglobulinemia in systemic lupus erythematosus: in vitro demonstration of multiple cellular defects. J Allergy Clin Immunol 1982;70:465.
133. Swaak AJG, van den Brink HG. Common variable immunodeficiency in a patient with systemic lupus erythematosus. Lupus 1996;5:242–6, I.K.
134. Tsokos GC, Smith PL, Balow JE. Development of hypogammaglobulinemia in a patient with systemic lupus erythematosus. Am J Med 1986;81:1081–4.
135. Cronin ME, Balow JE, Tsokos GC. Immunoglobulin deficiency in patients with systemic lupus erythematosus. Clin Exp Rheumatol 1989;7:359–64.
136. Stein A, Winkelstein A, Agarwal A. Concurrent systemic lupus erythematosus and common variable hypogammaglobulinemia. Arthritis Rheum 1985;28: 462–5.
137. Baum CG, Chiorazzi N, Frankel S, et al. Conversion of systemic lupus erythematosus to common variable hypogammaglobulinemia. Am J Med 1989;87: 449–56.
138. Sussman GL, Rivera VK, Kohler PF. Transition from systemic lupus erythematosus to common variable hypogammaglobulinemia. Ann Intern Med 1983;99: 32–5.
139. Fernandez-Castro M, Mellor-Pita S, Jesus CM, et al. Common variable immunodeficiency in systemic lupus erythematosus. Semin Arthritis Rheum 2007;36: 238–45.
140. Rankin EC, Isenberg DA. IgA deficiency and SLE: prevalence in a clinic population and a review of the literature. Lupus 2007;6:390–4.
141. Cassidy JT, Kitson RK, Selby CL. Selective IgA deficiency in children and adults with systemic lupus erythematosus. Lupus 2007;16(8):647–50.
142. Slepian SA, Schwartz Weiss JJ, et al. Immunodeficiency with hyper IgM after systemic lupus erythematosus. J Allergy Clin Immunol 1984;73:846–57.
143. Saiki O, Saeki Y, Tanaka T, et al. Development of selective IgM deficiency in systemic lupus erythematosus patients with disease of long duration. Arthritis Rheum 1987;30:1289–92.
144. Senaldi G, Ireland R, Bellingham AJ, et al. IgM reduction in systemic lupus erythematosus. Arthritis Rheum 1988;31:1213.

145. Takeuchi T, Nakagawa T, Maeda Y, et al. Functional defect of B lymphocytes in a patient with selective IgM deficiency associated with systemic lupus erythematosus. Autoimmunity 2001;34:115–22.
146. Goldstein MF, Goldstein AL, Dunsky EH, et al. Selective IgM immunodeficiency: retrospective analysis of 36 adult patients with review of the literature. Ann Allergy Asthma Immunol 2006;97:717–30.
147. Gluck T, Muller-Ladner U. Vaccination in patients with chronic rheumatic or autoimmune diseases. Clin Infect Dis 2008;46(9):1459–65.
148. Holvast B, Huckriede A, Kallenberg CG, et al. Influenza vaccination in systemic lupus erythematosus: safe and protective? Autoimmun Rev 2007;6:300–5.
149. Stojanovich L. Influenza vaccination of patients with systemic lupus erythematosus (SLE) and rheumatoid arthritis (RA). Clin Dev Immunol 2006;13(2–4):373–5.
150. O'Neill SG, Isenberg DA. Immunizing patients with systemic lupus erythematosus: a review of effectiveness and safety. Lupus 2006;15(11):778–83.

Parvovirus B19: Its Role in Chronic Arthritis

Ines Colmegna, MD*, Noah Alberts-Grill, BA

KEYWORDS

- Parvovirus B19 • B19 arthropathy • B19-associated arthritis
- Viral arthritis • Pathogenic mechanisms • Persistence

Parvovirus B19 (B19, B19 virus) was discovered serendipitously in 1975[1] and was first recognized as the cause of aplastic crisis in patients who had chronic hemolytic anemia in 1981,[2] and erythema infectiosum in 1983.[3] It was not until 1985 that B19 was linked to rheumatic manifestations.[4,5] B19 infection–associated joint symptoms occur most frequently in adults, usually presenting as a self-limited, acute symmetric polyarthritis affecting the small joints of the hands, wrists, and knees.[4,5] A small percentage of patients persist with chronic polyarthritis that mimics rheumatoid arthritis (RA) raising the question of whether B19 virus may have a role as a concomitant or precipitating factor in the pathogenesis of autoimmune conditions.[5] Comprehensive and updated reviews address different aspects of human parvovirus infection.[6,7,8,9,10,11,12,13,14] This article focuses on the evidence supporting the arthritogenic potential of the B19 virus and the proposed mechanisms that underlie it.

MICROBIOLOGIC AND MOLECULAR FEATURES OF B19 INFECTION

Parvovirus B19 is a member of the *Erythrovirus* genus of the Parvoviridae family. B19 is a non-enveloped icosahedral single-stranded DNA virus that encodes no DNA polymerase and therefore depends on cells undergoing division for viral replication.[15] The small genome and the absence of a lipid envelope make B19 relatively stable and resistant to many physicochemical procedures used for inactivating blood-borne viruses.[16]

Although B19 seroprevalence in adults exceeds 80%, isolates of the virus show very few differences in genetic sequence, which do not associate with distinct clinical manifestations.[17] B19 genome encodes two capsomer proteins (VP1 and VP2) and a nonstructural protein (NS1). All these structures have functions that can account for the arthritogenic potential of B19 (**Table 1**).

VP1 and VP2 originate from overlapping reading frames and are identical except for an extension of 227 additional amino acids at the VP1 N-terminal region known as the

Lowance Center for Human Immunology and Rheumatology, Emory University School of Medicine, 101 Woodruff Circle, Room 1014, Atlanta, GA 30322, USA
* Corresponding author.
E-mail address: icolmeg@emory.edu (I. Colmegna).

Rheum Dis Clin N Am 35 (2009) 95–110
doi:10.1016/j.rdc.2009.03.004
0889-857X/09/$ – see front matter © 2009 Elsevier Inc. All rights reserved.

Table 1
Functional implications of B19 structure

	Protein Name	Immunomodulatory Function	Proposed Mechanism of Arthropathy
Capsomer proteins	VP1 VP1u	Contains neutralizing Ab epitopes	Immune complex deposition
		Induces autoreactive Ab responses	Viral mimicry Alteration of cellular immunity
		Target of CD4/CD8 cellular response	Elevated inflammatory mediators by way of arachidonic acid
		Phospholipase A2-like activity	
	VP2	Targeted by humoral antiviral response	Alteration of cellular immunity
Nonstructural protein	NS1	Cell cycle arrest	Cytopathic effect
		Apoptosis induction through mitochondrial cell death pathway	
		P6 promoter *trans*-activation (B19 replication)	Viral replication
		Trans-activation of host genes: up-regulation of IL-6, TNF, and NF-κB	Elevated inflammatory cytokines
		Modulation of signaling pathways: STAT3 activation without SOCS1/SOCS3 activation	Elevated inflammatory and antiviral response factors
		ATPase, helicase, and endonuclease function	Unknown
		Target of CD8 cellular response	Alteration of cellular immunity

Abbreviations: Ab, antibody; IL, interleukin; NF, nuclear factor; STAT, signal transducer and activator of transcription; TNF, tumor necrosis factor.

VP1 "unique-region" (VP1u). VP1u is of central relevance to the immunogenicity and pathogenic potential of the B19 virus in that it contains the dominant neutralizing epitopes targeted by the host humoral immune response.[18,19,20,21] In addition to its immunodominant role, VP1u possesses a functional phospholipase A2-like activity that is involved in intracellular Ca^{2+} regulation and plays a critical role in viral infectivity.[22,23] Studies showing that synoviocytes are activated in vitro by secreted phospholipase A2 enzyme point toward a direct role of the phospholipase A2-like motif of VP1u in initiating or accelerating the inflammatory response in synovial tissue, thus contributing to B19-asociated arthropathy.[22,24,25]

VP2 is the main structural component of the B19 virus, accounting for more than 90% of total capsid protein.[26] When VP2 is expressed in insect cells, it self-assembles to form viruslike particles that are antigenically similar to native virions, but devoid of viral DNA.[19] A phase 1 study of a recombinant parvovirus B19 vaccine using these empty B19-capsid particles was capable of inducing a neutralizing antibody response.[27]

The nonstructural B19 protein NS1 is a multifunctional protein. It acts as a transcriptional *trans*-activator that regulates various viral and cellular promoters. Among them is the *trans*-activation of the viral P6 promoter, which being the sole promoter controlling B19 transcription, is crucial for viral replication.[28] Other cellular genes that are *trans*-activated by NS1 include interleukin 6 (IL-6), tumor necrosis factor alpha (TNF), NF-κB and the tumor suppressor p53.[29,30,31] The activation of the TNF and IL-6 promoter has been proposed as the mechanism for the production of these cytokines in inflammatory and autoimmune syndromes linked to B19.[32]

In addition to the direct modulation of inflammatory cytokine production, NS1 is also capable of influencing signaling pathways involved in the antiviral response. Signal transducer and activator of transcription (STAT) proteins are a family of latent transcription factors with a crucial immune-regulatory role in the activation of cytokine response genes. Although STAT1 is critical for the innate immune response, the dysregulation of STAT3 signaling in T cells and macrophages can lead to chronic inflammation through the uncontrolled production of interferons and other proinflammatory cytokines.[33] The STAT signaling is negatively regulated by suppressor of cytokine signaling (SOCS) proteins.[34] In human endothelial cells, B19 NS1 expression leads to the activation of STAT3 in the absence of SOCS1/SOCS3 activation, resulting in the up-regulation of STAT3 target genes involved in the immune response against viral infections.[35] In contrast, STAT1 is not targeted by NS1, which has been hypothesized to result in a reduced interferon (IFN) response.[35]

Unlike enveloped viruses, parvovirus B19 is incapable of budding mature virions from infected cells and instead must rely on lytic replication to spread from cell to cell.[36,37] This is accomplished in large part by NS1, which can initiate proapoptotic processes through the mitochondria cell death pathway.[38] This pathway involves p53-induced Bax expression and subsequent activation of caspases 3 and 9.[39] The NS1 protein also contains a nucleoside triphosphate (NTP)–binding motif that has been involved in the induction of apoptosis in erythroid lineage cells during B19 infection.[40]

In addition to its central role in the genomic replication and lytic release of B19 parvovirus, sequence homology studies have predicted that NS1 also possess ATPase, helicase, and site-specific endonuclease function.[41]

In contrast to the structural proteins targeted by the humoral response, in adults who have symptomatic B19 infection peptides within the NS1 protein are the targets of multispecific CD8 T cells.[42] Anti-B19 CD8 T cells possess strong effector function and proliferative capacity. These cells have an activated phenotype (CD38+), express perforin and CD57, and down-regulate CD27 and CD28.[43] That the anti-B19 CD8 response persists in some patients for months and even years despite the resolution of their clinical symptoms suggests a low level of antigen persistence over the postinfection period. In fact, differences in cellular immune responses have been proposed as an explanation for viral persistence in the presence of an intact humoral response.[42] In healthy seropositive patients, host IFN-γ responses are elicited by the viral NS1 protein, whereas in patients who have B19 persistence these responses are of lower magnitude and skewed toward a VP-directed response.[44]

VIRAL–HOST INTERACTIONS IN B19 INFECTION

The most common route of B19 infection is by way of the inhalation of aerosol droplets, although the virus can also be transmitted parenterally by infected blood and blood products,[15] vertically from mother to fetus,[45] and by solid-organ and hematopoietic stem cell transplantation.[46] Because most infections occur in children aged 5 to 15 years, adults at risk for infection are the parents of children in that age group and those working at day care centers or schools.[47] For those adults living with infected children the transmission rate is about 50%, whereas in susceptible teachers and day care workers the incidence of transmission is about 20% to 30%.[48]

Once an individual is infected, the virus multiplies in the throat leading to viremia by day 6. At this point, parvovirus B19 has a selective tropism for early erythroid progenitors[49] by way of interaction with a cellular receptor and blood-group P system antigen known as P antigen or globoside.[50] The level of P antigen expression in cells is not directly related to the efficiency of viral binding[7] but individuals lacking P antigen are naturally resistant to infection with B19.[51] This cellular receptor is expressed not only on erythrocytes and erythroid precursors (target cells) but also on a wide variety of other cell types, including platelets, granulocytes, endothelial cells, vascular smooth muscle cells, and placental trophoblast cells, as well as fetal liver cells and cells in the lung, kidney, heart, and synovium.[10,14,52] Save for erythroid precursors, other P antigen–positive cells are nonpermissive to B19 infection. Although the virus can bind and enter these cells, it is unable to produce complete virions. P antigen alone is thus insufficient to impart erythroid specificity to parvovirus B19, implicating the expression of a cell surface co-receptor necessary for successful infection.[53] Following binding of P antigen, there are changes in B19 capsid conformation leading to the externalization of VP1u sequences.[54] Early exposure of VP1u allows interaction with the co-receptor $\alpha 5\ \beta 1$ integrin on erythroid progenitors, which facilitates virus entry.[53,55,56] In addition, B19 can bind specifically to Ku80 autoantigen expressed on bone marrow cells and B and T lymphocytes. Binding to Ku80 has been shown to mediate efficient B19 entry in cooperation with P antigen, most likely using $\alpha 5\ \beta 1$ integrin as a co-receptor.[57] Once B19 infects the host cell, the parvovirus capsid follows a complex path from the cell surface to the nucleus where DNA replication occurs. The course of viral trafficking by way of the endosomal system, cytoplasm, and events leading to nuclear entry are still not defined (reviewed in[58]). Following nuclear entry, DNA replication, RNA transcription, capsid assembly, and packaging of the viral genome occur,[59] ending in cell lysis and the release of mature virions.[9]

CLINICAL ASPECTS OF B19 INFECTION

The clinical outcomes associated with B19 infection depend heavily on the age, hematologic, and immune status of the host. The natural history of B19 infection was characterized in experimental infections of healthy volunteers[60] with clinically distinct constellations of symptoms accompanying the "viremic phase" and the "antibody response phase."[14]

In natural infection, the incubation period typically is 6 to 18 days, but can run as long as 28 days in some outbreaks (**Fig. 1**). During viremia in naïve subjects the virus

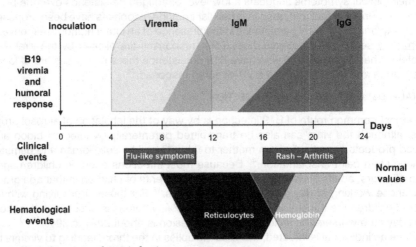

Fig. 1. Clinical aspects of B19 infection.

may be shed in nasal and oropharyngeal secretions but not urine or feces.[60,61] The viremic phase is asymptomatic in 25% to 68% of individuals, but can be accompanied by flulike symptoms, including transient fevers, malaise, myalgia, and headaches. A profound areticulocytosis coincides with peak viremia (10–12 days postinfection) and continues until several days after the appearance of specific anti-B19 IgM antibodies.[60,61] Erythropoietin shows a sharp increase following peak viremia, which coincides with the loss of erythroid precursors in the bone marrow.[61] During the second week postinfection, neutropenia, lymphopenia, and thrombocytopenia can also occur.[30,61] Save for reduced red cell survival and immunosuppression, it remains unknown what factors determine symptomatology following B19 infection.[30] In immunocompromised hosts who are unable to mount an adequate immune response against the virus, there is ongoing replication of B19 in erythroblasts[49] leading to chronic, pure red cell aplasia (reviewed in[62]). On the other hand, B19 infection is associated with transient aplastic crisis in patients who have sickle cell anemia or other hemolytic anemias (ie, beta thalassemia, hereditary spherocytosis, malaria, and autoimmune hemolytic anemias) (reviewed in[7]). B19 fetal infection can lead to aplastic crisis, high-output cardiac failure, and nonimmune hydrops fetalis (reviewed in[63]).

Rash, arthralgias, and arthritis may occur during the antibody response phase, 15 to 18 days after infection (see **Fig. 1**). The symptoms of this phase are temporally associated with the development of anti-B19 IgM.[4] By this time, patients are no longer infectious. Because the B19 IgM antibody response lasts for only 1 to 3 months, there is a brief window of opportunity to make a diagnosis of B19 infection based on IgM serology. B19-specific IgG directed against linear and conformational epitopes of viral capsid proteins VP1, VP2, and NS1 also arise within weeks of infection. With time, however, there is a loss of IgG responses against linear epitopes of the VP1, VP2, and NS1 proteins,[64] whereas antibodies against the capsid protein VP2 are maintained. The detection of B19-specific IgG against conformational epitopes is currently the most reliable method for the detection of prior infection because these antibody responses are maintained throughout life.[65] IgG studies show an increase in anti-B19 seroprevalence from 2% to 15% in children aged 1 to 5 years, which increases to 50% of 15-year-old adolescents, and to almost 80% of adults (reviewed in[9]).

EPIDEMIOLOGIC AND CLINICAL ASPECTS OF B19 ARTHROPATHY

Acute B19 arthropathy is similar in its epidemiology, distribution, and duration to the joint manifestations that follow rubella infection or immunization, and has been suggested to be immune complex mediated.[4,66] Arthralgias associated with B19 infection occur in about 5% of infected children and up to 80% of adults. Similarly, joint swelling is described in 3% of children and 60% of adults.[67] Joint involvement is more common in females than in males[3,5,68]; approximately 60% of females who have symptomatic disease have joint manifestations versus 30% of males.

The pattern of acute B19 arthropathy differs between children and adults. In children arthropathy is most often asymmetrical and pauciarticular, and commonly affects the knees. Arthropathy is either preceded or accompanied by the most common clinical manifestation of acute B19 infection, the "slapped-cheek" rash of erythema infectiosum, or fifth disease.[4] In adults this rubella-like rash is less frequent (~50%), and tends to be more subtle, lasting 3 to 4 days and producing mild itchiness.[4] Other prodromal symptoms include an influenza-like illness with malaise or pyrexia and gastrointestinal symptoms.[5] The most commonly affected joints in adults are the proximal interphalangeals and metacarpophalangeals, followed by the knees, wrists, and ankles. Joint stiffness is often associated with B19-induced arthritis.[5] Of interest is that some patients exhibit the transient expression of a low-to-moderate titer of autoanti-bodies during acute infection, which include rheumatoid factor,[69,70] anti-DNA, anti-neutrophil cytoplasmic antibodies, and antiphospholipid antibodies.

B19 viral infection is detected in 3.3% of patients examined for acute reactive arthritis[71] and in 0.4% of patients hospitalized with recent-onset inflammatory arthritis.[72] There is some validity in considering a role for B19 in these settings because B19 arthropathy can resemble early rheumatoid arthritis in the distribution of joint manifestations, symmetry of involvement, and incidence of morning stiffness. Further-more, persisting B19 arthritis can be erosive and followed by the development of rheu-matoid factor, which also likens it to RA presentation. A distinct characteristic of B19 arthropathy is that symptoms usually resolve within 2 weeks except for a small subset of patients (0%–17% according to different reports), in whom arthritis can persist for months or even years.[5] In patients who have prolonged arthritic symptoms there is no increase in the magnitude or duration of anti-B19 IgM response,[10] which suggests that the prolonged arthritis is not due to a failure in the anti-B19 humoral response to switch from IgM- to IgG-mediated immunity.

Although no definitive association between chronic arthritis and HLA type has been shown[73–76] some studies linked HLA-DR4 with the occurrence or severity of B19 arthritis. Kerr and colleagues[75] reported an association between HLA-DRB1*01, *04, *07, and HLA-B49 with acute B19 symptomatic infection and a higher frequency of shared epitope (64%) in symptomatic patients compared with control subjects (45%). Associations of shared epitope with particular clinical manifestations other than fatigue have not been demonstrated.

MECHANISMS UNDERLYING B19 ARTHROPATHY

Viruses are one of the environmental factors capable of initiating immunoreactivity leading to autoimmune diseases when infecting an individual who has genetic or epige-netic susceptibility to chronic immune activation.[77] Autoimmunity following viral infection can occur by several mechanisms that include: molecular mimicry (shared immunologic epitope between a microbe and the host), bystander activation (activation of antigen-presenting cells that can stimulate preprimed autoreactive T cells), and viral persistence (constant presence of viral antigen driving the immune response).[78] Parvo-virus B19 infection has been associated with immune-mediated syndromes,[6,11] including a great variety of rheumatic conditions (**Box 1**).[79–94] For some of these condi-tions the data in support of an association are insufficient, based on case reports or small cohorts without control groups, or conflicting with subsequent studies not con-firming the proposed association.

The evidence implicating B19 virus in the pathogenesis of rheumatoid arthritis is conflicting and in certain areas circumstantial. The proposed mechanisms responsible for B19-associated chronic arthritis include immune complex deposition mainly secondary to anti-VP1u humoral responses, viral persistence, cytotoxicity, and the up-regulation of inflammatory cytokines by NS1, phospholipase A2-like activity of VP1u, the production of autoantibodies, and the alteration of cellular immunity by viral or host-derived antiviral responses.[10,38]

Immune Complexes in B19-Associated Arthritis

In the clinical setting, the arthritogenic role of B19 is supported by the fact that B19 arthritis often meets clinical diagnostic criteria for rheumatoid arthritis.[10] Whether B19 is a culprit, concomitant, or precipitating factor in a subset of patients who have rheumatoid arthritis is still unproven.[5] Studies of B19 seroprevalence in patients

---

Box 1
Rheumatic conditions associated with B19 infection

Arthritis

    Rheumatoid arthritis

    Juvenile idiopathic arthritis

    Still disease

    Reactive arthritis

    Remitting seronegative symmetrical synovitis with pitting edema

Connective tissue diseases

    Systemic lupus erythematosus

    Dermatomyositis

    Polymyositis

    Progressive systemic sclerosis

    Sjögren syndrome

Vasculitis

    Leukocytoclastic vasculitis

    Schönlein-Henoch purpura

    Panarteritis nodosa

    Kawasaki disease

    Papular-purpuric "gloves and socks" syndrome

    Giant cell arteritis

    Wegener granulomatosis

Fibromyalgia

Chronic fatigue syndrome

Other

    Carpal tunnel syndrome

    Raynaud

---

who have RA and control patients have yielded conflicting results. Some reports show high levels of anti-B19 IgG and IgM in plasma and synovial fluid in RA.[95] Other groups failed to confirm these findings either in JIA or in RA.[96–98] Although the reported incidence of anti-B19 IgM in patients at the onset of RA is approximately 2% to 6%,[10,99] IgG seroprevalence is generally what would be expected for that particular age group.[10] Moreover, a recent study that looked at B19 seroprevalence in premorbid and postdiagnostic samples from patients who had rheumatoid arthritis found no difference in the rate of seroconversion in individuals who later on developed RA.[100]

The immune complex deposition believed to play a role in acute B19 arthropathy is also a mechanism implicated in the persistence of arthritis. This is suggested by case reports showing the reduction of joint symptoms following intravenous immunoglobulin therapy, which coincides with a decrease in B19-positive cells in the bone marrow.[101,102]

Viral Persistence in B19-Associated Arthritis

The presence of B19 products in synovial lymphocytes, macrophages, and follicular dendritic cells of patients who have RA has been investigated. In several studies, B19 persistence occurred at a higher frequency in the RA synovium compared with osteoarthritis, traumatic, or healthy control joints.[96,103–106] In contrast to these data, other authors found increased expression of B19 DNA in the synovial membranes of controls compared with children who had juvenile idiopathic arthritis (JIA), suggesting that the presence of B19 DNA in the synovial membrane is not sufficient etiologic evidence of B19 arthropathy and does not correlate with rheumatoid synovitis.[97,107,108] Another study looked at the persistence of B19 in RA using in vitro transwell coculture systems. The authors demonstrated the transfer of B19 gene products from B19 DNA-positive synoviocytes from patients who had RA to macrophage cell lines.[106] Although the mechanism for this transfer was not explained, expression of VP1 RNA and protein was found within cocultured macrophages and the enhanced production of IL-6 and TNF characteristic of NS1 activity. This effect was suppressed after the addition of neutralizing anti-VP1 antibodies, suggesting that the B19 DNA found in RA synoviocytes possesses infectious capability despite that synoviocytes are nonpermissive to B19 infection.[106]

Viral persistence has also been demonstrated in the bone marrow of patients who have RA[109] with an estimated frequency of 32%[103] compared with 2% of healthy seropositive individuals[9] and 4% of patients attending a hematology clinic.[110] RA characteristics, such as rheumatoid factor seropositivity and joint erosions, were less common in patients who had RA positive for B19 DNA than in those who were negative.[103] These data suggest that ubiquitous and lifelong persistence of B19 genomic DNA can occur in human tissues[111] and may lead to a dynamic interplay between viral replication and host immune surveillance. The mechanism that facilitates the persistence of B19 DNA products remains unclear.[112] Assessment of viral and host factors in patients persistently infected with B19 demonstrated B19-neutralizing antibodies with a normal epitope distribution, which suggests that persistence can occur despite an intact humoral and B19-specific CD8 response.[76] Polymorphisms in the viral genome also cannot explain this phenomenon because B19 strains isolated from persistently infected patients show high viral sequence homology to strains isolated from transient infections.[17,113]

Cytotoxicity, Up-Regulation of Inflammatory Cytokines, and Phospholipase A2-Like Activity in B19-Associated Arthritis

Cartilage degradation is a characteristic feature of RA synovial fibroblasts. It is noteworthy that B19-containing sera can induce invasive properties in synovial fibroblasts, allowing them to acquire the ability to degrade reconstituted cartilage matrix. That this effect can be abrogated by B19-neutralizing antibodies suggests that viral protein products play a role in this phenomenon.[114] This suggestion is further supported by recent findings that show that synoviocyte activation is mediated by phospholipase A2 activity of the B19 viral capsid.[24] The inflammatory events evoked by phospholipase A2 are associated with its enzymatic activity and the release of arachidonic acid metabolites, including prostaglandins such as PGE2.[24] It should be noted that synovial fibroblasts in vitro are nonpermissive for B19 replication.[24,66] It thus remains unknown whether productive infection of primary human synovial fibroblasts occurs or is even required for virus-induced activation.

In vitro and in vivo evidence implicates cytokine dysregulation as another mechanism involved in B19-associated chronic arthritis. Transfection of COS-7 endothelial cells with NS1 in vitro resulted in increased IL-6 production, which is a hallmark of RA.[29] Further evidence comes from transgenic expression of B19 NS1 onto a nonpermissive, arthritis-resistant C57BL/6 murine background, which rendered the mice susceptible to experimental type II collagen-induced arthritis.[115] Arthritic disease manifested as the formation of granulomatous lesions and pannus, resulting in the destruction of articular cartilage and bone that was qualitatively similar to human RA.[115] In this model TNF elevation was induced by NS1.[115] These data show that the B19 NS1 gene is capable of inducing cytokine dysregulation outside the context of B19 infection.[106]

Support for the viral modulation of inflammatory cytokines secondary to cell-mediated host responses to B19 infection come from experiments showing that lymphocytes from convalescent adults also produce high levels of IL-2 and IFN-γ in response to B19 VP1 and VP2 proteins, whereas in recently infected children there is a significant deficit in the IFN-γ response against capsid proteins. This defect in IFN-γ production is not an intrinsic feature of the T-cell population, because mitogen-specific responses are intact.[18] Cytokine profiling of sera from adults who have acute symptomatic B19 infection shows elevated levels of IL-6, IFN-γ, and TNF-α.[30] Although TNF and IFN remain elevated in patients who have persistent infection,[9] serum TNF was not associated with arthralgias either in acute B19 infection or at follow-up.[30] In fact, postinfectious B19 arthritis has been shown to be associated with lower levels of inflammatory cytokines, such as TNF-α, IL-6, and granulocyte monocyte colony-stimulating factor, than acute symptomatic infection,[68] in contrast to what occurs in RA.

Autoantibodies in B19-Associated Arthritis

B19 infection is associated with autoantibody production, including rheumatoid factor, antiphospholipids, anti–smooth muscle, antinuclear, antimitochondrial, and antineutrophil cytoplasmic antibodies.[77] In addition, chronic parvovirus B19 infection can induce antiviral antibodies with autoantigen binding properties.[11] In fact, anti-B19 VP1 IgG shows similarities with several human epitopes, including human collagen II, keratin, single-stranded DNA, and cardiolipin, implying that the persistence of the virus might induce autoimmunity through a mechanism of molecular mimicry.[116] In support of this idea, type II collagen immunization induced a destructive polyarthritis in transgenic mice expressing the NS1 gene.[115] On the other hand, antiviral antibodies cross-reacting with GATA1, a transcription factor essential for normal hematopoiesis, may arrest the maturation of erythroblasts and megakaryoblasts. This finding and the direct cytotoxicity of the NS1 protein are pathogenetic mechanisms underlying B19-induced cytopenias.[11]

Cellular Immunity in B19-Associated Arthritis

Alteration of cellular immunity is also a putative mediator of B19-induced arthropathy. In a small number of patients who had acute infection, serum IL-2 was a predictor of positive outcome; in fact, detection of IL-2 baseline was associated with clearance of the virus from peripheral blood and absence of symptoms at follow-up.[30] Recent evidence shows that CD8 T-cell responses to B19 NS1 peptides were sustained as mature "effector memory populations" up to 2 years postinfection.[43] Other support from antiviral T-cell responses comes from recent work showing that large populations of CD4 T cells reactive to tetramers loaded with peptide sequences spanning VP1 and VP2 proteins were involved in acute B19 infection. These cells exhibit a central memory phenotype and may play a role in those individuals who develop chronic arthritis by recognizing persisting B19 or cross-reactive self antigens.[117]

DIAGNOSTIC CONSIDERATIONS IN B19 INFECTION

There are two basic approaches to diagnosing B19 infection: application of serologic tests for antibody detection (specific antibody reactivity against viral capsid proteins or NS1) and the direct detection of viral products (polymerase chain reaction [PCR] for B19 DNA).[9] Anti-B19 humoral responses are directed to structural proteins with persistence of IgG antibodies directed to conformational epitopes. Immunoassays that only incorporate Escherichia coli–expressed B19 antigens that have undergone denaturation as part of the manufacturing process give false-negative results. B19 IgM and IgG detection seems to be optimal in immunoassays that use VP2 capsids for antibody detection.[65] IgM antibodies specific for the VP2 protein are present 10 to 12 days after infection and usually disappear within 3 to 4 months.[47] Shortly after the advent of the IgM response, there is a shift to IgG directed toward VP1 and VP2 with most linear epitopes located in the VP1u region and the junction between VP1 and VP2.[118]

Caution should be made when interpreting serology in immunodeficient patients and pregnant women because of their decreased capacity to mount an antibody response.[47] In these cases, serology should be complemented by PCR analysis of B19 DNA. Although PCR improves the sensitivity of detection, PCR results should be interpreted with caution for several reasons. First, false-positive results can occur because of B19 DNA products' persistence; therefore, DNA detection does not always indicate acute infection. In addition, technical considerations affect the quality and sensitivity of PCR analyses because some PCR assays use primers with an undefined sensitivity of detection.

SUMMARY

Although the link between parvovirus B19 infection and rheumatic manifestations has been suggested for almost 25 years, the evidence supporting a causal association between the virus and chronic arthritis remains circumstantial and inconclusive. The study of this virus and specifically of viral–host interactions have been hampered by the limitations in propagating B19 in vitro due in part to the cytotoxic nature of NS1.[7] In fact, only a handful of erythroid leukemic cell lines or megakaryoblastoid cell lines with erythroid characteristics support B19 replication,[53] and even these cells are only semipermissive to B19 infection supporting limited viral production. The recent report of CD36+ erythroid progenitor cells generated from CD34 hematopoietic progenitors provides a highly permissive cell lineage for B19 infection and replication[53] and offers a system that mimics infection in vivo.

B19 viral persistence seems to be a crucial factor related to the potential arthritogenic effect of the virus. How the virus escapes immune surveillance mechanisms and an efficient neutralizing antibody response remains unknown. Also unknown is how in some patients viral persistence is associated with the breaking of tolerance, leading to autoimmunity. Answering these questions not only is critical for the understanding of B19 pathogenesis but also will provide a greater overall understanding of the rheumatoid arthritis syndrome and viral triggering of autoimmune processes in general.

ACKNOWLEDGMENT

The authors acknowledge Carlos E. Perandones, MD, for helpful suggestions.

REFERENCES

1. Cossart YE, Field AM, Cant B, et al. Parvovirus-like particles in human sera. Lancet 1975;1:72–3.

2. Pattison JR, Jones SE, Hodgson J, et al. Parvovirus infections and hypoplastic crisis in sickle-cell anaemia. Lancet 1981;1:664–5.

3. Anderson MJ, Jones SE, Fisher-Hoch SP, et al. Human parvovirus, the cause of erythema infectiosum (fifth disease)? Lancet 1983;1:1378.

4. Reid DM, Reid TM, Brown T, et al. Human parvovirus-associated arthritis: a clinical and laboratory description. Lancet 1985;1:422–5.

5. White DG, Woolf AD, Mortimer PP, et al. Human parvovirus arthropathy. Lancet 1985;1:419–21.

6. Aslanidis S, Pyrpasopoulou A, Kontotasios K, et al. Parvovirus B19 infection and systemic lupus erythematosus: activation of an aberrant pathway? Eur J Intern Med 2008;19:314–8.

7. Corcoran A, Doyle S. Advances in the biology, diagnosis and host-pathogen interactions of parvovirus B19. J Med Microbiol 2004;53:459–75.

8. Franssila R, Hedman K. Infection and musculoskeletal conditions: viral causes of arthritis. Best Pract Res Clin Rheumatol 2006;20:1139–57.

9. Heegaard ED, Brown KE. Human parvovirus B19. Clin Microbiol Rev 2002; 15:485–505.

10. Kerr JR. Pathogenesis of human parvovirus B19 in rheumatic disease. Ann Rheum Dis 2000;59:672–83.

11. Lunardi C, Tinazzi E, Bason C, et al. Human parvovirus B19 infection and autoimmunity. Autoimmun Rev 2008;8:116–20.

12. Meyer O. Parvovirus B19 and autoimmune diseases. Joint Bone Spine 2003;70: 6–11.

13. Moore TL. Parvovirus-associated arthritis. Curr Opin Rheumatol 2000;12: 289–94.

14. Naides SJ. Rheumatic manifestations of parvovirus B19 infection. Rheum Dis Clin North Am 1998;24:375–401.

15. Brown KE, Simmonds P. Parvoviruses and blood transfusion. Transfusion 2007; 47:1745–50.

16. Mani B, Gerber M, Lieby P, et al. Molecular mechanism underlying B19 virus inactivation and comparison to other parvoviruses. Transfusion 2007;47: 1765–74.

17. Gallinella G, Venturoli S, Manaresi E, et al. B19 virus genome diversity: epidemiological and clinical correlations. J Clin Virol 2003;28:1–13.

18. Corcoran A, Doyle S, Waldron D, et al. Impaired gamma interferon responses against parvovirus B19 by recently infected children. J Virol 2000;74:9903–10.

19. Kajigaya S, Fujii H, Field A, et al. Self-assembled B19 parvovirus capsids, produced in a baculovirus system, are antigenically and immunogenically similar to native virions. Proc Natl Acad Sci USA 1991;88:4646–50.

20. Musiani M, Manaresi E, Gallinella G, et al. Immunoreactivity against linear epitopes of parvovirus B19 structural proteins. Immunodominance of the amino-terminal half of the unique region of VP1. J Med Virol 2000;60:347–52.

21. Zuffi E, Manaresi E, Gallinella G, et al. Identification of an immunodominant peptide in the parvovirus B19 VP1 unique region able to elicit a long-lasting immune response in humans. Viral Immunol 2001;14:151–8.

22. Dorsch S, Liebisch G, Kaufmann B, et al. The VP1 unique region of parvovirus B19 and its constituent phospholipase A2-like activity. J Virol 2002;76: 2014–8.

23. Filippone C, Zhi N, Wong S, et al. VP1u phospholipase activity is critical for infectivity of full-length parvovirus B19 genomic clones. Virology 2008;374: 444–52.

24. Lu J, Zhi N, Wong S, et al. Activation of synoviocytes by the secreted phospholipase A2 motif in the VP1-unique region of parvovirus B19 minor capsid protein. J Infect Dis 2006;193:582–90.

25. Zadori Z, Szelei J, Lacoste MC, et al. A viral phospholipase A2 is required for parvovirus infectivity. Dev Cell 2001;1:291–302.

26. Ozawa K, Young N. Characterization of capsid and noncapsid proteins of B19 parvovirus propagated in human erythroid bone marrow cell cultures. J Virol 1987;61:2627–30.

27. Ballou WR, Reed JL, Noble W, et al. Safety and immunogenicity of a recombinant parvovirus B19 vaccine formulated with MF59C.1. J Infect Dis 2003;187: 675–8.

28. Gareus R, Gigler A, Hemauer A, et al. Characterization of cis-acting and NS1 protein-responsive elements in the p6 promoter of parvovirus B19. J Virol 1998;72:609–16.

29. Hsu TC, Tzang BS, Huang CN, et al. Increased expression and secretion of interleukin-6 in human parvovirus B19 non-structural protein (NS1) transfected COS-7 epithelial cells. Clin Exp Immunol 2006;144:152–7.

30. Kerr JR, Barah F, Mattey DL, et al. Circulating tumour necrosis factor-alpha and interferon-gamma are detectable during acute and convalescent parvovirus B19 infection and are associated with prolonged and chronic fatigue. J Gen Virol 2001;82:3011–9.

31. Moffatt S, Yaegashi N, Tada K, et al. Human parvovirus B19 nonstructural (NS1) protein induces apoptosis in erythroid lineage cells. J Virol 1998;72:3018–28.

32. Fu Y, Ishii KK, Munakata Y, et al. Regulation of tumor necrosis factor alpha promoter by human parvovirus B19 NS1 through activation of AP-1 and AP-2. J Virol 2002;76:5395–403.

33. O'Shea JJ, Murray PJ. Cytokine signaling modules in inflammatory responses. Immunity 2008;28:477–87.

34. Croker BA, Kiu H, Nicholson SE. SOCS regulation of the JAK/STAT signalling pathway. Semin Cell Dev Biol 2008;19:414–22.

35. Duechting A, Tschope C, Kaiser H, et al. Human parvovirus B19 NS1 protein modulates inflammatory signaling by activation of STAT3/PIAS3 in human endothelial cells. J Virol 2008;82:7942–52.

36. Bruggeman LA. Viral subversion mechanisms in chronic kidney disease pathogenesis. Clin J Am Soc Nephrol 2007;2(Suppl 1):S13–9.

37. Yaegashi N, Niinuma T, Chisaka H, et al. Parvovirus B19 infection induces apoptosis of erythroid cells in vitro and in vivo. J Infect 1999;39:68–76.

38. Tsay GJ, Zouali M. Unscrambling the role of human parvovirus B19 signaling in systemic autoimmunity. Biochem Pharmacol 2006;72:1453–9.

39. Hsu TC, Wu WJ, Chen MC, et al. Human parvovirus B19 non-structural protein (NS1) induces apoptosis through mitochondria cell death pathway in COS-7 cells. Scand J Infect Dis 2004;36:570–7.

40. Moffatt S, Tanaka N, Tada K, et al. A cytotoxic nonstructural protein, NS1, of human parvovirus B19 induces activation of interleukin-6 gene expression. J Virol 1996;70:8485–91.

41. Raab U, Beckenlehner K, Lowin T, et al. NS1 protein of parvovirus B19 interacts directly with DNA sequences of the p6 promoter and with the cellular transcription factors Sp1/Sp3. Virology 2002;293:86–93.

42. Norbeck O, Isa A, Pohlmann C, et al. Sustained CD8+ T-cell responses induced after acute parvovirus B19 infection in humans. J Virol 2005;79:12117–21.

43. Isa A, Kasprowicz V, Norbeck O, et al. Prolonged activation of virus-specific CD8+T cells after acute B19 infection. PLoS Med 2005;2:e343.
44. Isa A, Norbeck O, Hirbod T, et al. Aberrant cellular immune responses in humans infected persistently with parvovirus B19. J Med Virol 2006;78:129–33.
45. Harger JH, Adler SP, Koch WC, et al. Prospective evaluation of 618 pregnant women exposed to parvovirus B19: risks and symptoms. Obstet Gynecol 1998;91:413–20.
46. Eid AJ, Brown RA, Patel R, et al. Parvovirus B19 infection after transplantation: a review of 98 cases. Clin Infect Dis 2006;43:40–8.
47. Broliden K, Tolfvenstam T, Norbeck O. Clinical aspects of parvovirus B19 infection. J Intern Med 2006;260:285–304.
48. Gillespie SM, Cartter ML, Asch S, et al. Occupational risk of human parvovirus B19 infection for school and day-care personnel during an outbreak of erythema infectiosum. JAMA 1990;263:2061–5.
49. Srivastava A, Lu L. Replication of B19 parvovirus in highly enriched hematopoietic progenitor cells from normal human bone marrow. J Virol 1988;62:3059–63.
50. Brown KE, Anderson SM, Young NS. Erythrocyte P antigen: cellular receptor for B19 parvovirus. Science 1993;262:114–7.
51. Brown KE, Hibbs JR, Gallinella G, et al. Resistance to parvovirus B19 infection due to lack of virus receptor (erythrocyte P antigen). N Engl J Med 1994;330:1192–6.
52. Cooling LL, Koerner TA, Naides SJ. Multiple glycosphingolipids determine the tissue tropism of parvovirus B19. J Infect Dis 1995;172:1198–205.
53. Wong S, Zhi N, Filippone C, et al. Ex vivo-generated CD36+ erythroid progenitors are highly permissive to human parvovirus B19 replication. J Virol 2008;82:2470–6.
54. Bonsch C, Kempf C, Ros C. Interaction of parvovirus B19 with human erythrocytes alters virus structure and cell membrane integrity. J Virol 2008;82:11784–91.
55. Weigel-Kelley KA, Yoder MC, Chen L, et al. Role of integrin cross-regulation in parvovirus B19 targeting. Hum Gene Ther 2006;17:909–20.
56. Weigel-Kelley KA, Yoder MC, Srivastava A. Alpha5beta1 integrin as a cellular coreceptor for human parvovirus B19: requirement of functional activation of beta1 integrin for viral entry. Blood 2003;102:3927–33.
57. Munakata Y, Saito-Ito T, Kumura-Ishii K, et al. Ku80 autoantigen as a cellular coreceptor for human parvovirus B19 infection. Blood 2005;106:3449–56.
58. Harbison CE, Chiorini JA, Parrish CR. The parvovirus capsid odyssey: from the cell surface to the nucleus. Trends Microbiol 2008;16:208–14.
59. Zhi N, Mills IP, Lu J, et al. Molecular and functional analyses of a human parvovirus B19 infectious clone demonstrates essential roles for NS1, VP1, and the 11-kilodalton protein in virus replication and infectivity. J Virol 2006;80:5941–50.
60. Anderson MJ, Higgins PG, Davis LR, et al. Experimental parvoviral infection in humans. J Infect Dis 1985;152:257–65.
61. Potter CG, Potter AC, Hatton CS, et al. Variation of erythroid and myeloid precursors in the marrow and peripheral blood of volunteer subjects infected with human parvovirus (B19). J Clin Invest 1987;79:1486–92.
62. Florea AV, Ionescu DN, Melhem MF. Parvovirus B19 infection in the immunocompromised host. Arch Pathol Lab Med 2007;131:799–804.
63. Ergaz Z, Ornoy A. Parvovirus B19 in pregnancy. Reprod Toxicol 2006;21:421–35.

64. Corcoran A, Mahon BP, Doyle S. B cell memory is directed toward conformational epitopes of parvovirus B19 capsid proteins and the unique region of VP1. J Infect Dis 2004;189:1873–80.
65. Peterlana D, Puccetti A, Corrocher R, et al. Serologic and molecular detection of human Parvovirus B19 infection. Clin Chim Acta 2006;372:14–23.
66. Miki NP, Chantler JK. Non-permissiveness of synovial membrane cells to human parvovirus B19 in vitro. J Gen Virol 1992;73(Pt 6):1559–62.
67. Anderson MJ, Lewis E, Kidd IM, et al. An outbreak of erythema infectiosum associated with human parvovirus infection. J Hyg (Lond) 1984;93:85–93.
68. Kerr JR, Cunniffe VS, Kelleher P, et al. Circulating cytokines and chemokines in acute symptomatic parvovirus B19 infection: negative association between levels of pro-inflammatory cytokines and development of B19-associated arthritis. J Med Virol 2004;74:147–55.
69. Luzzi GA, Kurtz JB, Chapel H. Human parvovirus arthropathy and rheumatoid factor. Lancet 1985;1:1218.
70. Sasaki T, Takahashi Y, Yoshinaga K, et al. An association between human parvovirus B-19 infection and autoantibody production. J Rheumatol 1989;16:708–9.
71. Hannu T, Hedman K, Hedman L, et al. Frequency of recent parvovirus infection in patients examined for acute reactive arthritis. A study with combinatorial parvovirus serodiagnostics. Clin Exp Rheumatol 2007;25:297–300.
72. Zerrak A, Bour JB, Tavernier C, et al. Usefulness of routine hepatitis C virus, hepatitis B virus, and parvovirus B19 serology in the diagnosis of recent-onset inflammatory arthritides. Arthritis Rheum 2005;53:477–8.
73. Dykmans BA, Breedveld FC, de Vries RR. HLA antigens in human parvovirus arthropathy. J Rheumatol 1986;13:1192–3.
74. Gendi NS, Gibson K, Wordsworth BP. Effect of HLA type and hypocomplementaemia on the expression of parvovirus arthritis: one year follow up of an outbreak. Ann Rheum Dis 1996;55:63–5.
75. Kerr JR, Mattey DL, Thomson W, et al. Association of symptomatic acute human parvovirus B19 infection with human leukocyte antigen class I and II alleles. J Infect Dis 2002;186:447–52.
76. Isa A, Lundqvist A, Lindblom A, et al. Cytokine responses in acute and persistent human parvovirus B19 infection. Clin Exp Immunol 2007;147:419–25.
77. Kerr JR. Pathogenesis of parvovirus B19 infection: host gene variability, and possible means and effects of virus persistence. J Vet Med B Infect Dis Vet Public Health 2005;52:335–9.
78. Fujinami RS, von Herrath MG, Christen U, et al. Molecular mimicry, bystander activation, or viral persistence: infections and autoimmune disease. Clin Microbiol Rev 2006;19:80–94.
79. Buyukkose M, Kozanoglu E, Basaran S, et al. Seroprevalence of parvovirus B19 in fibromyalgia syndrome. Clin Rheumatol 2009;28:305–9.
80. Challine-Lehmann D, Mauberquez S, Pawlotsky J, et al. Parvovirus B19 and Schonlein-Henoch purpura in adults. Nephron 1999;83:172.
81. Cohen BJ. Human parvovirus B19 infection in Kawasaki disease. Lancet 1994; 344:59.
82. Corman LC, Dolson DJ. Polyarteritis nodosa and parvovirus B19 infection. Lancet 1992;339:491.
83. Ferguson PJ, Saulsbury FT, Dowell SF, et al. Prevalence of human parvovirus B19 infection in children with Henoch-Schonlein purpura. Arthritis Rheum 1996;39:880–1.

84. Ferri C, Azzi A, Magro CM. Parvovirus B19 and systemic sclerosis. Br J Dermatol 2005;152:819–20.

85. Grilli R, Izquierdo MJ, Farina MC, et al. Papular-purpuric "gloves and socks" syndrome: polymerase chain reaction demonstration of parvovirus B19 DNA in cutaneous lesions and sera. J Am Acad Dermatol 1999;41:793–6.

86. Harel L, Straussberg R, Rudich H, et al. Raynaud's phenomenon as a manifestation of parvovirus B19 infection: case reports and review of parvovirus B19 rheumatic and vasculitic syndromes. Clin Infect Dis 2000;30:500–3.

87. Lehmann HW, Kuhner L, Beckenlehner K, et al. Chronic human parvovirus B19 infection in rheumatic disease of childhood and adolescence. J Clin Virol 2002; 25:135–43.

88. Nikkari S, Mertsola J, Korvenranta H, et al. Wegener's granulomatosis and parvovirus B19 infection. Arthritis Rheum 1994;37:1707–8.

89. Perandones CE, Colmegna I, Arana RM. Parvovirus B19: another agent associated with remitting seronegative symmetrical synovitis with pitting edema. J Rheumatol 2005;32:389–90.

90. Ramos-Casals M, Cervera R, Garcia-Carrasco M, et al. Cytopenia and past human parvovirus B19 infection in patients with primary Sjogren's syndrome. Semin Arthritis Rheum 2000;29:373–8.

91. Samii K, Cassinotti P, de Freudenreich J, et al. Acute bilateral carpal tunnel syndrome associated with human parvovirus B19 infection. Clin Infect Dis 1996;22:162–4.

92. Schwarz TF, Roggendorf M, Suschke H, et al. Human parvovirus B19 infection and juvenile chronic polyarthritis. Infection 1987;15:264–5.

93. Staud R, Corman LC. Association of parvovirus B19 infection with giant cell arteritis. Clin Infect Dis 1996;22:1123.

94. Yazici AC, Aslan G, Baz K, et al. A high prevalence of parvovirus B19 DNA in patients with psoriasis. Arch Dermatol Res 2006;298:231–5.

95. Chen YS, Chou PH, Li SN, et al. Parvovirus B19 infection in patients with rheumatoid arthritis in Taiwan. J Rheumatol 2006;33:887–91.

96. Kozireva SV, Zestkova JV, Mikazane HJ, et al. Incidence and clinical significance of parvovirus B19 infection in patients with rheumatoid arthritis. J Rheumatol 2008;35:1265–70.

97. Peterlana D, Puccetti A, Beri R, et al. The presence of parvovirus B19 VP and NS1 genes in the synovium is not correlated with rheumatoid arthritis. J Rheumatol 2003;30:1907–10.

98. Weissbrich B, Suss-Frohlich Y, Girschick HJ. Seroprevalence of parvovirus B19 IgG in children affected by juvenile idiopathic arthritis. Arthritis Res Ther 2007;9:R82.

99. Cohen BJ, Buckley MM, Clewley JP, et al. Human parvovirus infection in early rheumatoid and inflammatory arthritis. Ann Rheum Dis 1986;45:832–8.

100. Jorgensen KT, Wiik A, Pedersen M, et al. Cytokines, autoantibodies and viral antibodies in premorbid and postdiagnostic sera from patients with rheumatoid arthritis: case-control study nested in a cohort of Norwegian blood donors. Ann Rheum Dis 2008;67:860–6.

101. Murai C, Munakata Y, Takahashi Y, et al. Rheumatoid arthritis after human parvovirus B19 infection. Ann Rheum Dis 1999;58:130–2.

102. Ogawa E, Otaguro S, Murata M, et al. Intravenous immunoglobulin therapy for severe arthritis associated with human parvovirus B19 infection. J Infect Chemother 2008;14:377–82.

103. Lundqvist A, Isa A, Tolfvenstam T, et al. High frequency of parvovirus B19 DNA in bone marrow samples from rheumatic patients. J Clin Virol 2005; 33:71–4.
104. Mehraein Y, Lennerz C, Ehlhardt S, et al. Detection of parvovirus B19 capsid proteins in lymphocytic cells in synovial tissue of autoimmune chronic arthritis. Mod Pathol 2003;16:811–7.
105. Saal JG, Steidle M, Einsele H, et al. Persistence of B19 parvovirus in synovial membranes of patients with rheumatoid arthritis. Rheumatol Int 1992;12:147–51.
106. Takahashi Y, Murai C, Shibata S, et al. Human parvovirus B19 as a causative agent for rheumatoid arthritis. Proc Natl Acad Sci USA 1998;95:8227–32.
107. Nikkari S, Roivainen A, Hannonen P, et al. Persistence of parvovirus B19 in synovial fluid and bone marrow. Ann Rheum Dis 1995;54:597–600.
108. Soderlund M, von Essen R, Haapasaari J, et al. Persistence of parvovirus B19 DNA in synovial membranes of young patients with and without chronic arthropathy. Lancet 1997;349:1063–5.
109. Foto F, Saag KG, Scharosch LL, et al. Parvovirus B19-specific DNA in bone marrow from B19 arthropathy patients: evidence for B19 virus persistence. J Infect Dis 1993;167:744–8.
110. Lundqvist A, Tolfvenstam T, Brytting M, et al. Prevalence of parvovirus B19 DNA in bone marrow of patients with haematological disorders. Scand J Infect Dis 1999;31:119–22.
111. Norja P, Hokynar K, Aaltonen LM, et al. Bioportfolio: lifelong persistence of variant and prototypic erythrovirus DNA genomes in human tissue. Proc Natl Acad Sci USA 2006;103:7450–3.
112. Mitchell LA, Leong R, Rosenke KA. Lymphocyte recognition of human parvovirus B19 non-structural (NS1) protein: associations with occurrence of acute and chronic arthropathy? J Med Microbiol 2001;50:627–35.
113. Tolfvenstam T, Lundqvist A, Levi M, et al. Mapping of B-cell epitopes on human parvovirus B19 non-structural and structural proteins. Vaccine 2000;19:758–63.
114. Ray NB, Nieva DR, Seftor EA, et al. Induction of an invasive phenotype by human parvovirus B19 in normal human synovial fibroblasts. Arthritis Rheum 2001;44:1582–6.
115. Takasawa N, Munakata Y, Ishii KK, et al. Human parvovirus B19 transgenic mice become susceptible to polyarthritis. J Immunol 2004;173:4675–83.
116. Lunardi C, Tiso M, Borgato L, et al. Chronic parvovirus B19 infection induces the production of anti-virus antibodies with autoantigen binding properties. Eur J Immunol 1998;28:936–48.
117. Kasprowicz V, Isa A, Tolfvenstam T, et al. Tracking of peptide-specific CD4+ T-cell responses after an acute resolving viral infection: a study of parvovirus B19. J Virol 2006;80:11209–17.
118. Saikawa T, Anderson S, Momoeda M, et al. Neutralizing linear epitopes of B19 parvovirus cluster in the VP1 unique and VP1-VP2 junction regions. J Virol 1993; 67:3004–9.

Hepatitis C–Associated Rheumatic Disorders

Dan Buskila, MD

KEYWORDS

- Hepatitis C virus • Rheumatic disorders
- Musculoskeletal manifestations • Autoimmunity
- Arthritis

Hepatitis C virus (HCV), an RNA flavivirus with six major genotypes and several subtypes, is an important causative agent of liver diseases. However, HCV infection is more than just a liver disease and has been associated with numerous hematologic, renal, dermatologic, rheumatic, and autoimmune disorders.[1–3]

Much interest has been expressed in rheumatic disorders in HCV-infected patients. The many rheumatologic manifestations associated with HCV infection include arthralgia, myalgia, arthritis, vasculitis, sicca symptoms, mixed cryoglobulinemia (MC), and fibromyalgia.[4,5]

Associations have been reported between HCV infection and other autoimmune diseases including systemic lupus erythematosus, Sjogren's syndrome, and antiphospholipid antibody syndrome (APS).[5,6]

The purpose of this article is to review the prevalence and spectrum of rheumatic disorders and autoimmune phenomena in HCV-infected patients and current treatment options.

PREVALENCE AND CLINICAL MANIFESTATIONS OF HEPATITIS C-ASSOCIATED RHEUMATIC DISORDERS

Rheumatic manifestations were found in 31% (28 of 90) subjects infected with HCV in an Israeli study, and included arthralgias (9%), arthritis (4%), cryoglobulinemia (11%), sicca symptoms (8%), cutaneous vasculitis (2%), polymyositis (1%), myalgia (24%).[7] Rheumatic complications were not associated with liver disease severity or a subject's gender.

Nissen and colleagues,[8] retrospectively studied the clinical, radiological, and biologic data on 21 rheumatology patients (Group I) presenting symptoms consistent with a chronic inflammatory arthritis with a known HCV infection and compared them with 41 members of an HCV-support association (Group II). Symptoms of myalgia,

Division of Internal Medicine, Department of Medicine H, Soroka Medical Center, Faculty of Health Sciences, Ben Gurion University, Beer Sheva, P.O.B 151, Israel 84101
E-mail address: dbuskila@bgu.ac.il

Rheum Dis Clin N Am 35 (2009) 111–123
doi:10.1016/j.rdc.2009.03.005
0889-857X/09/$ – see front matter © 2009 Elsevier Inc. All rights reserved.

sicca syndrome, Raynaud phenomenon, or paresthesias were similarly frequent in the two groups. However, inflammatory joint pain and joint swelling were more common in Group I. It was concluded that rheumatological symptoms are common in patients chronically infected with HCV.

A Bulgarian study found a high prevalence of extrahepatic manifestations in 136 chronically infected HCV patients.[9] This included arthralgia (18.4%), palpable purpura (17.6%), Raynaud phenomenon (11.8%), and sicca syndrome (6.6%). All extrahepatic manifestations showed an association with cryoglobulin positivity, with the exception of thyroid dysfunction, sicca syndrome, and lichen planus.

Lovy and colleagues[10] provided a case study of 19 consecutive patients—referred because of polyarthritis, polyarthralgia, or positive rheumatoid factor (RF)—who were subsequently found to have hepatitis C. Carpal tunnel syndrome (8 patients), palmar tenosynovitis (7 patients), fibromyalgia (FM) (6 patients), and nonerosive, nonprogressive arthritis typified the articular manifestations. Fifteen patients fulfilled diagnostic criteria for rheumatoid arthritis. Three patients had small vessel skin vasculitis. It was concluded that HCV infection can present with rheumatic manifestations indistinguishable from rheumatoid arthritis.[10]

A high prevalence of rheumatologic symptoms was documented in Korean patients infected with HCV.[11] The clinical features were arthralgia or arthritis (35%), cutaneous manifestations (37%), Raynaud phenomenon (8%), paresthesias (44%), dry eyes (22%), dry mouth (10%), and oral ulcers (33%).

Moder and Lindor[12] reported musculoskeletal complaints in 69% of 42 HCV-infected patients, most of which were myalgias and arthralgias. In another study, the most common rheumatic manifestations in chronic hepatitis C-infected patients were arthralgias (52%), myalgias (16%), xerostomia (28.5%), and xerophthalmia (14%).[13]

Thus, rheumatic disorders are common in HCV infection. An investigation for HCV infection is pertinent in a patient presenting with new rheumatic manifestations (**Table 1**).

Arthritis

Arthralgias are relatively common in HCV. In a prospective study of 1614 patients with HCV infections, the prevalence of arthralgia was 23%.[14] Rivera and colleagues[15]

Table 1
Rheumatic and serologic manifestations associated with hepatitis C virus infection

Clinical Manifestation	Serologic Markers (Autoantibodies)
Arthralgia	RF
Arthritis	ANA
Sjogren's syndrome	ANCA
MC syndrome	Anti-LKM-1
Myalgia	Antiplatelet
Inflammatory myopathy	Anti-Ro/SSA and Anti-La/SSB
Fibromyalgia	Antineuronal
SLE	—
APS	—

Abbreviations: ANA, antinuclear antibody; ANCA, antineutrophil cytoplasmic autoantibody; anti-LKM-1, anti–liver-kidney microsome antibodies; SLE, systemic lupus erythematosus.

described the clinical picture of arthritis in patients with chronic infection by HCV. Two patient populations were studied. Patients with arthritis and evidence of serum elevation of alanine aminotransferase at the consultation were checked for HCV infection. A second group of 303 consecutive patients with rheumatoid arthritis (RA) was also checked for the presence of HCV antibodies. A group of 315 first-time blood donors served as controls. Twenty-eight patients with arthritis and chronic HCV infection were identified.

Seven fulfilled criteria for rheumatoid arthritis, psoriatic arthritis was found in 1 patient, systemic lupus erythematosus in 1, gout in 2, chondrocalcinosis in 2, osteoarthritis in 7, and tenosynovitis in 1. In 7 patients with a clinical picture of intermittent arthritis, a definite diagnosis could not be made. In these patients, MC was present in 6 of 7 (86%), whereas MC was found in 6 of 21 (28%) of the other patients. It was concluded that there is not a single clinical picture of arthritis in patients with chronic HCV infection. Arthritis associated with cryoglobulinemia consisted of an intermittent monoarticular or oligoarticular nondestructive arthritis affecting large- and medium-sized joints.[15]

Zuckerman and collegues[16] studied 28 HCV-infected patients with arthritis. Nineteen patients (68%) had symmetric polyarthritis; none of the patients had erosive disease or subcutaneous nodules. Fourteen patients (50%) had greater than or equal to four American College of Rheumatology criteria for the diagnosis of RA. Of these, 9 were mistakenly diagnosed and previously treated as RA patients. Complete or partial response of arthritis-related symptoms in interferon-α (INF-α)–treated patients was observed in 44% and 32%, respectively.

Rosner and colleagues[17] summarized the clinical characteristics of HCV-associated arthritis. Arthritis, not otherwise explained, has been noted in 2% to 20% of HCV patients. This arthritis was rheumatoid-like in two thirds of the cases and a waxing-waning oligoarthritis in the rest. Cryoglobulinemia alone did not explain the arthritis, and there was difficulty in differentiating it from RA. The arthropathy was nonerosive and nondeforming. It was concluded that HCV arthropathy should be considered in the differential diagnosis of new onset arthritis.[17] It was suggested that HCV-related arthritis might preset in two clinical pictures:

RA-like presentation, involving mainly small joints in which the RF is often present and rheumatoid nodules are absent.
A less common mono-oligoarthritis usually of the large joints.[18,19]

As mentioned earlier, HCV-associated arthritis may mimic RA. The existence of morning stiffness, rheumatoid nodules, and erosive arthritis, and the presence of antibodies to cyclic citrullinated peptide (CCP) may be useful to diagnose a true coexistence of RA and HCV.[2,16]

The pathogenesis of HCV-related arthritis is not entirely clear, but three possible mechanisms have been suggested, namely: synovial tissue damage by direct viral invasion, synovial autoimmune response induced by the virus, and immune complexes or cryoglobulins deposition.[18,19]

Sjogren's Syndrome

Sialadenitis and sicca symptoms are seen frequently in patients with HCV infection.[20] A lymphocytic sialadenitis suggestive of Sjogren's syndrome has been described in patients with chronic HCV infection.[21] Ramos-Casals and colleagues[21] studied the clinical and immunologic pattern of expression of Sjogren's syndrome associated with chronic HCV infection in 137 cases. Seventy-nine (58%) patients presented a systemic process with diverse extraglandular manifestations, with articular involvement (44%), vasculitis (20%), and neuropathy (16%) being the most frequent features observed.

The main immunologic features were antinuclear antibodies (ANA) (65%), hypocomplementemia (51%), and cryoglobulinemia (50%). Cryoglobulins were associated with a higher frequency of cutaneous vasculitis, RF, and hypocomplementemia.

Thirty-two (23%) patients had positive anti–Ro/SS-A or anti–La/SS-B antibodies. These patients were predominantly women and had a higher prevalence of some extraglandular features and a lower frequency of liver involvement. It was concluded that HCV-associated Sjogren's syndrome is indistinguishable in most cases from the primary form. Circulating monoclonal immunoglobulins were detected in nearly 20% of patients with primary Sjogren's syndrome, with monoclonal IgG being the most frequent type of immunoglobulin detected.[22]

In patients with HCV-associated Sjogren's syndrome, the prevalence of monoclonal immunoglobulins was higher (43%) with monoclonal IgM being the most frequent type of band found. Patients with HCV-associated Sjogren's syndrome presented a more restrictive monoclonal expression compared with patients with primary Sjogren's syndrome.[22]

An association was found between chronic HCV infection and sicca syndrome and HLA-DQB1*02.[23] DQB1*02 was highly significantly associated with viral persistence. Nineteen of 21 patients with sicca syndrome were HCV polymerase chain reaction positive, demonstrating a strong association with viral persistence and the development of the syndrome. Human leukocyte antigen DQB1*02 was significantly associated with the development of sicca syndrome.[23]

Ramos-Casals and colleagues[24] have suggested that HCV may be considered the most important etiopathogenetic causal agent for Sjogren's syndrome identified to date, with Sjogren's syndrome HCV being indistinguishable in most cases from the primary form using the most recent sets of classification criteria.

Mixed Cryoglobulinemia

MC is a systemic vasculitis of small- to medium-sized vessels due to the vascular deposition of circulating immune complexes and complement. The association between HCV infection and MC is firmly established. Lunel and colleagues[25] prospectively evaluated the prevalence of cryoglobulins in 226 patients with chronic liver disease. Of the 127 with chronic-HCV infection, cryoglobulins were found in 69 (54%), frequently with anti-HCV antibody and HCV RNA concentrated in the cryoprecipitates. Bryce and colleagues[26] examined the cases of 66 patients with type II MC. Among the causes of type II cryoglobulinemia, HCV was the most common—found in 61% of the cases, a rate similar to other reports. Indeed, circulating mixed cryoglobulins are detected in 40% to 60% of HCV-infected patients, whereas overt cryoglobulinemia vasculitis develops in only 5% to 10% of the cases.[27]

An effect of the HCV virus on the B cell line has been suggested in the pathogenesis of HCV-associated cryoglobulinemia. The association of MC with HCV infection may be linked to the ability of the HCV to bind to B lymphocytes by way of CD81.[28] It was suggested that anti-apoptotic mechanisms in the B cell compartment through B lymphocyte stimulator upregulation might be implicated in a fraction of patients with MC syndrome.[29]

Higher serum levels of chemokines (CXCL10 and CCL2) have been reported in patients with HCV-associated MC.[30] It was suggested that future studies in larger series are needed to evaluate the potential usefulness of serum CXCL10 and CCL2 determination as a prognostic marker in follow-up of MC—also in relation to the presence of autoimmune thyroiditis. High CXCL10 and tumor necrosis factor α (TNF-α) serum levels have been demonstrated in patients with HCV-associated cryoglobuline-mia.[31] Moreover, in MC-positive HCV patients, increased CXCL10 levels were significantly associated with the presence of active vasculitis.[31] Circulating CXCL10 were higher overall in cryoglobulinemic patients with active vasculitis suggesting a prevalence of the TH1 immune response in this phase.[32]

MC syndrome followed a relatively benign clinical course in over 50% of cases, whereas a moderate-severe clinical course was observed in one third of patients whose prognosis was severely affected by renal or liver failure.[33] In 15% of the individuals, the disease was complicated by a malignancy, B cell lymphoma, and less frequently by hepatocellular carcinoma or thyroid cancer.[33]

Fibromyalgia

FM syndrome, a condition characterized by widespread pain and diffuse tenderness, is considered a multifactorial disorder. Certain infections, including hepatitis C, have been associated with the development of FM.[34,35] The prevalence of FM was evaluated in 90 patients with HCV, 128 healthy anti-HCV negative controls, and 32 patients with non–HCV-related cirrhosis.[36] The diagnosis of FM was established in 16% (14 of 90) of HCV-infected patients, in 3% (1) with non–HCV-related cirrhosis, and in none of the healthy controls. Similarly, Rivera and colleagues[37] provided evidence for an association between FM and active HCV infection in some patients. Another study, revealed a moderate increase in prevalence of FM in HCV patients.[38] A Turkish study demonstrated FM in 18.9% of 95 HCV patients and 5.3% in healthy controls.[39]

Two studies could not find an increased prevalence of HCV infection in FM patients.[40,41] Fatigue is one of the ancillary symptoms associated with FM. Fatigue was present in 53% of 1614 HCV-infected patients.[42] In 17% of patients, fatigue was severe and impaired activity. Fatigue was independently associated with female gender, age over 50 years, cirrhosis, depression, and purpura.[42]

AUTOIMMUNITY AND HEPATITIS C VIRUS INFECTION

HCV-infected subjects express a high prevalence of a variety of autoantibodies, usually in low titers.[43] Lenzi and colleagues[44] explored the prevalence of non–organ-specific autoantibodies (NOSAs), their relation to different HCV genotypes, and the presence and severity of chronic liver disease in the general population of northern Italy. The sera of 226 anti–HCV-positive and 87 hepatitis B surface antigen-positive patients were tested for the presence of different NOSAs, and compared with 226 gender- and age-matched cases negative for both viruses. It was found that in the general population the prevalence of NOSAs is higher in anti–HCV-positive subjects than in normal or disease controls. The author and colleagues[7] have reported that 69% of 90 HCV-infected subjects had at least one autoantibody in their serum.

Some of the autoantibodies were more frequently expressed—especially RF, antinuclear antibodies, and anticardiolipin antibodies. At least one serologic marker was found in 75% of 80 patients with chronic viral hepatitis, 60 of whom had HCV infection.[45] RF was present in 31%, anticardiolipin antibodies in 34%, P-ANCA in 27%, and circulating immunologic complexes in 20% of the patients. ANA, antimitochondrial antibodies, anti–liver-kidney microsome antibodies (anti-LKM-1), and cryoglobulins were less frequently observed.[45]

Anti-LKM-1 has been detected in HCV-infected patients in Europe but not in the United States.[46] It was suggested that the absence of anti-LKM-1 in United States sera compared with French sera may be due to differences in induction of anti-LKM-1 related to environmental or host genetic factors, or genomic variation in the HCV.[46] An increased prevalence of anti–C-reactive protein antibodies was manifested in HCV-infected patients; and correlated with the presence of RF, cryoglobulinemia, and severity of liver disease.[47] Antiplatelet antibodies were detected in 20% (8 in 40) of patients with chronic hepatitis C before and after IFN-α therapy.[48]

It was concluded that thrombocytopenia observed during IFN-α therapy was not due to the development of antiplatelet antibodies. Anti-SSA/Ro and anti-SSB/La antibodies were detected in 12.8% and 9.7% of HCV-infected patients.[49] Anti-SSB/La antibody was negatively associated with HLA-DR2 in HCV-infected patients in Taiwan.[49] A significant increase in plasma titers of antineuronal antibodies (anti-GM1 ganglioside and antisulfatide) was observed in patients with HCV-related MC.[50] It was suggested that antineuronal reactivity could be a direct trigger of neurologic injury in this disorder.[50]

The presence of autoantibodies in the sera of HCV-infected patients may pose diagnostic dilemmas. Thus, a patient presenting with symmetric polyarthritis and positive RF may be misdiagnosed as having rheumatoid arthritis. Antibodies against CCP may be helpful to solve this diagnostic dilemma. In contrast to rheumatoid arthritis, CCP antibodies were not increased in HCV infection.[51] In another study anti-CCP antibodies were rarely found in HCV-infected patients with rheumatological manifestations or Sjogren's syndrome.[52]

It was concluded that they are reliable serologic markers to distinguish these from patients with rheumatoid arthritis. Interestingly, autoantibodies may first become detectable or increase in titer during interferon treatment in HCV-infected patients. Indeed, a strong correlation was demonstrated between INF-α treatment and autoimmune phenomena, notably the emergence of thyroid antibodies in chronic HCV-infected subjects.[52]

Autoimmune Diseases and Hepatitis C Virus

Ramos-Casals and colleagues[6] analyzed 180 patients diagnosed with systemic autoimmune diseases associated with chronic HCV infection. Of the 180 HCV patients: 77 had Sjogren's syndrome, 43 systemic lupus erythematosus (SLE), 14 RA, 14 APS, 8 polyarteritis nodósa (PAN), and 24 had other systemic autoimmune diseases. The main immunologic features were ANA in 69% of patients, cryoglobulinemia in 62%, hypocomplementemia in 56%, and RF in 56%. In comparison with a systemic autoimmune diseases-matched, HCV-negative population, autoimmune patients with HCV were older and more likely to be male, with a higher frequency of vasculitis, cryoglobulinemia, and neoplasia.

It was concluded that this complex pattern of disease expression is generated by a chronic viral infection that induces both liver and autoimmune disease. Different degrees of association between systemic autoimmune diseases and HCV have been stressed.[6] A high degree of association was found for Sjogren's syndrome, SLE, and RA; an intermediate degree of association for PAN, APS, inflammatory myopathies; and a low degree of association for systemic sclerosis, Wegener granulomatosis, giant cell arteritis, polymyalgia rheumatica, and ankylosing spondylitis.[6]

A subset of HCV patients with positive antimitochondrial antibodies who presented a broad spectrum of clinical features including liver, autoimmune, and neoplastic manifestations was described.[53] Two thirds of these patients presented an associated systemic autoimmune disease, mainly Sjogren's syndrome or systemic sclerosis, together with a high frequency of cytopenias and multiple autoantibodies.[53] Cervera and colleagues[54] analyzed the clinical characteristics of 100 patients with APS associated with infections. HCV infection was documented in 13% of the patients. The spectrum of clinical features related to APS was analyzed in 45 HCV-infected patients.

In comparison with unselected APS patients, APS-HCV patients had a lower frequency of typical APS features but a higher prevalence of some atypical or infrequent features such as myocardial infarction or intra-abdominal thrombotic events. It was suggested that the HCV might act in some patients as a chronic triggering agent that induce a heterogeneous, atypical presentation of APS.[55] The prevalence of HCV infection in SLE patients was higher than in blood donors from the same geographic area.[56] SLE HCV-positive patients showed a lower frequency of cutaneous SLE features and anti-double stranded DNA antibodies; and a higher prevalence of liver involvement, hypocomplementemia, and cryoglobulinemia. It was suggested that HCV testing should be considered in the diagnosis of SLE—especially in patients who lack the typical cutaneous features of SLE or who have low titers of autoantibodies, cryoglobulinemia, or liver involvement.[56] SLE in HCV-positive patients showed higher prevalence of cryoglobulin without MC syndrome.[57] SLE by itself or treated with steroids did not seem to worsen HCV infection.[57] The prevalence of HCV infection was significantly higher in SLE patients in Louisiana, United States, than in blood donors from the same area.[58]

Few cases of PAN-like vasculitis have been reported in HCV-infected individuals. The prevalence of anti-HCV antibodies among patients suffering from PAN ranges from 5% to 12%.[59] PAN without cryoglobulins has been described, although as an exception.[60] PAN may also occur with INF-α therapy.[61]

TREATMENT OF HEPATITIS C VIRUS-ASSOCIATED RHEUMATIC DISORDERS

Treatment of HCV-associated rheumatic disorders has largely been empiric and based on a few studies analyzing this topic.[62] The use of glucocorticoids or immunosuppressant agents for treating HCV-associated autoimmune or rheumatic manifestations may lead to worsening of the clinical outcome of HCV. Under these conditions, the viral infection often needs to be treated with antiviral agents, mainly pegylated (polyethylene glycol attached) INF-α (PEG INF-α) combined with ribavirin.[63]

Coxibs, nonsteroidal antiinflammatory drugs, low doses of corticosteroids, and hydroxychloroquine are used in the treatment of HCV-related arthritis, whereas penicillamine and methotrexate have been used less frequently.[62] Nissen and colleagues[8] reported that treatment with methotrexate in HCV-associated arthritis was usually effective and well tolerated.

The clinical effect of INF-α was, however, markedly more variable with manifestations aggravated or induced in a high proportion. It was concluded that to most effectively treat these patients it is essential to individualize the effect of treatment with agents such as INF-α, and in certain cases methotrexate could be added to the therapeutic armamentarium.[8] There is emerging evidence suggesting that combined antiviral therapy, namely INF-α, or PEG INF-α and ribavirin, is beneficial in patients with HCV-associated cryoglobulinemia.[64–66] Mazzaro and colleagues[65] treated 18 patients with HCV-associated MC with PEG INF-α 2b plus ribavirin for 48 weeks. At the end of the treatment, HCV RNA became undetectable in 83% and most patients improved clinically. It was concluded that PEG INF-α 2b in combination with ribavirin seems safe and useful for patients affected by MC, but not as effective as in patients with HCV-positive chronic hepatitis without cryoglobulinemia.[65] In another study,[66] 9 patients with HCV-related MC were treated with a combination of PEG INF-α 2b and ribavirin for at least 6 months. It was concluded that treatment with this antiviral combination therapy can achieve a complete clinical response in most patients with HCV-related MC.

Complete clinical response correlated with the eradication of HCV and required a shorter treatment period than that previously reported for IFN-α plus ribavirin.[66] Joshi and colleagues[67] assessed the symptomatic and virological response to antiviral therapy in patients with HCV-associated complications of cryoglobulinemia. Symptomatic cryoglobulinemia responded well to antiviral therapy even when virological response was not achieved.[67] Cyclosporin A (CsA) seems to be safe and effective in treating autoimmune diseases in HCV-infected patients as is documented by the reduction in viremia and transaminases, particularly in patients with high baseline levels.[63] Galeazzi and colleagues[68] summarized the experience with CsA in patients affected by rheumatological disorders and concomitant HCV infection. It was concluded that recent reports, although limited in number, suggest the safety of CsA in the treatment of patients with autoimmune disorders and concomitant HCV infection. These authors also described two cases of RA patients and concomitant HCV infection, treated with combination therapy of CsA and anti–TNF-α agents.[69] In both cases the combined therapy proved to be safe and efficacious for the treatment of HCV-infected RA patients.

High levels of TNF-α are associated with HCV infection and TNF-α may have a role in the pathogenesis of this infection.[70] Indeed, some data have been recently reported on the experience with anti–TNF-α treatment in HCV-associated arthritis. Linardaki and colleagues[70] reported on a patient with HIV-HCV coinfection who developed psoriasis and severe psoriatic arthritis not responding to combination treatment with methotrexate and CsA. Treatment with etanercept was followed by remission of the joint inflammation and improvement of the exanthem. Romero-Maté and colleagues[71] have concluded that treatment of patients infected with HCV or HIV with etanercept does not increase viral load, affect liver function tests, or increase the risk or infections. Thirty-one HCV-positive patients with active RA unresponsive to conventional therapies were treated with anti-α blockers.[72] A significant clinical serologic improvement was recorded at the 3-month reevaluation. Mean values of transaminases and HCV viral load showed no significant variations. It was concluded that the results support the safety of TNF-α blockers in patients with HCV, provided there is close monitoring of clinical and virological data.[72] Finally, treatment with etanercept in six patients with chronic HCV infection and systemic autoimmune diseases showed it to be effective, safe, and well tolerated.[73] A recent report however, demonstrated reactivation of HCV infection in two of four patients while they were receiving etanercept without antiviral prophylaxis.[74]

The use of rituximab in HCV-associated MC has been reported recently. Five patients with active biopsy-proven glomerulonephritis in hepatitis C-related type II MC syndrome were treated with four weekly infusions of rituximab in monotherapy, without steroid whenever possible.[75] A rapid and sustained renal response was observed in all patients. No major side effects occurred and steroids were not required in the follow-up. It was concluded that rituximab may provide effective and safe therapy in MC-related glomerulonephritis—possibly as first line therapy, avoiding steroids and hazardous immunosuppressive treatments.[75] Fifteen patients with type II MC (HCV-related in 12 of 15) were treated with rituximab weekly for 4 weeks.[76] Rituximab proved effective on skin vasculitis, subjective symptoms of peripheral neuropathy, low grade B cell lymphoma, arthralgias, and fever. Treatment was well tolerated with no infectious complications.[76] It was suggested that rituximab may represent a safe and effective therapeutic option for type II MC syndrome.

However, controlled randomized trials are needed to clearly define drug indications, the cost efficacy profile, and treatment schedules in the different features of the disease if compared with standard available treatment.[77]

SUMMARY

HCV is associated with a variety of rheumatic disorders and autoimmune phenomena. This includes arthralgia, arthritis, vasculitis, sicca syndrome, myalgia, and fibromyalgia. Arthralgia is the most common rheumatic manifestation. Arthritis is less common and may present as a rheumatoid arthritis-like, nondeforming arthritis mainly involving small joints with RF and absence of rheumatoid nodules, and, less commonly, a mono-oligoarthritis usually of large joints. MC is most often induced by HCV infection and follows a chronic smoldering course. HCV-infected subjects express a high prevalence of a variety of autoantibodies. The absence of anti-CCP antibodies may help to distinguish HCV-related arthritis from true rheumatoid arthritis. There is a paucity of data concerning the optimal treatment of HCV-associated arthritis. Nonsteroidal anti-inflammatory drugs, low-dose corticosteroids, hydroxychloroquine, and, less frequently, methotrexate and penicillamine have been used.

Combined antiviral therapy including PEG INF-α and ribavirin may be effective in the treatment of HCV-associated cryoglobulinemia. Recent evidence confirms the efficacy and safety of cyclosporin A and anti–TNF-α agents in HCV-associated rheumatic disorders. Rituximab may represent a safe and effective therapeutic option for MC. Larger, controlled studies are needed to further establish the treatment indications, efficacy, and safety of these agents.

REFERENCES

1. Cacoub P, Renou C, Rosenthal E, et al. Extrahepatic manifestations associated with hepatitis C virus infection. A prospective multicenter study of 321 patients. The GERMIVIC. Medicine (Baltimore) 2000;79(1):47–56.
2. Ramos-Casals M, Font J. Extrahepatic manifestations in patients with chronic hepatitis C virus infection. Curr Opin Rheumatol 2005;17(4):447–55.
3. Sterling RK, Bralow S. Extrahepatic manifestations of hepatitis C virus. Curr Gastroenterol Rep 2006;8(1):53–9.
4. Buskila D. Hepatitis C-associated arthritis. Curr Opin Rheumatol 2000;12(4): 295–9.
5. Lormeau C, Falgarone G, Roulot D, et al. Rheumatologic manifestations of chronic hepatitis C infection. Joint Bone Spine 2006;73(6):633–8.
6. Ramos-Casals M, Jara LJ, Medina F, et al. Systemic autoimmune diseases coexisting with chronic hepatitis C virus infection (the HIS PAMEC Registry): patterns of clinical and immunological expression in 180 cases. J Intern Med 2005;257(6): 549–57.
7. Buskila D, Shnaider A, Neumann L, et al. Musculoskeletal manifestations and autoantibody profile in 90 hepatitis C virus-infected Israeli patients. Semin Arthritis Rheum 1998;28(2):107–13.
8. Nissen MJ, Fontanges E, Allam Y, et al. Rheumatological manifestations of hepatitis C: incidence in a rheumatology and non-rheumatology setting and the effect of methotrexate and interferon. Rheumatology 2005;44(8):1016–20.
9. Stefanova-Petrova DV, Tzvetanska AH, Naumova EJ, et al. Chronic hepatitis C virus infection: prevalence of extrahepatic manifestations and association with cryoglobulinemia in Bulgarian patients. World J Gastroenterol 2007;13(48): 6518–28.

10. Lovy MR, Starkebaum G, Uberoi S. Hepatitis C infection presenting with rheumatic manifestations: a mimic of rheumatoid arthritis. J Rheumatol 1996;23(6): 979–83.
11. Lee YH, Ji JD, Yeon JE, et al. Cryoglobulinemia and rheumatic manifestations in patients with hepatitis C virus infection. Ann Rheum Dis 1998;57(12):728–31.
12. Moder KG, Lindor K. Musculoskeletal symptoms associated with hepatitis C. [abstract]. Arthritis Rheum 1995;38(Suppl):S200.
13. Romero Portales M, De Diego Lorenzo A, Rivera J, et al. Rheumatologic and autoimmune manifestations in patients with chronic hepatitis C virus infection. Rev Esp Enferm Dig 1997;89(8):591–8.
14. Cacoub P, Poynard T, Ghillani P, et al. Extrahepatic manifestations of chronic hepatitis C. MULTIVIRC Group. Arthritis Rheum 1999;42(10):2204–12.
15. Rivera J, Garcia-Monforte A, Pineda A, et al. Arthritis in patients with chronic hepatitis C virus infection. J Rheumatol 1999;26(9):420–4.
16. Zuckerman E, Keren D, Rosenbaum M, et al. Hepatits C virus-related arthritis: characteristics and response to therapy with interferon alpha. Clin Exp Rheumatol 2000;18(5):579–84.
17. Rosner I, Rosenbaum M, Toubi E, et al. The case for hepatitis C arthritis. Semin Arthritis Rheum 2004;33(6):375–87.
18. Zuckerman E, Yeshurun D, Rosner I. Management of hepatitis C virus-related arthritis. BioDrugs 2001;15(9):573–84.
19. Oliveri I, Palazzi C, Padula A. Hepatitis C virus and arthritis. Rheum Dis Clin North Am 2003;29(1):111–22.
20. Haddad J, Deny P, Munz-Gotheil C, et al. Lymphocytic sialadenitis of Sjogren's syndrome associated with chronic hepatitis C virus liver disease. Lancet 1992; 339(8789):321–3.
21. Ramos-Casals M, Loustaud-Rati V, Devita S, et al. Sjogren syndrome associated with hepatitis C virus: a multicenter analysis of 137 cases. Medicine (Baltimore) 2005;84(2):81–9.
22. Brito-Zeron P, Ramos-Casals M, Nardi N, et al. Circulating monoclonal immunoglobulins in Sjogren syndrome: prevalence in 237 patients. Medicine (Baltimore) 2005;84(2):90–7.
23. Smyth CM, McKiernan SM, Hagan R, et al. Chronic hepatitis C infection and sicca syndrome: a clear association with HLA DQB1*02. Eur J Gastroenterol Hepatol 2007;19(6):493–8.
24. Ramos-Casals M, De Vita S, Tzioufas AG. Hepatitis C virus, Sjogren's syndrome and B-cell lymphoma: linking infection, autoimmunity and cancer. Autoimmun Rev 2005;4(1):8–15.
25. Lunel F, Musset L, Caccoub P, et al. Cryoglobulinemia in chronic liver diseases: role of hepatitis C virus and liver damage. Gastroenterology 1994;106(5): 1291–300.
26. Bryce AH, Kyle RA, Dispenzieri A, et al. Natural history and therapy of 66 patients with mixed cryoglobulinemia. Am J Hematol 2006;81(7):511–8.
27. Saadoun D, Landau DA, Calabrese LH, et al. Hepatitis C-associated mixed cryoglobulinemia: a crossroad between autoimmunity and lymphoproliferation. Rheumatology 2007;46(8):1234–42.
28. Pileri P, Umematsu Y, Campagnoli S, et al. Binding of hepatitis C virus to CD81. Science 1998;282(5390):938–41.
29. De Vita S, Quartuccio L, Fabris M. Hepatitis C virus infection, mixed cryoglobulinemia and BLyS upregulation: targeting the infectious trigger, the autoimmune response, or both? Autoimmun Rev 2008;8(2):95–9.

30. Antonelli A, Ferri C, Fallahi P, et al. Alpha-chemokine CXCL10 and beta-chemokine CCL2 serum levels in patients with hepatitis C-associated cryoglobulinemia in the presence or absence of autoimmune thyroiditis. Metabolism 2008;57(9):1270–7.
31. Antonelli A, Ferri C, Fallahi P, et al. High values of CXCL10 serum levels in mixed cryoglobulinemia associated with hepatitis C infection. Am J Gastroenterol 2008; 103(10):2488–94.
32. Antonelli A, Ferri C, Fallahi P, et al. CXCL10 and CCL2 serum levels in patients with mixed cryoglobulinemia and hepatitis C. Dig Liver Dis 2009;41(1):42–8.
33. Ferri C, Sebastiani M, Giuqqioli D, et al. Mixed cryoglobulinemia: demographic, clinical, and serologic features and survival in 231 patients. Semin Arthritis Rheum 2004;33(6):355–74.
34. Buskila D, Atzeni F, Sarzi Puttini P. Etiology of fibromyalgia: the possible role of infection and vaccination. Autoimmun Rev 2008;8(1):41–3.
35. Ablin JN, Shoenfeld Y, Buskila D. Fibromyalgia, infection and vaccination: two more parts in the etiological puzzle. J Autoimmun 2006;27(3):145–52.
36. Buskila D, Shnaider A, Neumann L, et al. Fibromyalgia in hepatitis C virus infection. Another infectious disease relationship. Arch Intern Med 1997;157(21): 2497–500.
37. Rivera J, de Diego A, Trinchet M, et al. Fibromyalgia-associated hepatitis C virus infection. Br J Rheumatol 1997;36(9):981–5.
38. Goulding C, O' Connell P, Murray FE. Prevalence of fibromyalgia, anxiety and depression in chronic hepatitis C virus infection: relationship to RT-PCR status and mode of acquisition. Eur J Gastroenterol Hepatol 2001;13(5):507–11.
39. Kozanoglu E, Canataroglu A, Abayli B, et al. Fibromyalgia syndrome in patients with hepatitis C infection. Rheumatol Int 2003;23(5):248–51.
40. Narvaez J, Nolla JM, Valverde-Garcia J. Lack of association of fibromyalgia with hepatitis C virus infection. J Rheumatol 2005;32(6):1118–21.
41. Palazzi C, D'Amico E, D'Angelo S, et al. Hepatitis C virus infection in Italian patients with fibromyalgia. Clin Rheumatol 2008;27(1):101–3.
42. Poynard T, Caccoub P, Ratziu V, et al. Fatigue in patients with chronic hepatitis C. J Viral Hepat 2002;9(4):295–303.
43. Buskila D, Sikuler E, Shoenfeld Y. Hepatitis C virus, autoimmunity and rheumatic disease. Lupus 1997;6(9):685–9.
44. Lenzi M, Bellentani S, Saccoccio G, et al. Prevalence of non-organ specific auto-antibodies and chronic liver disease in the general population: a nested case control study of the Dionysos cohort. Gut 1999;45(3):435–41.
45. Dudek A, Dudziak M, Sulek M, et al [Serological markers of arthritis in patients with chronic viral hepatitis]. Pol Merkur Lekarski 2006;20(118):404–7 [in Polish].
46. Reddy KR, Krawitt EL, Homberg JC, et al. Absence of anti-LKM-1 antibody in hepatitis C viral infection in the United States of America. J Viral Hepat 1995; 2(4):175–9.
47. Kessel A, Elias G, Pavlotzky E, et al. Anti –C-reactive protein antibodies in chronic hepatitis C infection: correlation with severity and autoimmunity. Hum Immunol 2007;68(10):844–8.
48. Christodoulou D, Christou L, Zervou E, et al. Antiplatelet antibodies in patients with chronic viral hepatitis receiving interferon-alpha. Hepatogastroenterology 2007;54(78):1761–5.
49. Wu CS, Hu CY, Hsu PN. Anti SSB/La antibody is negatively associated with HLA-DR2 in chronic hepatitis C infection. Clin Rheumatol 2008;27(3):365–8.
50. Alpa M, Ferrero B, Cavallo R, et al. Anti-neuronal antibodies in patients with HCV-related mixed cryoglobulinemia. Autoimmun Rev 2008;8(1):56–8.

51. Lienesch D, Morris R, Metzger A, et al. Absence of cyclic citrullinated peptide antibody in nonarthritic patients with chronic hepatitis C infection. J Rheumatol 2005;32(3):489–93.

52. Gehring S, Kullmer U, Koeppelmann S, et al. Prevalence of autoantibodies and the risk of autoimmune thyroid disease in children with chronic hepatitis C virus infection treated with interferon-alpha. World J Gastroenterol 2006;12(36): 5787–92.

53. Ramos-Casals M, Pares A, Jara LJ, et al. Antimitochondrial antibodies in patients with chronic hepatitis C virus infection: description of 18 cases and review of the literature. J Viral Hepat 2005;12(6):648–54.

54. Cervera R, Asherson RA, Acevedo ML, et al. Antiphospholipid syndrome associated with infections: clinical and microbiological characteristics of 100 patients. Ann Rheum Dis 2004;63(10):1312–7.

55. Ramos-Casals M, Cervera R, Laqrutta M, et al. Clinical features related to antiphospholipid syndrome in patients with chronic viral infection (hepatitis C virus/HIV infection): description of 82 cases. Clin Infect Dis 2004;38(7):1009–16.

56. Ramos-Casals M, Font J, Garcia-Carrasco M, et al. Hepatitis C virus infection mimicking systemic lupus erythematosus: study of hepatitis C virus infection in a series of 134 Spanish patients with systemic lupus erythematosus. Arthritis Rheum 2000;43(12):2801–6.

57. Perlemuter G, Cacoub P, Sbai A, et al. Hepatitis C virus infection in systemic lupus erythematosus: a case control study. J Rheumatol 2003;30(7):1473–8.

58. Ahmed MM, Berney SM, Wolf RE, et al. Prevalence of active hepatitis C virus infection in patients with systemic lupus erythematosus. Am J Med Sci 2006; 331(5):252–6.

59. Sene D, Limal N, Cacoub P. Hepatitis C virus-associated extrahepatic manifestations: a review. Metab Brain Dis 2004;19(3–4):357–81.

60. Cacoub P, Maisonobe T, Thibault V, et al. Systemic vasculitis in patients with hepatitis C. J Rheumatol 2001;28(1):109–18.

61. de Dios Garcia-Diaz J, Garcia-Sanchez M, Arcos P, et al. Polyarteritis nodosa after interferon treatment for chronic hepatitis C. J Clin Virol 2005;32(2):181–2.

62. Palazzi C, D'Angelo S, Olivieri I. Hepatitis C virus-related arthritis. Autoimmun Rev 2008;8(1):48–51.

63. Antonelli A, Ferri C, Galeazzi M, et al. HCV infection: pathogenesis, clinical manifestations and therapy. Clin Exp Rheumatol 2008;26(1 Suppl 48):S39–47.

64. Zuckerman E, Keren D, Slobodin G, et al. Treatment of refractory symptomatic hepatitis C virus related mixed cryoglobulinemia with ribavirin and interferon alpha. J Rheumatol 2000;27(9):2172–8.

65. Mazzaro C, Zorat F, Caizzi M, et al. Treatment with peg-interferon alfa-2b and ribavirin of hepatitis C virus-associated mixed cryoglobulinemia: a pilot study. J Hepatol 2005;42(5):632–8.

66. Cacoub P, Saadoun D, Limal N, et al. PEGylated interferon alfa-2b and ribavirin treatment in patients with hepatitis C virus-related systemic vasculitis. Arthritis Rheum 2005;52(3):911–5.

67. Joshi S, Kuczynski M, Heathcote EJ. Symptomatic and virological response to antiviral therapy in hepatitis C associated with extrahepatic complications of cryoglobulinemia. Dig Dis Sci 2007;52(9):2410–7.

68. Galeazzi M, Bellisai F, Giannitti C, et al. Safety of cyclosporin A in HCV-infected patients: experience with cyclosporin A in patients affected by rheumatological disorders and concomitant HCV infection. Ann N Y Acad Sci 2007;1110(9): 544–9.

69. Bellisai F, Giannitti C, Donvito A, et al. Combination therapy with cyclosporine A and anti TNF-alpha agents in the treatment of rheumatoid arthritis and concomitant hepatitis C virus infection. Clin Rheumatol 2007;26(7):1127–9.
70. Linardaki G, Katsarou O, Ioannidou P, et al. Effective etanercept treatment for psoriatic arthritis complicating concomitant human immunodeficiency virus and hepatitis C virus infection. J Rheumatol 2007;34(6):1353–5.
71. Romero-Maté A, Garcia Donoso C, Cordoba-Guijarro S. Efficacy and safety of etanercept in psoriasis/psoriatic arthritis: an updated review. Am J Clin Dermatol 2007;8(3):143–55.
72. Ferri C, Ferraccioli G, Ferrari D, et al. Safety of anti-tumor necrosis factor-alpha therapy in patients with rheumatoid arthritis and chronic hepatitis C virus infection. J Rheumatol 2008;35(10):1944–9.
73. Cavazzana I, Ceribelli A, Cattaneo R, et al. Treatment with etanercept in six patients with chronic hepatitis C infection and systemic autoimmune diseases. Autoimmun Rev 2008;8(2):104–6.
74. Cansu DU, Kalifoglu T, Korkmaz C. Short-term course of chronic hepatitis B and C under treatment with etanercept associated with different disease modifying antirheumatic drugs without antiviral prophylaxis. J Rheumatol 2008;35(3):421–4.
75. Quartuccio L, Soardo G, Romano G, et al. Rituximab treatment for glomerulonephritis in HCV-associated mixed cryoglobulinemia: efficacy and safety in the absence of steroids. Rheumatology (oxford) 2006;45(7):842–6.
76. Zaja F, Devita S, Mazzaro C, et al. Efficacy and safety of rituximab in type II mixed cryoglobulinemia. Blood 2003;101(10):3827–34.
77. De Vita S, Quartuccio L, Fabris M, et al. Rituximab in mixed cryoglobulinemia: increased experience and perspectives. Dig Liver Dis 2007;39(Suppl 1):S122–8.

Hepatitis B-Related Autoimmune Manifestations

Patrice Cacoub, MD[a,b,*], Benjamin Terrier, MD[a,b]

KEYWORDS

- Hepatitis B virus • Autoimmune manifestation
- Polyarteritis nodosa • Vasculitis

There is a high incidence of hepatitis B virus (HBV) infection, with about 400 million individuals infected worldwide.[1,2] Extrahepatic manifestations, though they occur less frequently than in hepatitis C virus (HCV) infections, may be observed in patients infected with HBV in both acute and chronic infections. Approximately 20% of patients with HBV infection develop extrahepatic manifestations. The best described and the most severe are the polyarteritis nodosa (PAN) form of vasculitis and glomerulonephritis. In terms of less severe manifestations however, no large study has been done and there are only a few sporadic studies available.[3,4]

A recent, multicenter, French study including 190 patients with chronic hepatitis B estimated the incidence of clinical and biologic extrahepatic manifestations to be 16% and 15%, respectively (**Table 1**).[5] The most common clinical manifestations are sensorimotor neuropathies (5%), myalgia (3%), arthralgia (3%), Sjögren's syndrome (3%), glomerulonephritis (3%), uveitis (2%), Raynaud syndrome (2%), psoriasis (1%), and pruritus (1%). The most common biologic manifestations are the presence of anti-smooth muscle (7%); antinuclear (3%), antinucleosome (2%), and anti–liver-kidney microsomal (2%) antibodies (Ab); cryoglobulinemia (2%); and rheumatoid factor (2%) (**Box 1** and **Table 2**; see **Table 1**).

PATHOPHYSIOLOGY

The pathophysiology of HBV-associated extrahepatic manifestations is not completely understood, and there is no animal model capable of reproducing these manifestations. Two main hypotheses have been proposed. The first, which is most often suggested, is that of a disease of immune-complex deposits comprised of HBs or HBe antigens, according to the type of clinical manifestations. These complexes may be responsible for classical local activation of the complement

[a] Service de Médecine Interne, AP, HP Pitié-Salpêtrière Hospital Group, 75651 Paris Cedex 13, France
[b] CNRS UMR 7087, Université Pierre et Marie Curie, Paris VI, 75005 Paris, France
* Corresponding author. Service de Médecine Interne, Groupe Hospitalier Pitié-Salpêtrière, 47 Boulevard de l'Hôpital, 75651 Paris Cedex 13, France.
E-mail address: patrice.cacoub@psl.aphp.fr (P. Cacoub).

Rheum Dis Clin N Am 35 (2009) 125–137
doi:10.1016/j.rdc.2009.03.006
0889-857X/09/$ – see front matter © 2009 Elsevier Inc. All rights reserved.

Table 1
Main clinical and biologic extrahepatic manifestations associated with chronic hepatitis B virus infection

Extra hepatic manifestation		n (%)
Clinical manifestations	None	160 (84)
	At least one	30 (16)
Sensorimotor deficits	—	10 (5)
Myalgia	—	6 (3)
Sjögren's syndrome	—	6 (3)
Arthralgia-arthritis	—	5 (3)
Glomerulonephritis	—	5 (3)
Raynaud syndrome	—	3 (2)
Uveitis	—	3 (2)
Pruritis	—	2 (1)
Cutaneous vasculitis	—	1 (1)
Cutaneous psoriasis	—	1 (1)
Biologic manifestations	None	161 (85)
	At least one	29 (15)
Anti-smooth muscle Ab	—	14 (7)
Antinuclear Ab	—	6 (3)
Anti-nucleosome Ab	—	4 (2)
Cryoglobulinemia	—	3 (2)
Rheumatoid factor	—	3 (2)
Anti–liver-kidney microsomal Ab	—	3 (2)
Anti-DNA Ab	—	0 (0)
Soluble antinuclear antigen antibodies	—	0 (0)
Antihistone Ab	—	0 (0)
Antimitochondrial Ab	—	0 (0)

Abbreviation: Ab, antibodies.
Data from Cacoub P, Saadoun D, Bourlière M, et al. Hepatitis B virus genotypes and extrahepatic manifestations. J Hepatol 2005;43:764–70.

cascade and the recruitment of inflammatory cells. High viral replication or a persistent infection can promote the production of these soluble immune complexes, which are deposited at specific sites such as the medium- or small-sized arteries of the kidney and the skin. This is the mechanism implicated in the occurrence of PAN-systemic vasculitis and membranous glomerulonephritis (MGN). However, the presence of circulating immune complexes is not always pathogenic, and some extrahepatic manifestations of HBV occur in their absence.[6]

The second hypothesis was suggested in a study done on two patients with chronic hepatitis B in whom viral replication was demonstrated in the vascular endothelium of targeted tissues.[7] This observation suggested the role of viral replication in extrahepatic tissue in the genesis of certain extrahepatic manifestations of HBV,[7] though this remains to be substantiated. Regardless of these hypotheses (which are not, in fact, exclusive of each other), it is necessary to emphasize that suppression of viral replication, whether spontaneous or due to the influence of antiviral treatments, is often associated with the resolution of extrahepatic manifestations.[6]

It is striking to note that over a 20-year period, there has been a progressive but continuous decrease of HBV-associated PAN vasculitis and a simultaneous increase

Box 1
Main extrahepatic manifestations during hepatitis B infection
Systemic manifestations
Flu-like syndrome
Serum sickness
Polyarteritis nodosa
Rheumatological manifestations
Polyarticular pain
Polyarthritis
Neurological manifestations
Polyradiculoneuritis
Renal manifestations
Membranous glomerulonephritis
Membranoproliferative glomerulonephritis
IgA nephropathy
Skin manifestations
Papular acrodermatitis of childhood
Acute urticaria
Oral lichen planus
Pitted keratolysis
Leukocytoclastic vasculitis
Rheumatoid purpura
Ophthalmological manifestations
Uveitis
Hematological manifestations
Non-Hodgkin's lymphoma

of HBeAg-positive infections. Thus, in the 1980s, up to 40% of PAN cases were secondary to HBV infection,[8] while this proportion is currently less than 10% according to the data of the French vasculitis study group (GFEV). In parallel, chronic HBV infections related to HBeAg-negative mutant viruses, which were rare in the 1980s, are currently the most common form in France (70%). These findings might suggest that the pre-C variant of HBV generates fewer extrahepatic manifestations than the wild virus. Though this hypothesis cannot be ruled out, the reduced incidence of HBV-associated PAN is in fact greater probably because of the great decline in the incidence of HBV viral infection over these last 20 years.

The role of HBV genotypes in the occurrence of extrahepatic manifestations has been studied recently. In fact, no correlation has been found between the type of extrahepatic manifestations and HBV genotypes.[5]

GENERAL MANIFESTATIONS

A flu-like syndrome including headaches, arthralgia, and myalgia, and sometimes associated with urticarial skin lesions, was observed in approximately half of the

Table 2
Factors associated with biologic extrahepatic manifestations during chronic hepatitis B infection (n=129)

Factors		Number Patients	None	At Least One	P
Male gender	—	190	127 (79%)	20 (69%)	0.240
Age (mean)	—	186	41 (15)	43 (13)	0.555
Age	—	186	—	—	—
	<50 years	—	117 (74%)	17 (61%)	0.147
	>50 years	—	41 (26%)	11 (39%)	—
Ethnicity	—	187	—	—	—
	African	—	18 (11%)	6 (21%)	0.402
	Asian	—	25 (16%)	4 (14%)	—
	Caucasian	—	115 (73%)	19 (66%)	—
Alcohol abuse	—	181	10 (7%)	1 (3%)	1
HIV +	—	177	13 (9%)	0 (0%)	0.227
HCV +	—	177	4 (3%)	2 (7%)	0.242
HBV genotype	—	185	—	—	—
	A	—	40 (25%)	4 (14%)	0.189
	B	—	6 (4%)	2 (7%)	0.354
	C	—	18 (11%)	2 (7%)	0.744
	D	—	45 (28%)	8 (28%)	0.953
	E	—	16 (10%)	3 (10%)	1
	F	—	1 (1%)	0 (0%)	1
	G	—	3 (2%)	0 (0%)	1
HBV phenotype	—	171	—	—	—
	HBe Ag-positive	—	67 (47%)	5 (19%)	0.007
	HBe Ag-negative	—	77 (53%)	22 (81%)	—
HBV DNA	—	171	—	—	—
	Detectable	—	104 (69%)	20 (69%)	0.969
	Undetectable	—	46 (31%)	9 (31%)	—
Increased ALT	—	179	110 (73%)	21 (72%)	0.918
Increased AST	—	179	95 (63%)	17 (59%)	0.631
Platelets (.10^3/μl)	—	167	179 (62%)	218 (67%)	0.003
Hepatic fibrosis (METAVIR)	—	150	—	—	—
	F0	—	6 (5%)	2 (9%)	0.303
	F1	—	34 (27%)	9 (41%)	—
	F2	—	24 (19%)	5 (23%)	—
	F3	—	28 (22%)	2 (9%)	—
	F4	—	36 (28%)	4 (18%)	—
	F0, F1, or F2	—	64 (50%)	16 (73%)	0.048
	F3 or F4	—	64 (50%)	6 (27%)	—
Hepatic activity (METAVIR)	—	106	—	—	—
	A0	—	6 (7%)	1 (7%)	0.710
	A1	—	25 (27%)	5 (36%)	—
	A2	—	46 (50%)	5 (36%)	—
	A3	—	15 (16%)	3 (21%)	—
	A0 or A1	—	31 (34%)	6 (43%)	0.554
	A2 or A3	—	61 (66%)	8 (57%)	—

Modified from Cacoub P, Saadoun D, Bourlière M, et al. Hepatitis B virus genotypes and extrahepatic manifestations. J Hepatol 2005;43:764–70.

patients with acute hepatitis from HBV (but also from other hepatotropic viruses) during the preicteric phase.[9] It lasts from 3 to 8 days and disappears with the appearance of icterus.

A smaller proportion of hepatitis B cases (5% to 10%) may occur with a serum sickness-like syndrome caused by the deposit of circulating immune complexes and complement activation.[9] The clinical manifestations may include a skin rash, cutaneous vasculitis with purpura, arthralgia, and glomerulonephritis; each of these manifestations (described later in this article) may also occur alone.

POLYARTERITIS NODOSA

The close relationship between HBV infection and the occurrence of PAN has been demonstrated since the 1970s[10,11] and confirmed by many studies.[8] Some epidemiologic studies have found a higher incidence of PAN in populations with endemic HBV infection: 4.6 cases per one million inhabitants annually in England[12] and 31 cases per one million inhabitants annually in France[13] versus 77 cases per one million inhabitants annually in a population of Eskimos from Alaska, a region where the B virus is highly endemic.[14]

In a study of HBV-associated PAN cases followed for 30 years by the GFEV, out of the 341 PAN cases from all causes, the overall frequency of HBV infection was 33.7%.[8] However, HBV infection in patients with PAN has been consistently declining for 20 years in France (41% in 1980–1984, 48% in 1984–1989, 28% in 1990–1994, 12% in 1995–1999, < 10% after 2000, according to GFEV data), probably because of better transfusion safety measures, and the effects of universal hygiene precautions and HBV vaccination.

Vasculitis manifests early in the course of HBV infection, generally in the first 6 months following the onset of the infection.[8,10,15,16] It is not uncommon for it to reveal the viral infection. The main differences compared with the clinical manifestations of primary PAN are a greater frequency of gastrointestinal disorders (46%), orchitis-like testicular disorders (26%), severe arterial hypertension (27%), and renal infarction.[15] The onset of PAN is usually sudden and the disease is severe from the beginning. The prognosis is usually favorable if the appropriate treatment is started early. Liver biopsy shows signs of chronic hepatitis, even in cases of recent B virus infection.

In chronic HBeAg-positive hepatitis, HBe antigen seroconversion generally occurs with recovery from the vasculitis. Relapses are seen in 8% of HBV-associated PAN cases versus 19% of PAN cases that are not related to HBV.[15,17,18]

Standard PAN treatment (which includes the combination of corticosteroids and cyclophosphamide) is not appropriate for HBV-associated PAN since it promotes the persistence and replication of the virus, thereby leaving the antigen-triggering factor of the disease intact and subjecting the patient to the risk of worsening liver lesions. The treatment of HBV-associated PAN is based on the combination of plasma exchanges, which enable the clearance of immune complexes, antiviral treatments,[15,19–21] and a short course of corticosteroid therapy, which is prescribed in cases of life-threatening organ involvement. Several studies have been done to test the efficacy of this therapeutic plan through the use of different antiviral drugs, specifically vidarabine (at the start of trials), interferon alfa-2a and (more recently) lamivudine (**Table 3**).[15,19–21] A long-term analysis on the treated diseases (35 with vidarabine and 6 with interferon alfa-2b), which was derived from the first studies, found an HBe antigen seroconversion rate of 51% and a vasculitis recovery rate of 81%.[15] In addition to the antiviral treatment, the treatment plan that was used included a short course of corticosteroid treatment (1 mg/kg/day for one week, followed by tapering and

Table 3
Efficacy of the therapeutic strategy for hepatitis B virus-associated polyarteritis nodosa according to the antiviral drug used

Year, Reference	1993[19]	1994[20]	2004[21]
Number of patients	33	6	10
Anti-viral drug used	Vidarabine	Interferon alfa-2b	Lamivudine
HBe antigen seroconversion	45%	67%	66%
Clinical recovery of vasculitis	73%	100%	90%

discontinuation for 1 week), and plasma exchanges (3 per week for 3 weeks, then 2 per week for 2 weeks, then 1 per week until HBe seroconversion or persistent clinical remission was achieved).

In the GFEV study of 115 observations of HBV-associated PAN followed since 1972,[8] there was an overall PAN remission rate of 80.9%, a relapse rate of 9.7% and a death rate of 35.7%. Among the patients who did not receive an antiviral agent but were treated with corticosteroids alone or in combination with cyclophosphamide or plasma exchanges (n=35), the analysis showed a vasculitis relapse rate of 14.3%, death rate of 48.6%, and HBe seroconversion rate of 14.7%. Among the patients treated with an antiviral agent (n=80), the analysis showed a relapse rate of 5%, death rate of 30%, and HBe seroconversion rate of 49.3% (40.8% for vidarabine, 64.3% for interferon alfa-2b and 64.3% for lamivudine).[8] All the patients with HBe seroconversion had a complete remission without relapse.[8]

Therefore, although this disease has become extremely rare, the optimal therapeutic management of HBV-associated PAN includes the combination of a short-term course of corticosteroids according to the organ involvement, plasma exchanges, and antiviral therapy (based currently on potent nucleoside analogs), with the aim of achieving HBe seroconversion and an end to viral replication.

RENAL MANIFESTATIONS

HBV-associated glomerulonephritis was first described in 1971 by Combes and colleagues.[22] Several types of glomerulonephritis have been associated with HBV, including MGN, which is the most common type, membranoproliferative glomerulonephritis (MPGN), and immunoglobulin (Ig) A nephropathies.[23–29]

The association between chronic HBV infection and the occurrence of glomerulonephritis has been found in several epidemiologic studies.[23,24,30] In these cases, glomerulonephritis occur mainly in male children residing in HBV-endemic areas, with most of them being asymptomatic carriers of HBV and with no active liver disease. It is relatively rare.

The analysis of renal biopsies in patients with HBV-associated glomerulonephritis usually finds MGN, followed by MPGN (less frequently) and proliferative glomerulonephritis (more rarely). There are no significant tubulointerstitial nephropathy alterations, but glomerular immunoglobulin deposits (mainly IgG) and complement fraction deposits (C3, C4, and C1q) can be observed. Viral antigens (HBs, HBc, and HBe) are shown in the deposits with the acid elution technique.[24,31] In one study, HBcAg was found in 100% of biopsies, HBeAg in 88%, and HBs in a minority of cases.[32]

The pathophysiological mechanism implicated in HBV-associated glomerulonephritis (mainly MGN) is the formation and deposit of circulating immune complexes, with HBeAg as the triggering antibody.[33,34] The pathogenic mechanism of other forms of glomerulonephritis is less clear, but viral antigens are also found in renal lesions.

HBV-associated MGN is generally accompanied by proteinuria with otherwise normal renal function. The majority of patients that develop MGN are HBeAg-positive.[32,35] The severity of the liver disease is not correlated with the development of MGN. The course of HBV-associated glomerulonephritis varies according to the population under study. Renal disease in children usually has a benign course, with a 64% cumulative probability of spontaneous remission at 4 years and only very rare cases of progression to renal insufficiency.[36] The membrane deposits disappear after spontaneous remission of the nephrotic syndrome.[37] HBe seroconversion frequently accompanies remission[38] but does not occur consistently. The course in adults is not as favorable. Progression to chronic renal insufficiency may occur. One study done in an endemic country found a low prevalence of spontaneous remissions, with progressive renal insufficiency in 29% of cases and an indication for dialysis in 10% of patients after 60 months of follow-up.[35]

The treatment of HBV-associated glomerulonephritis is based on antiviral agents. The use of immunosuppressant drugs subjects the patient to the risk of additional viral replication and exacerbation of the liver disease.[39] Interferon-alfa has been the most studied molecule. A controlled, randomized study done in 40 children analyzed the benefits of interferon-alfa in the treatment of HBV-associated MGN that was refractory to corticosteroid therapy. All the children treated with interferon-alfa had regression of the proteinuria after 3 months of treatment, and HBe seroconversion occurred in 80% of cases. However, 50% of the children treated with a placebo continued to have high proteinuria and 50% had low proteinuria; no HBe seroconversion was observed.[40] As for adults, in a study done on 5 patients treated with interferon-alfa, only one case was noted to have a complete response associated with HBe seroconversion.[35] Another study analyzed the response to interferon-alfa in 15 patients. Eight of them had a virological response with HBe seroconversion and an end to viral replication. Seven of these 8 virological responder patients had a significant reduction of proteinuria. Renal involvement persisted, however, in the 7 virological nonresponder patients. The 8 responder patients had MGN, whereas 4 of the 7 nonresponder patients had MPGN.[41] Lamivudine was tested in 10 patients with HBV-associated MGN. It was associated with complete remission of proteinuria in 60% of patients after 12 months of treatment.

A recent meta-analysis analyzed the data from six therapeutic trials (three of which were controlled studies) that studied the efficacy of interferon-alfa and lamivudine in the treatment of HBV-associated glomerulonephritis.[35,40–45] Out of the 82 patients studied (interferon-alfa in 72 patients, lamivudine in 10 patients), the overall remission rate of the proteinuria was 65.2% and the HBe seroconversion rate was 62.0%. There was a significant relationship between the HBe seroconversion rate and the proteinuria remission rate.[45]

RHEUMATOLOGICAL MANIFESTATIONS

Clinical features of polyarticular pain or polyarthritis may occur during the preicteric phase of acute hepatitis,[1] which are usually incorporated as part of a flu-like syndrome.

Polyarthritis that is associated with HBV infection usually affects finger joints and can mimic rheumatoid arthritis, with the rheumatoid factor sometimes present. It is distinguished by the absence of joint destruction on radiographs in a very large majority of cases. The pathophysiological hypothesis is that the complement cascade is activated by a disease of intrasynovial deposits of immune complexes comprised of HBsAg and anti-HBs antibodies.[46,47]

NEUROLOGIC MANIFESTATIONS

Some extremely rare cases of acute polyradiculoneuritis have been reported with HBV infection, acute and chronic, though it is not possible to officially rule out the possibility of chance association.[48–51] There have been immune complexes containing HBs antigen in patient serum and cerebrospinal fluid found contemporaneously with the neurologic episode, suggesting the role of such immune complex deposits along the nerve structures.[49,51] Some cases of sensorimotor neuropathy other than PAN have been reported in isolation.[5,52]

SKIN MANIFESTATIONS

Papular acrodermatitis of childhood and urticaria are the most common HBV-associated skin manifestations.

Papular acrodermatitis of childhood or Gianotti-Crosti syndrome is a papular skin rash with a rapid onset, which is sometimes pruriginous and affects children 1 to 6 years old. The lesions are located on the palms and backs of the hands, the soles of the feet, legs, forearms, elbows, knees, face, and buttocks. The rash resolves spontaneously in 1 to 6 weeks. Signs other than dermatologic may also occur, such as splenomegaly, hepatomegaly, weakness, anorexia and weight loss, and diarrhea. Papular acrodermatitis of childhood is generally viral in origin and HBV infection is one of the most common causes.[53–55]

Acute urticaria, occurring in isolation or as part of the Caroli triad (urticaria, headaches, arthralgias), can occur during the preicteric phase of acute hepatitis B or in about 15% to 20% of patients. It appears 1 to 6 weeks before the jaundice and resolves in the icteric phase.[56] Skin biopsy shows vasculitis lesions associated with deposits of C3 complement fraction, IgM, and HBsAg in the blood vessel walls,[57] suggesting the role of immune complex deposits containing HBsAg.[57,58] Urticaria is not specific to viral hepatitis B and can occur during the preicteric phase of other types of viral hepatitis.

Oral lichen planus, especially in its erosive form, has been found to be associated with chronic HBV infection.[59–63] An Italian study group confirmed this association by finding the relative risk of developing lichen planus to be 1.8 (95% CI, 1.0-3.2) in patients with hepatitis B.[64] This association was not seen by others.[65] The pathophysiology of lichen planus involves HBV-induced antibodies that are directed against the basal cells of the epidermis.[63,66]

Other skin manifestations, pitted keratolysis[59] and leukocytoclastic vasculitis,[67–69] have been described more rarely and are most often manifest by purpura, rheumatoid purpura,[70–72] and erythema nodosum.[73]

Although much rarer than during HCV infection, mixed cryoglobulinemia with skin involvement has been described.[74–76] This HBV–cryoglobulinemia association is controversial.[77]

OPHTHALMOLOGIC MANIFESTATIONS

Uveitis, mainly the acute anterior form, may also be a manifestation of HBV infection. A Swiss study suggested HBV as a possible cause of uveitis, with a 13% prevalence of HBs antigen in patients with uveitis.[78] These results are controversial. An English study found only 2% prevalence in such patients.[79] A French study reported the occurrence of uveitis in 2% of patients infected with HBV.[5]

HEMATOLOGICAL MANIFESTATIONS

There are solid arguments demonstrating a link, at least epidemiologically, between certain chronic viral infections and non-Hodgkin's B lymphoma (BNHL), particularly infections with the Epstein-Barr virus, HTLV-1, and hepatitis C virus. Some recent data also suggest the role of HBV.

The first studies on the relationship between HBV and BNHL infection were performed in high HBV endemic areas, notably in Asia. Chronic HBV infection was found two to five times more frequently in patients with BNHL than in hospitalized control patients without BNHL[80] or in the general population.[81,82] However, several methodological limitations have been pointed out: the small sample size of the cohorts (cases and controls), the retrospective nature of the studies, and the case definition based only on the presence of serum HBsAg.

A more recent study without these limitations appears to support the possibility of such an association. Yood and colleagues[83] compared the incidence of non-Hodgkin's lymphoma (NHL) in patients with (case) and without (control) chronic HBV infection; the study analyzed two North American patient databases, one on chronic HBV infection and the other on malignant tumors. Based on HBV-infection cases, previously diagnosed between 1995 and 2001, and newly diagnosed cases of NHL infection, calculations for the incidence of NHL were done in 3,888 HBV-positive patients and 205,203 HBV-negative patients. They demonstrated a relative risk of 2.80 (95% CI, 1.16–6.75) after adjustment for age, sex, ethnicity, income, comorbidities, and HBV or HCV infection. Even if this large-scale study also presents some methodological limitations, these results, if confirmed, will have potentially important implications for the medical management and follow-up of patients with hepatitis B virus infection and those with BNHL.

SUMMARY

The manifestations of HBV infection, although occurring less frequently than those seen in hepatitis C, are varied. The best described and the most severe are polyarteritis nodosa and membranous glomerulonephritis. These manifestations, as with many others related to HBV, are the consequence of circulating immune complex deposits. Although severe, they seem to be much less common than they once were, undoubtedly due to the effect of HBV vaccination. Treatment of these manifestations is mainly based on the use of antiviral drugs (with the current availability of potent agents) for control of the viral infection.

REFERENCES

1. Lee WM. Hepatitis B virus infection. N Engl J Med 1997;337:1733–45.
2. Lai CL, Ratziu V, Yuen MF, et al. Viral hepatitis B. Lancet 2003;362:2089–94.
3. Han SH. Extrahepatic manifestations of chronic hepatitis B. Clin Liver Dis 2004;8: 403–18.
4. Pyrsopoulos NT, Reddy KR. Extrahepatic manifestations of chronic viral hepatitis. Curr Gastroenterol Rep 2001;3:71–8.
5. Cacoub P, Saadoun D, Bourlière M, et al. Hepatitis B virus genotypes and extrahepatic manifestations. J Hepatol 2005;43:764–70.
6. Mason A. Role of viral replication in extrahepatic syndromes related to hepatitis B virus infection. Minerva Gastroenterol Dietol 2006;52:53–66.

7. Mason A, Theal J, Bain V, et al. Hepatitis B virus replication in damaged endothelial tissues of patients with extrahepatic disease. Am J Gastroenterol 2005;100: 972–6.

8. Guillevin L, Mahr A, Callard P, et al. Hepatitis B virus-associated polyarteritis nodosa: clinical characteristics, outcome, and impact of treatment in 115 patients. Medicine (Baltimore) 2005;84:313–22.

9. Caroli J. Serum-sickness-like prodromata in viral hepatitis: Caroli's triad. Lancet 1972;1:964–5.

10. Trépo C, Thivolet J. Antigène Australia, hépatite virale et périartérite noueuse. Presse Med 1970;78:1575.

11. Gocke DJ, Hsu K, Morgan C, et al. Association between polyarteritis and Australia antigen. Lancet 1970;2:1149–53.

12. Scott DG, Bacon PA, Elliott PJ, et al. Systemic vasculitis in a district general hospital 1972–1980: clinical and laboratory features, classification and prognosis of 80 cases. Q J Med 1982;51:292–311.

13. Mahr A, Guillevin L, Poissonnet M, et al. Prevalences of polyarteritis nodosa, microscopic polyangiitis, Wegener's granulomatosis, and Churg-Strauss syndrome in a French urban multiethnic population in 2000: a capture-recapture estimate. Arthritis Rheum 2004;51:92–9.

14. McMahon BJ, Heyward WL, Templin DW, et al. Hepatitis B-associated polyarteritis nodosa in Alaskan Eskimos: clinical and epidemiologic features and long-term follow-up. Hepatology 1989;9:97–101.

15. Guillevin L, Lhote F, Cohen P, et al. Polyarteritis nodosa related to hepatitis B virus. A prospective study with long-term observation of 41 patients. Medicine (Baltimore) 1995;74:238–53.

16. Prince AM, Trépo C. Role of immune complexes involving SH antigen in pathogenesis of chronic active hepatitis and polyarteritis nodosa. Lancet 1971;1:1309–12.

17. Guillevin L, Lhote F. Treatment of polyarteritis nodosa and microscopic polyangiitis. Arthritis Rheum 1998;41:2100–5.

18. Gayraud M, Guillevin L, le Toumelin P, et al. Long-term followup of polyarteritis nodosa, microscopic polyangiitis, and Churg-Strauss syndrome: analysis of four prospective trials including 278 patients. Arthritis Rheum 2001;44:666–75.

19. Guillevin L, Lhote F, Léon A, et al. Treatment of polyarteritis nodosa related to hepatitis B virus with short term steroid therapy associated with antiviral agents and plasma exchanges. A prospective trial in 33 patients. J Rheumatol 1993; 20:289–98.

20. Guillevin L, Lhote F, Sauvaget F, et al. Treatment of polyarteritis nodosa related to hepatitis B virus with interferon-alpha and plasma exchanges. Ann Rheum Dis 1994;53:334–7.

21. Guillevin L, Mahr A, Cohen P, et al. Short-term corticosteroids then lamivudine and plasma exchanges to treat hepatitis B virus-related polyarteritis nodosa. Arthritis Rheum 2004;51:482–7.

22. Combes B, Shorey J, Barrera A, et al. Glomerulonephritis with deposition of Australia antigen-antibody complexes in glomerular basement membrane. Lancet 1971;2:234–7.

23. Johnson RJ, Couser WG. Hepatitis B infection and renal disease: clinical, immunopathogenetic and therapeutic considerations. Kidney Int 1990;37:663–76.

24. Bhimma R, Coovadia HM. Hepatitis B virus-associated nephropathy. Am J Nephrol 2004;24:198–211.

25. Ozdamar SO, Gucer S, Tinaztepe K. Hepatitis-B virus associated nephropathies: a clinicopathological study in 14 children. Pediatr Nephrol 2003;18:23–8.

26. Lai KN, Lai FM, Chan KW, et al. The clinico-pathologic features of hepatitis B virus-associated glomerulonephritis. Q J Med 1987;63:323–33.
27. Lai KN, Ho RT, Tam JS, et al. Detection of hepatitis B virus DNA and RNA in kidneys of HBV-related glomerulonephritis. Kidney Int 1996;50:1965–77.
28. Wang NS, Wu ZL, Zhang YE, et al. Role of hepatitis B virus infection in pathogenesis of IgA nephropathy. World J Gastroenterol 2003;9:2004–8.
29. Lai KN, Lai FM, Tam JS. IgA nephropathy associated with chronic hepatitis B virus infection in adults: the pathogenetic role of HBsAg. J Pathol 1989;157:321–7.
30. Kleinknecht C, Levy M, Peix A, et al. Membranous glomerulonephritis and hepatitis B surface antigen in children. J Pediatr 1979;95:946–52.
31. Venkataseshan VS, Lieberman K, Kim DU, et al. Hepatitis-B-associated glomerulonephritis: pathology, pathogenesis, and clinical course. Medicine (Baltimore) 1990;69:200–16.
32. Lin CY. Hepatitis B virus-associated membraneous nephropathy: clinical features, immunological profiles and outcome. Nephron 1990;55:37–44.
33. Ito H, Hattori S, Matusda I, et al. Hepatitis B e antigen-mediated membranous glomerulonephritis. Correlation of ultrastructural changes with HBeAg in the serum and glomeruli. Lab Invest 1981;44:214–20.
34. Hirose H, Udo K, Kojima M, et al. Deposition of hepatitis B e antigen in membranous glomerulonephritis: identification by F(ab')2 fragments of monoclonal antibody. Kidney Int 1984;26:338–41.
35. Lai KN, Li PK, Lui SF, et al. Membranous nephropathy related to hepatitis B virus in adults. N Engl J Med 1991;324:1457–63.
36. Gilbert RD, Wiggelinkhuizen J. The clinical course of hepatitis B virus-associated nephropathy. Pediatr Nephrol 1994;8:11–4.
37. Gonzalo A, Mampaso F, Barcena R, et al. Membranous nephropathy associated with hepatitis B virus infection: long-term clinical and histological outcome. Nephrol Dial Transplant 1999;14:416–8.
38. Wiggelinkhuizen J, Sinclair-Smith C, Stannard LM, et al. Hepatitis B virus associated membranous glomerulonephritis. Arch Dis Child 1983;58:488–96.
39. Lai KN, Tam JS, Lin HJ, et al. The therapeutic dilemma of the usage of corticosteroid in patients with membranous nephropathy and persistent hepatitis B virus surface antigenaemia. Nephron 1990;54:12–7.
40. Lin CY. Treatment of hepatitis B virus-associated membranous nephropathy with recombinant alpha-interferon. Kidney Int 1995;47:225–30.
41. Conjeevaram HS, Hoofnagle JH, Austin HA, et al. Long-term outcome of hepatitis B virus-related glomerulonephritis after therapy with interferon alfa. Gastroenterology 1995;109:540–6.
42. Chung DR, Yang WS, Kim SB, et al. Treatment of hepatitis B virus associated glomerulonephritis with recombinant human alpha interferon. Am J Nephrol 1997;17:112–7.
43. Bhimma R, Coovadia HM, Kramvis A, et al. Treatment of hepatitis B virus-associated nephropathy in black children. Pediatr Nephrol 2002;17:393–9.
44. Tang S, Lai FM, Lui YH, et al. Lamivudine in hepatitis B-associated membranous nephropathy. Kidney Int 2005;68:1750–8.
45. Fabrizi F, Dixit V, Martin P. Meta-analysis: anti-viral therapy of hepatitis B virus-associated glomerulonephritis. Aliment Pharmacol Ther 2006;24:781–8.
46. Guéroult N, Dorfmann H, Etienne JP. L'arthrite au cours de l'hépatite virale. Ann Med Interne (Paris) 1972;123:561–71.
47. Inman RD. Rheumatic manifestations of hepatitis B virus infection. Semin Arthritis Rheum 1982;11:406–20.

48. Ray G, Ghosh B, Bhattacharyya R. Acute hepatitis B presenting as Guillain-Barré syndrome. Indian J Gastroenterol 2003;22:228.

49. Penner E, Maida E, Mamoli B, et al. Serum and cerebrospinal fluid immune complexes containing hepatitis B surface antigen in Guillain-Barré syndrome. Gastroenterology 1982;82:576–80.

50. Chroni E, Thomopoulos C, Papapetropoulos S, et al. A case of relapsing Guillain-Barré syndrome associated with exacerbation of chronic hepatitis B virus hepatitis. J Neurovirol 2003;9:408–10.

51. Tsukada N, Koh CS, Inoue A, et al. Demyelinating neuropathy associated with hepatitis B virus infection. Detection of immune complexes composed of hepatitis B virus surface antigen. J Neurol Sci 1987;77:203–16.

52. Caniello M, Baxter P, Lino AM, et al. Confluent peripheral multiple mononeuropathy associated to acute hepatitis B: a case report. Rev Inst Med Trop Sao Paulo 2002;44:171–3.

53. Gianotti F. Papular acrodermatitis of childhood. An Australia antigen disease. Arch Dis Child 1973;48:794–9.

54. De Gaspari G, Bardare M, Costantino D. AU antigen in Crosti-Gianotti acrodermatitis. Lancet 1970;1:1116–7.

55. Konno M, Kikuta H, Ishikawa N, et al. A possible association between hepatitis-B antigen-negative infantile papular acrodermatitis and Epstein-Barr virus infection. J Pediatr 1982;101:222–4.

56. Gocke DJ. Extrahepatic manifestations of viral hepatitis. Am J Med Sci 1975;270: 49–52.

57. Dienstag JL, Rhodes AR, Bhan AK, et al. Urticaria associated with acute viral hepatitis type B: studies of pathogenesis. Ann Intern Med 1978;89:34–40.

58. Neumann HA, Berretty PJ, Folmer SC, et al. Hepatitis B surface antigen deposition in the blood vessel walls of urticarial lesions in acute hepatitis B. Br J Dermatol 1981;104:383–8.

59. Dogan B. Dermatological manifestations in hepatitis B surface antigen carriers in east region of Turkey. J Eur Acad Dermatol Venereol 2005;19:323–5.

60. Denli YG, Durdu M, Karakas M. Diabetes and hepatitis frequency in 140 lichen planus cases in Cukurova region. J Dermatol 2004;31:293–8.

61. Jorge J Jr, Lopes MA, de Almeida OP, et al. Oral lichen planus and chronic active hepatitis B: a salutary tale. Dent Update 1994;21:335–7.

62. Rebora A, Robert E, Rongioletti F. Clinical and laboratory presentation of lichen planus patients with chronic liver disease. J Dermatol Sci 1992;4:38–41.

63. Rebora A. Hepatitis viruses and lichen planus. Arch Dermatol 1994;130: 1328–9.

64. Gruppo Italiano Studi Epidemiologici in Dermatologia (GISED). Lichen planus and liver diseases: a multicentre case-control study. Br Med J 1990;300:227–30.

65. Bokor-Bratic M. Lack of evidence of hepatic disease in patients with oral lichen planus in Serbia. Oral Dis 2004;10:283–6.

66. Rebora A, Rongioletti F, Grosshans E. Syndrome lichen plan-hépatite. Revue générale à propos d'un cas. Ann Dermatol Venereol 1985;112:27–32.

67. Bonkovsky HL, Liang TJ, Hasegawa K, et al. Chronic leukocytoclastic vasculitis complicating HBV infection. Possible role of mutant forms of HBV in pathogenesis and persistence of disease. J Clin Gastroenterol 1995;21:42–7.

68. Surmali Onay O, Baskin E, Ozcay F, et al. Successful treatment of hepatitis B-associated leukocytoclastic vasculitis with lamivudine treatment in a child patient. Rheumatol Int 2007;27:869–72.

69. Gluck T, Weber P, Wiedmann KH. Hepatitis-B-associated vasculitis. Clinical course with glucocorticoid and alpha-interferon therapy. Dtsch Med Wochenschr 1994;119:1388–92.
70. Ergin S, Sanli Erdogan B, Turgut H, et al. Relapsing Henoch-Schonlein purpura in an adult patient associated with hepatitis B virus infection. J Dermatol 2005;32: 839–42.
71. Maggiore G, Martini A, Grifeo S, et al. Hepatitis B virus infection and Schonlein-Henoch purpura. Am J Dis Child 1984;138:681–2.
72. Shin JI, Lee JS. Hepatitis B virus infection and Henoch-Schonlein purpura. J Dermatol 2007;34:156.
73. Cervia M, Parodi A, Rebora A. Chronic active hepatitis and erythema nodosum. Arch Dermatol 1982;118:878.
74. Garcia-Bragado F, Genesca J, Allende H, et al. Etude de la réplication du virus de l'hépatite B dans cinq cas de cryoglobulinémie mixte essentielle. Gastroenterol Clin Biol 1986;10:772.
75. Lohr H, Goergen B, Weber W, et al. Mixed cryoglobulinemia type II in chronic hepatitis B associated with HBe-minus HBV mutant: cellular immune reactions and response to interferon treatment. J Med Virol 1994;44:330–5.
76. Levo Y, Gorevic PD, Kassab HJ, et al. Association between hepatitis B virus and essential mixed cryoglobulinemia. N Engl J Med 1977;296:1501–4.
77. Galli M, Monti G, Invernizzi F, et al. Hepatitis B virus-related markers in secondary and in essential mixed cryoglobulinemias: a multicentric study of 596 cases. The Italian Group for the Study of Cryoglobulinemias (GISC). Ann Ital Med Int 1992;7: 209–14.
78. Grob PJ, Martenet AC, Witmer R. Nonspecific immune parameters and hepatitis B antigens in patients with uveitis. Mod Probl Ophthalmol 1976;16:254–8.
79. Murray PI, Waite J, Rahi AH, et al. Acute anterior uveitis and hepatitis B virus infection. Br J Ophthalmol 1984;68:595–7.
80. Kim JH, Bang YJ, Park BJ, et al. Hepatitis B virus infection and B-cell non-Hodgkin's lymphoma in a hepatitis B endemic area: a case-control study. Jpn J Cancer Res 2002;93:471–7.
81. Kuniyoshi M, Nakamuta M, Sakai H, et al. Prevalence of hepatitis B or C virus infections in patients with non-Hodgkin's lymphoma. J Gastroenterol Hepatol 2001;16:215–9.
82. Cucuianu A, Patiu M, Duma M, et al. Hepatitis B and C virus infection in Romanian non-Hodgkin's lymphoma patients. Br J Haematol 1999;107:353–6.
83. Yood MU, Quesenberry CP Jr, Guo D, et al. Incidence of non-Hodgkin's lymphoma among individuals with chronic hepatitis B virus infection. Hepatology 2007;46:107–12.

HIV Infection and Rheumatic Diseases: The Changing Spectrum of Clinical Enigma

Nirupa Patel, MD[a], Neej Patel, BS[a,b], Luis R. Espinoza, MD[a,*]

KEYWORDS

- HIV infection • Rheumatic diseases • Spondyloarthropathy
- Osteonecrosis • Hyperuricimia

HIV infection has been diagnosed for approximately 3 decades, and rheumatic diseases have been recognized along with it since the mid-1980s. Antiretroviral therapy has continued to change over time. It started as a single agent (zidovudine), then as a combination therapy (highly active antiretroviral therapy [HAART]), and now even newer agents have emerged (fusion therapy and anti-CCR5 antibody). Particular ensuing rheumatic diseases have emerged with each respective change in antiretroviral therapy (**Table 1**). Clinicians, especially rheumatologists, need to be aware of this changing spectrum of diseases. Although long-established rheumatic manifestations are still prevalent in developing countries, systemic inflammatory response syndrome and morbid conditions have emerged since HAART treatment. The newer treatments may lead to different rheumatic vignettes in the future.

In this article, the authors discuss the occurrence and prevalence of rheumatic syndromes in the pre-HAART and HAART eras. The immunologic, environmental, and genetic factors behind the combination of HIV infection and rheumatic manifestation contribute to the complexity of these diseases. Miscellaneous case reports are briefly discussed in relation to HIV infection.

Staging of HIV infection is somewhat helpful, but rheumatic conditions can occur at any stage of the disease. The simplified stages are as follows:

Stage I: acute infection
Stage II: CD4+ > 200/μl
Stage III: onset of AIDS
Stage IV: HAART treatment

[a] Section of Rheumatology, Louisiana State University Health Sciences Center, 2020 Gravier Street, 7th Floor, Rm 719/7D4, New Orleans, LA 70065, USA
[b] College of Arts and Sciences, University of Pennsylvania, Philadelphia, PA, USA
* Corresponding author.
E-mail address: lespin@lsuhsc.edu (L.R. Espinoza).

Rheum Dis Clin N Am 35 (2009) 139–161
doi:10.1016/j.rdc.2009.03.007
0889-857X/09/$ – see front matter © 2009 Published by Elsevier Inc.

Table 1
Rheumatic conditions in HIV infection (United States)

Treatment Era	Rheumatic Manifestation	Prevalence (%)
pre-HAART	–	Overall: 11–72[17,159]
	Arthralgias	5–45[11,17,65]
	Arthritis	10–12[11,17,19,160]
	Reactive arthritis (Reiter syndrome)	0.4–10[11,17,19,29]
	Psoriatic arthritis	1.3–5.7[17,19,21,29]
	Undifferentiated spondyloarthropathy	NA
	DILS	3[52]
	Myopathy—PM, dermatomyositis, inclusion body myositis, nemaline rod	2–7[17,29,65,73]
	Vasculitis	–
	Gout, hyperuricemia	0.5,[123]42[11,122]
	Septic conditions—septic arthritis osteomyelitis, pyomyositis	<1[34,108]
HAART	IRIS—DILS, sarcoidosis, RA, systemic lupus erythematosus	25[161]
	Drug induced conditions: zidovudine myopathy nemaline rod rhabdomyolysis gout, hyperuricemia lipodystrophy Osseous conditions: osteoporosis, osteomyelitis, osteonecrosis	NA

Abbreviations: DILS, diffuse infiltrative lymphocytosis syndrome; IRIS, immune reconstitution inflammatory syndrome; NA, not available; PM, polymyositis; RA, rheumatoid arthritis.

Stages I, II, and IV have concurrent autoimmune diseases. Stage III exhibits immunosuppression and has the least autoimmune phenomenon. During Stage III, opportunistic infections and septic arthritis can occur.

The following pathogenetic mechanisms are involved in HIV infection and rheumatic diseases:

HIV-1 infects CD4+ T cells that express different chemokines. Chemokine CCR5 (coreceptor for HIV-1) and CXCR4 (fusin) are chemokines that aid HIV viral entrance and replication in host cells.[1,2] Newer agents are being investigated to antagonize these mechanisms.[3] CD4+ T cells have several populations, and the depletion of them results in immune alterations.[4]

Depletion or imbalance of Th_1 and Th_2 leads to a heightened susceptibility to different infections. Increased Th_1 cells lead to a decrease in IFNγ and an increase in viral infection. An increase in Th_2 activity causes an increase in interleukin (IL)-10 and IL-4 levels, and keeps the virus under control.[5] Nonprogressors of HIV infection cause vigorous Th_1 and moderate Th_2 responses; this keeps HIV infection in balance.

Decreased regulatory T cells (Treg) along with viremia lead to CD4 and CD8 activation.[6] CD4+/CD25+ Treg cells express CCR5, which makes them prone to HIV-1 infection.

HIV particles show a similarity to host antigens, thereby exhibiting molecular mimicry. This results in autoimmune responses such as reactive arthritis, psoriatic arthritis, diffuse infiltrative lymphocytosis syndrome (DILS), myopathy, and vasculitis. Human leukocyte antigens (HLA)-DR4, DR2, Fas protein, IgG, and IgA are homologous to the envelope protein in HIV.[7]

B-cell proliferation (**Table 2**).

Cytotoxic T cell responses to HIV infection are caused by the direct killing and inhibition of the virus through cytokines and chemokines. This phenomenon is HLA dependent; genetic haplotypes also play a role. HLA-B14, B27, B51, B57, C8, and DR6 haplotypes were nonprogressors, while HLA-A24, A29, A35, C4, DR1, and DR3 were rapid progressors of HIV disease.[8] Reveille shows that HLA-A29, A23, B8, B22, B35, and C4 null alleles are rapid progressors, while HLA-A32, B13, B14, B27, B51, B57, DQ B1*0302, and DQ B1*0303 are long-term survivors.[9]

Macrophage tropism (M-tropism) and T-lymphocyte tropism (T-tropism) occur in early and late phases of HIV infection, respectively. Chemokine CCR5 is involved in M-tropism, while CXCR4 is involved in T-tropism. The homozygosity and heterozygosity of the host, in combination with these tropisms, may determine the rate of the disease's progression.[10]

Apoptosis is a possible mechanism involved in HIV-infected cells.[7]

Direct effect of HIV on CD4+ T cells is well documented. Direct effect of HIV on endothelial, synovial, and hematopoietic cells occurs, resulting in decreased CD4+ and increased CD8+ counts and autoantibodies.[11,12]

Possible pathogenetic mechanisms in HIV-AIDS patients with rheumatic diseases are outlined in **Box 1**.

The antibodies in **Table 2** were found in low titers and were of no clinical significance. However, they do bear a prognostic significance in that they were associated with lower CD4 count, late HIV stage, and increased mortality.[13]

Table 2
Different autoantibodies found in HIV infection

Type of Condition	Autoantibodies Related to Condition
Rheumatologic	ANA
	RF (Polyclonal, IgG, IgA, IgM)
	Cardiolipin (IgG, IgM)
	Phospholipids
	$AntiB_2GP-1$
	Antinuclear cytoplasmic antibody (P and C)
	DsDNA
	Histone
	Sm U1RNP
	SSA
Hematologic	Antiplatelet
	Anti-RBC
	Antilymphocyte surface antigen
	Antiprothrombin
Neurologic	Antineuronal
	Anti-neurotransmitters
	Antimyelin-associated proteins
Endocrinologic	Antithyroid
General	Circulating immune complexes
	Hypergammaglobulinemia

Data from Refs. [11,13,134,136]

Box 1
Possible pathogenetic mechanisms in HIV-AIDS patients with rheumatic diseases
HIV-1 interaction with chemokines
CCR5
CXCR4 (fusin)
Th_1/Th_2 depletion or imbalance (switch)
Decreased T-regulatory cells
Molecular mimicry
B-cell proliferation (see Table 2)
Cytotoxic T cell response—HLA haplotypes
M- and T-tropism
Apoptosis—TNF-α
Direct CD4+ destruction by HIV
Abbreviations: Th, T-helper cells; TNF-α, tumor necrosis factor α

Antiphospholipids antibodies (APLA) are found in systemic lupus erythematosus (SLE) and HIV infection. In HIV infection, both types of APLA, nonpathogenic (non–2 glycoprotein-1 dependent) and pathogenic (2 glycoprotein-1 dependent) antibodies, are detected.[14] Coinfection of HIV and HCV demonstrates high frequency of thrombotic episodes.[15] Otherwise, thrombotic events in HIV monoinfection and APLA are seldom.

DISCUSSION
Rheumatic Diseases in the Pre-Highly Active Antiretroviral Therapy Era

Arthralgias
Acute HIV viral syndrome is associated with arthralgias (see **Table 1**). It occurs as a part of flu-like illness.[16] Fever, malaise, and arthralgias, though common, rarely exist beyond 2 weeks when associated with HIV. Knees, shoulders, and elbows are commonly involved joints. Arthralgias and myalgias tend to recur in advanced stages of HIV infection.[17] Treatment with analgesics usually suffices.

Acute intermittent painful articular syndrome
Acute intermittent painful articular syndrome occurs in initial stages of HIV infection. Even though it requires opioid analgesics, it ameliorates rapidly.[18]

Arthritis
Arthritis can occur at any of the four stages of HIV infection. It can also occur in advanced HIV infections.[17] It is usually nonerosive, pauciarticular, and favors lower extremities. It is mostly self-limited and does not exceed durations of 6 weeks.[19] Synovial fluid analysis is usually noninflammatory and cultures are negative. Tubulo-reticular inclusions have been found and suggest direct viral etiology.[19–21] In patients with arthritis, HIV-$_p$24 antigen has been detected in the synovial tissue and the CD4 and CD8 lymphocytes.[22] Njobvu and colleagues'[23] study from Zambia supports the fact that HIV-related arthropathy is a distinct entity. In this study, one group of patients had no extra-articular or infectious manifestations.

Treatment of arthritis is usually nonsteroidal antiinflammatory agents (NSAIDS). Low-dose steroids can be used with caution in severe cases. Hydroxychloroquine[24] and sulfasalazine[25] have been effective in seronegative arthritis.

Jaccoud arthritis

Jaccoud arthritis has been reported in HIV infection. Two case reports found Jaccoud arthritis to be associated with reactive arthritis.[26] In a third instance, a patient had poorly controlled HIV infection.[27] Jaccoud arthritis does not respond well to any traditional therapy.

Spondyloarthropathies

Spondyloarthropathies include reactive arthritis (ReA; Reiter-like syndrome), psoriatic arthritis (PsA), and undifferentiated spondyloarthropathy (SpA). ReA is prevalent in HIV-positive pediatric and adult patients.[28] It presents as asymmetric oligoarthritis. Enthesopathy is prevalent, but sacroiliitis and axial disease, though uncommon, can occur.[11,17,19,29] Extra-articular symptoms of conjunctivitis, circinate balanitis, urethritis, keratoderma blenorrhagicum, and psoriasiform skin rashes are frequent.[17] ReA in HIV-positive patients can be explained by severe immunosuppression, which predisposes to invasion by various microorganisms. AIDS and HIV-infected patients are also prone to gastrointestinal and genitourinary infections, which cause ReA.[30,31] HIV positivity increases the susceptibility of developing ReA in HLA-B27-positive patients.[32] The clinical overlap between ReA and PsA makes one wonder if they are a continuum of the same disease. More severe ReA with erosive changes and ankylosis can occur in African black patients.[33] Severe psoriasis vulgaris, pustular, or papulosquamous dermopathy with arthritis should alert one to look for HIV infection.[34,35] Different patterns of psoriasis—vulgaris, inverse, guttate, palmo-plantar, erythrodermic, and pustular—coexist with ReA.[36,37]

Cytotoxic CD8 cells predominate in HIV-positive ReA and PsA patients.[32] Treg cells are deficient in psoriasis,[38] and these expand when patients are placed on HAART.[39,40] Cytokines such as tumor necrosis factor (TNF)-α play a great role in HIV replication and psoriasis. This response is blunted by HAART[41] and anti-TNF agents such as etanercept, infliximab, and adalimumab. There are case reports showing successful treatment of PsA with the use of anti-TNF agents.[42–44] PsA is usually asymmetrical and may coexist with distal interphalangeal joint involvement. Dactylitis and enthesitis do occur. The course is usually explosive, resulting in erosive changes and deformities developing in a very short period.[30] Undifferentiated SpA has incomplete stigmata of ReA and PsA.

Treatment of PsA and ReA with NSAIDS is usually not successful. Sulfasalazine (1–3 grams/day) has been helpful in ReA. Intra-articular steroid injections are effective.[30,45] Etretinate is effective for ReA.[46] It has been useful in pustular psoriasis, PsA, and skin or joint manifestations of ReA.[37,46,47] Cyclosporine is another agent partially helpful in some patients, yet has a total response in others.[45] Hydroxychloroquine has been effective in ReA since it has shown to reduce HIV viral load.[48] Methotrexate can be used with caution.[49] Anti-TNF agents and HAART have some success in ReA and PsA, as discussed earlier.

Sub-Saharan Africa is home to HIV infection. A recent increase in SpA has kindled interest in research and HLA haplotyping. In a Zambian study, 64 HIV-positive SpA patients were found to have increased HLA-B*5703 frequency.[50] HLA-B27 is rarely associated with these Africans.[28,51]

Diffuse infiltrative lymphocytosis syndrome

Among HIV patients, diffuse infiltrative lymphocytosis syndrome is a syndrome of bilateral, painless, parotid, and lacrimal gland enlargement, peripheral CD8 lymphocytosis, and sicca symptoms.[52] It is often confused with primary Sjögren's syndrome (SS) (**Table 3**). The diagnostic criteria for DILS includes persistence for

Table 3
Comparison between diffuse infiltrative lymphocytosis syndrome (in HIV patients) and primary Sjögren's syndrome

Features	DILS	Primary SS
Parotid enlargement	Massive	Mild to moderate
Lymphocytic infiltrate, biopsy	CD8+ in periductal area	CD4+ in perivascular area
Auto-antibodies	Usually negative (low titers)	Anti-SSA, SSB, RF
Sicca symptoms	Common	Very common
HLA-MHCII	DRB1*0102, 1301, 1302, DRB5, B6,45,49,50	DRB1*0301,B8, DR2, DR3
Extra-glandular features	Predominant LIP, neurologic features	Uncommon
Treatment	Steroids: use with caution DMARDS: not helpful Anti-TNF agents: no HAART: helps symptoms and parotid cysts Low-dose radiation—reduces gland size	Steroids: may help DMARDS: helpful Anti-TNF agents: useful HAART: NA Not recommended

Abbreviations: DMARDS, disease modifying anti-rheumatic drugs; NA, not available.

6 months, positive salivary gland biopsy (lip preferred), and intense bilateral uptake on gallium citrate 67 scintigraphy (in hemophiliacs and unequivocal cases).[53,54] Parotid lipomatosis occurring in patients on protease inhibitors (PI) have no uptake on gallium scan.[55] CT scanning helps to evaluate parotid cysts and malignancy. Extraglandular features of DILS prior to antiretroviral therapy are lymphocytic interstitial pneumonia (LIP), which occurs in 25% to 50% of patients, and facial palsy, which occurs in about 30% of patients. Peripheral neuropathy, renal tubular acidosis, polymyositis (PM), lymphocytic hepatitis, and lymphoma have all occurred with DILS.[55–58]

Pathogenesis of DILS may have a genetic basis. HLA-DRB1*1102 has been found in African American children with DILS. In adults, DILS is associated with HLA-DR5, DR6, and some others.[59] CD8+ and CD29-lymphocytes are found in different organs—such as lungs, salivary glands, GI tract, and meninges (homing mechanism) —where HIV suppression is needed.[60] T-tropic strains rapidly evolve into AIDS; M-tropic strains progress slowly.[61] Pathologically, salivary glands have CD8+ lymphocytosis,[60] while primary SS has CD4+ cells. Parotid glands in DILS have lymphoepithelial cysts, which contain high levels of HIV-1 messenger RNA. This proves that there is ongoing active HIV infection and viral shedding.[62]

Treatment of DILS is usually symptomatic. HAART and high-dose steroids help extraglandular features such as LIP and neuropathy. Patients in different geographic regions present with different patterns of DILS. In a study, 77 Greek female patients, who were HIV positive, were found to have a high prevalence of sicca symptoms (at 7.8%).[63] Also, African Americans are more afflicted with DILS.[52] DILS has a higher prevalence in West Africa than in the United States. Forty-eight percent of Cameroonians were affected as compared with only 6% of the United States patients. The United States patients were treated with HAART, yet none of the West Africans were; this could be a factor contributing to their higher prevalence of DILS.[64]

Myopathy of the pre-highly active antiretroviral therapy era

Myalgias, PM, dermatomyositis, inclusion body myositis, Nemaline rod myopathy, rhabdomyolysis, wasting syndrome, and pyomyositis are muscular conditions associated with HIV infection. Some HAART-induced myopathies are discussed later.

Myalgias

Myalgias occur in the early stages of HIV infection (33%).[17,65] They are part of a flu-like illness.[16] They can occur in late stages of HIV infection.[17]

Polymyositis

Polymyositis is the most common myopathy in HIV-positive patients. It usually occurs in early stages of HIV infection, but it can also be found at any stage. It is an inflammatory myopathy with increased creatine kinase (CK), myositis, and microvasculitis.[66] The predominant cells in HIV-positive muscle biopsies were CD8+ T cells. Endomysial infiltrates showed reduction in CD4+ T cells.[67] Viral antigens and nucleic acids have also been found in endomysial lymphocytes.[68,69] The clinical course, laboratory, and electromyographic findings are identical to idiopathic PM.[70] The cause of PM in HIV infection is unclear. Nutritional factors, such as selenium deficiency, may be causative.[71,72] Treatment usually involves moderate to high doses of corticosteroids. Methotrexate and azathioprine can be used with caution, monitoring CD4 counts and viral load. It responds well to therapy, and its prognosis is good with spontaneous resolution in some instances.[73] PM can be associated with DILS in 50% of patients in some series of studies.[73,74]

Dermatomyositis

Dermatomyositis is very rarely seen in HIV infection.[75]

Inclusion body myositis

In HIV-positive patients, the surfaces of muscle cells act as antigens to CD8+ T cells.[76]

Nemaline rod myopathy

Although it rarely occurs in HIV infection, patients with nemaline rod myopathy (NRM) present with painless muscle weakness, wasting, and elevated muscle enzymes.[77,78] Nemaline rods stain red or purple on the Gomori trichrome stain, and they are related to Z bands. They are electron dense,[79] and α-actinin is a constituent of nemaline rods and Z bands.[80] On light microscopy, HIV-associated NRM showed intracellular abnormalities. The type I fibers that were affected had granular rod material and were smaller. They also contained vacuoles. The sarcoplasmic pattern was disturbed. HIV infection can occur after NRM. If light microscopy shows typical features of NRM, HIV testing should be done.[78] Patients may respond to steroids or plasmapheresis. This may suggest an autoimmune mechanism in NRM.[81]

Rhabdomyolysis

Rhabdomyolysis can occur in HIV infection.[82,83] Drug-induced rhabdomyolysis is reviewed later.

Wasting syndrome

Wasting syndrome is associated with the AIDS complex. The syndrome involves severe muscle atrophy, 10% weight loss, diarrhea, weakness, and fever. In the HAART era, this is a rare occurrence.

Pyomyositis

Tropical pyomyositis occurs in HIV-positive patients during Stage 3 of the infection. It can simulate septic arthritis of proximal joints.[84–86] The most common organism in pyomyositis is *Staphylococcus aureus*. *Salmonella enteritides*, *Microsporum*, and *Toxoplasma* have also been found. Young males with low CD4+ counts were prone to pyomyositis. Pain, swelling, fever, and leukocytosis were presenting symptoms. Drainage of muscles or blood cultures was diagnostic. MRI of muscle can be helpful in diagnosis. Treatment involves long-term antibiotics and drainage of muscle abscess.[34]

Fibromyalgia

HIV infection is associated with fibromyalgia in the pre-HAART and HAART eras.[87] Depression is associated with fibromyalgia and treatment is the same as in non-HIV population[88] (**Box 2**).

Vasculitis

Small-, medium-, and large-sized vessels can be involved in vasculitis. It can occur at early and late stages of HIV infection. In a study of 145 muscle, nerve, and skin biopsies, 34 had vasculitis.[89]

Polyarteritis nodosa

PAN can occur at any stage of HIV disease. It occurs commonly in young males. PAN can present as viral-like syndrome; therefore, it can be often unrecognized. Myalgias, muscular atrophy, mononeuritis, and sensory motor polyneuropathy are common manifestations. Systemic involvement is rare. Associated hepatitis C infection and intravenous drug (IVD) use were features in reported patients.[90] In contrast to classical PAN, hepatitis B infection with HIV-related PAN is not a common occurrence. The cause of PAN is obscure. Instead of HbS antigen, HIV capsid antigen and HIV RNA were found in vascular lesions. This may suggest a direct role of HIV in the pathogenesis of PAN.[89,91] Histopathology reveals necrotizing vasculitis in muscle biopsy. Most patients do well on low-dose corticosteroids. Unlike classical PAN, HIV-related PAN is

---

Box 2
Different vasculitides in HIV infection

Polyarteritis nodosa (PAN)

Hypersensitivity angiitis

Henoch-Schönlein purpura

Giant cell arteritis

Takayasu arteritis

Kawasaki disease

Behçet-like disease

Churg-Strauss vasculitis

Wegener granulomatosis

Central nervous system (CNS) angiitis

    isolated

    granulomatous

Cryoglobulinemias (types 2 and 3)

less aggressive. In systemic involvement, immunosuppressives such as cyclophosphamide and high-dose steroids can be used with caution.[92] Anti-CD-25 therapy has bee successful in cerebral vasculitis.[93]

Hypersensitivity angiitis, Henoch-Schönlein purpura,[89] giant cell arteritis of aortic root,[94] Takayasu-like arteritis with aneurysms among Africans and North Americans have been described.[95–97] Kawasaki disease with presence of anticardiolipin antibodies has been observed in HIV-positive adults and children.[98] This has been reported with immune reconstitution inflammatory syndrome (IRIS).[99] Behçet-like disease is common in China, where hepatitis C infection is widespread. Blood transfusion was the route of HIV infection in 75% of patients. Orogenital ulcers were found in 60% to 70% of patients, and they had negative pathergy tests. These patients were IVD users.[100] Churg-Strauss vasculitis, Wegener granulomatosis, and central nervous system (CNS) angiitis rarely occur in HIV infection. Neurologic deficits and organic brain syndrome occur in isolated CNS angiitis.[101,102] Brain biopsy may be necessary, and perivascular mononuclear infiltration has been found from autopsies in five out of six children.[103] CNS vasculitis can occur with varicella zoster, cytomegalovirus infections, or lymphoma.[101] Granulomatous necrotizing vasculitis of CNS usually responds to combined antiretroviral therapy.[104] Acute coronary vasculitis with fatal myocardial infarction in HIV infection is reported.[105] Cryoglobulinemias (types 2 and 3) occur with HCV and HIV coinfections.[106] In the HAART era, HIV-infected patients have decreased levels of cryoglobulins.[107]

Septic arthritis

The prevalence of septic arthritis is less than 1% in most series.[34,108,109] It is extremely rare considering the propensity to different infections in HIV-positive patients. S aureus is the most common organism followed by Streptococcus, Salmonella, atypical Mycobacterium, and many others. Any acute monoarthritis should alert one to the possibility of infectious etiology. Its presentation, etiology, and therapy are, in all respects, like that those seen in HIV-negative patients.[34] There is preponderance of septic arthritis in IVD users. S aureus is the most common organism in IVD users and hemophiliacs.[34,65,110] Acute monoarthritis of large joints such as hips and knees are common in males. In IVD users, hip, sacroiliac, and sternoclavicular joints are frequently affected.[34,65,111] Salmonella organisms are quite prevalent in HIV-infected hemophiliacs.[112,113] Hemophiliacs with HIV infection and hemarthrosis should raise a suspicion of septic arthritis. These patients are febrile and have elevated sedimentation rates despite low white counts. Polyarticular septic arthritis is common when there is preexisting rheumatoid arthritis (RA) and hemophilia.[114] Candida septic arthritis has been reported in 15 cases of IVD users.[113] Gonococcal arthritis in HIV-positive homosexuals and African heterosexuals has been reported.[113]

Histoplasma capsulatum, Cryptococcus neoformans, Sporothrix schenkii, and Mucor species can cause septic arthritis.[34] Salmonella organisms have been offending pathogens in Thai patients, mostly in advanced stages of HIV infection.[115,116] Pyogenic organisms cause arthritis at CD4 counts greater than 250 cells/mm^3, while opportunistic organisms occur at CD4 counts less than 200 cells/mm^3.[108] Forty-one percent of HAART-era patients had septic involvement (arthritis, bursitis, cellulitis, osteomyelitis, disciitis, or pyomyositis) in a study involving 75 patients.[87]

Osteomyelitis

Osteomyelitis (OM) is a serious sequelae of HIV infection. Staphylococcus is the most common pathogen in IVD users. Mycobacterium tuberculosis was causative in 33% of OM in a large series.[34] Atypical Mycobacteria were a common occurrence in other series.[117] *M haemophilum, M kansasii, M avium-intracellulare, M terrae,* and *M fortuitum* with arthritis and OM have been reported in the HIV population.[118] Bone biopsy and open drainage are diagnostic in OM. MRI is the common radiographic modality used to diagnose depth, extent, and variety of septic conditions.[119] Surgical drainage and long-term (4–6 weeks) antibiotics usually results in full recovery.[35] Tuberculous myositis[120] and myositis due to trichinosis[121] have occurred also.

Gout and hyperuricemia

Gout and hyperuricemia have a high prevalence in the HIV population.[11,122–124] Increased cell turnover with HIV replication leads to elevated levels of serum urate.[115,122]

Rheumatic conditions in the highly active antiretroviral therapy era

HAART has revolutionized the natural history, long-term outcome, morbidity, and mortality of the HIV population (see **Table 1**). The pattern of rheumatic diseases has changed since HAART has been used. A longitudinal study from Cleveland showed decline in ReA, PsA, and other connective tissue diseases.[125] Decline in the incidence of DILS has been reported by some investigators[126] but not by others.[127] A study from New Orleans reported a rise in septic conditions and malignancies (non-Hodgkin lymphoma and Kaposi sarcoma of bone) and a decline in SpA after HAART.[87]

Immune reconstitution inflammatory syndrome

IRIS syndrome results from exacerbation of pre-existing conditions (RA, SLE, and sarcoidosis) or the emergence of new conditions (Graves' disease, SS, diabetes mellitus, ReA, subacute cutaneous lupus, tumid lupus).[128] In IRIS, different pathogenetic mechanisms that occur include: increase in CD4+ cells, CD4+/CD8+ ratio, and cytokines (IL-6, interferon gamma); imbalance of Th1/Th2, expression of CCR-3 and CCR-5 on monocytes and granulocytes.[129] In most cases IRIS occurs 3 to 27 months after HAART.[125] Concurrent occurrence of RA, SLE, and sarcoidosis with HIV is rare. These conditions flare in IRIS as CD4+ counts rise. Several months of HAART has resulted in flares of sarcoidosis.[130,131] In HIV infection, RA is prevented by a mechanism where reduced CD4+ counts and increased Th2 cytokines (IL4, IL-10) suppress TNF and IL-1 production. IRIS results in RA flares.[132] SLE has flared after the institution of HAART.[125,133] SLE and HIV infection have many clinical and laboratory similarities (see **Table 1**).[134,135] Anti–double-stranded-DNA may help in distinction (present in SLE).[134,136] An HIV test may be false-positive in SLE. HIV antigen or nucleic acid detection should be performed.[137] Management of IRIS is usually conservative, since it is self-limited in most instances. HAART can also be continued.

Drug-Induced Conditions

Zidovudine myopathy

Polymyositis, like myopathy, usually occurs in HIV patients after a year of therapy. It is dose-related and duration-dependent. It is associated with myalgia, proximal muscle weakness, and tenderness. It is thought to be due to mitochondrial dysfunction in myocytes. It is reversible on discontinuation of zidovudine (AZT) within 4 to 8 weeks. CK returns to normal and muscle biopsy improves.[138] Light microscopy of muscle biopsy shows "ragged red fibers," when stained with Gomori trichrome stain. This happens because of the toxic effect of AZT on muscle mitochondria and inhibition of muscle mitochondrial DNA polymerase gamma. Electron microscopy shows reduced abnormal mitochondrial DNA in cytochrome-negative muscle fibers. HAART also causes hyperlactatemia, which in turn leads to mitochondrial respiratory chain dysfunction. AZT-induced myopathy can be prevented by uridine supplementation or by stopping the drug.

Rhabdomyolysis

Rhabdomyolysis can be induced by PI. Statin drugs, when combined with PIs, can culminate into acute renal failure and rhabdomyolysis. Indinavir is known to cause several soft tissue problems such as adhesive capsulitis, Dupuytren contracture, temporomandibular joint dysfunction, de Quervain's tendinitis, arthralgias, and paronychia. Nephrolithiasis and alopecia are also observed with indinavir.[139] Indinavir crystals are found in the joint fluid of frozen-shoulder patients and in the urine.[140–143] Either switching to another class of antiretroviral drug or temporarily withdrawing the drug ameliorates the problem. Corticosteroid-induced lipodystrophy is associated with features of metabolic syndrome.[144] PIs also induce insulin resistance, hypertriglyceridemia, and lead to low levels of high-density-lipoprotein cholesterol.[145] These metabolic changes increase cardiovascular risk in HIV patients on PIs.[146]

Gout and hyperuricemia

Didanosine and stavudine are culprits in causing hyperuricemia and gout.[147] These antiretroviral drugs cause mitochondrial toxicity leading to ATP depletion[148] and hyperlactatemia.[149] Hyperuricemia occurs as a result.

Osseous Conditions

Osteoporosis and osteopenia

Osteoporosis and osteopenia bear multifactorial etiologies in HIV infection.[150] PIs,[151] wasting syndrome,[152,153] and lactic acidemia[152] accelerate the bone loss. Dual-energy x-ray absorptiometry showed that osteopenia and osteoporosis occurred commonly in men receiving PIs.[151] Bisphosphonate (alendronate) has shown an increase in bone-mass density in HIV individuals.[154,155]

Osteomalacia

Fanconi syndrome, with phosphate loss, is reported with Tenofovir.[156] Bone scans reveals pseudo-fractures (Looser transformation zones). Phosphate substitution and discontinuation of tenofovir reverses osteomalacia.

Osteonecrosis

HIV-infected individuals exhibit a very high risk of osteonecrosis (ON) compared to the general population. Using MRIs, investigators showed that ON occurred in hip joints at a prevalence of 4.4%.[55] Etiologic factors attributed to ON are PIs, use of high-dose corticosteroids, and APLA syndrome.[157]

Rheumatic diseases differ in their presentation not only in the pre-HAART and HAART eras, but also in different geographic areas as shown in **Table 4**. Genetics, environment, HIV-risk factors, and background diseases (malaria, tuberculosis, and HCV) vary in the clinical vignettes of HIV patients. The practices that lead to HIV infection play a definitive role in type of rheumatic presentations observed in different populations. This is depicted, and some of the larger studies are compared, in **Table 4**.

Newer antiretroviral agents

The CCR5 coreceptor antagonists are on the horizon (maraviroc was approved by the US Food and Drug Administration in 2007). They inhibit fusion of HIV with the host cell by blocking gp120 (viral glycoprotein) and CCR5 chemokine interaction. These drugs have shown greater and more efficient decline in large viral loads—and greater increases in CD4 counts than previous HAART. Intravenous and subcutaneous forms and greater dosing intervals will change the quality of life for HIV patients.[3,158]

Table 4
Geographic comparisons of different HIV-associated rheumatic diseases (large series)

Geographic Area (Number of HIV-Positive Patients)	Rheumatic Manifestations
United States: Texas (458 patients)[9]	DILS (21%), Tenosynovitis or bursitis (19%), ReA/PsA (4%) and other rheumatic conditions occurred with 0.5 to 7% prevalence.
United States: Ohio (31 patients—literature review)[125]	31 patients on HAART and IRIS demonstrated sarcoidosis as most common, then autoimmune thyroid disease, followed by inflammatory arthritis and connective tissue diseases. Most patients did well, except those with thyroid dysfunction-required replacement therapy.
United States (395 patients-longitudinal cohort study)	317 patients revealed homosexual transmission. The study revealed remarkable drop in rheumatic complications with exception of DILS.
United States: Georgia (4000 patients)[34]	30 patients with musculoskeletal infections in HIV-positive patients were studied. IVD use and homosexuality were risk factors. Septic arthritis was the most common, Staphylococcus being the common pathogen. OM was serious infection with high mortality (20%). This affected young individuals with low CD4 counts. Pyomyositis occurred in males with advanced disease. S aureus was common pathogen. Drainage of muscle and antibiotics resulted in full recovery in most cases.
United States: Louisiana (75 patients)[87]	Risk factors were heterosexual transmission, IVD use. Septic complications were the most common. Septic arthritis, bursitis, cellulites, OM, disciitis, and pyomyositis occurred in 31 patients. All patients were on HAART. Bone malignancy (Kaposi sarcoma) occurred in 2 patients.
United States: California (19 patients)[162]	11 of 19 patients had AIDS. S aureus was the most common organism (6 patients), mycobacterial infection (3 patients). There were no fungal infections reported.
African countries: Cameroon(West) (SS) (164 patients)[64]	48% of HIV-positive Cameroonians had severe salivary gland fibrosis and collagen 1 deposits (none of the patients received antiretrovirals). In comparison, only 6% of United States patients had SS with less fibrosis or collagen 1 deposits (76% on antiretroviral therapy)
African countries: Congo-Brazzaville (83 patients)[51]	83 patients with HIV infection were studied. Arthritis (poly-Articular) was the most common and it was different from ReA, PsA, and enteropathic type. HIV-associated arthritis is a separate entity.

(continued on next page)

Table 4
(continued)

Geographic Area (Number of HIV-Positive Patients)	Rheumatic Manifestations
African countries: Zambia (61 patients)[163]	61 of 170 patients tested HIV positive in Zambian population. Arthritis in these patients was polyarticular, involved lower extremities, and was progressive. HIV-associated ReA followed accelerated course, with relapsing nature. They had early erosions, deformities, and chronicity. Uveitis, keratoderma, and onycholysis were very frequent. HLA B*5703 association occurred with SpA. Heterosexual transmission was the common mode for HIV risk.
African countries: Zambia (120 patients)[164]	Young age and high erythrocyte sedimentation rate were indicative of HIV positivity. Enthesitis occurred as early form or as part of Spa in these patients.
African countries: Rwanda (19 patients)[112]	Prevalence of septic arthritis was not statistically different in HIV-positive and HIV-negative patients. It can occur at any stage of HIV infection.
African countries: Durban (South) (35 children)[28]	Arthritis was present in 78% of patients. SpA-like features were found in 34% of children, while only 5% of HIV patients had SpA. Male children predominated in arthritic symptoms. HIV-AIDS occurred in children through vertical transmission.
China (98 patients)[165]	98 patients from Hennan province were studied. Vasculitis (Behçet-like), SS, DILS, lupus-like syndrome were dominating rheumatic conditions. Articular features and Spa were rare. Contaminated blood transfusion (74), sexual transmission (6), and IVD use (2) were modes of HIV infection. Behçet disease is prevalent along Silk Route.
Spain (556 patients)[65]	HIV risks were IVD use (86%), homosexual (9%), heterosexual (3%), hemophilia (0.4%), unknown (2%). Rheumatic disorders occurred in 11%, myalgias/arthralgias (4.5%), skeletal infections (3.6%), myositis (1%), ReA (0.5%). septic arthritis (hip commonly involved) and OM were common in IVD users (*S aureus* in 60% and *Candida albicans* in 20%), whereas ReA occurred in homosexual patients.

(continued on next page)

Table 4
(continued)

Geographic Area (Number of HIV-Positive Patients)	Rheumatic Manifestations
Argentina (89 patients)[12]	HIV-positive patients had 66.1% rheumatic manifestations. Arthralgias (polyarticular), ReA, myalgias, painful articular syndrome were predominant. Homosexuals (53), IVD users (28), hemophiliacs (5), homosexuals plus IVD users (3) were not on AZT therapy. They were compared with 80 HIV-negative patients.
Argentina (270 patients)[160]	21/270 patients presented HIV-associated arthritis. The pattern was of acute onset, short duration, nonerosive, and nonrecurrent, as observed in other viral conditions.
Greece (SS) (77 patients)[63]	77 HIV-positive Greek patients presented with SLS (prevalence 7.79%). Greek adult HIV-positive females had 2.5 times higher prevalence of SLS than normal population. They had hypergammaglobulinemia but no SSA or SSB ANA. HIV risk factors were homosexual or bisexual (58), heterosexual (120), homosexual or IVD user (2).
Mexico (358 patients)[166]	173 pre-HAART and 185 HAART-era HIV-positive patients are compared. Arthralgias or arthritis, myalgias, and ReA declined while ON, TB, and osteoporosis were on the rise.
Thailand (62 patients)[167]	54 of 62 patients had heterosexual transmission of HIV. Myalgias was the most common finding followed by photosensitivity, arthralgias, vasculitis, sicca complex, arthritis, and ReA. Photosensitivity occurred in 1 of 3 and hair loss in 1 of 5 of the patients. The presentation mimicked SLE.
Israel (86 patients)[110]	4 of 86 patients were diagnosed with septic arthritis. They were hemophiliacs and hepatitis B and C infected. *S aureus, Streptococcal pneumoniae* and *Salmonella* are found in septic arthritis when they compared with other 39 cases in the literature. The response to antibiotics is good. High sedimentation rate, fever, and absence of leukocytosis, should lead to suspect infection in a patient who has hemarthrosis.

SUMMARY

Differences in HIV risk factors, geographic regions, genetic factors, and access to therapy have great bearing on rheumatic presentations. As clinicians, we will face chronic and morbid HIV conditions. Geriatric care of HIV patients is on the horizon as more people will have access to newer therapy and mortality is on the decline. Younger HIV patients will be committed to a lifetime of therapy to address bone disease and other chronic problems. In the future, newer agents may steer the clinical scenario in unforeseen directions.

REFERENCES

1. Bruhl H, Cihak J, Stangassinger M, et al. Depletion of CCR5-expressing cells with bispecific antibodies and chemokine toxins: a new strategy in the treatment of chronic inflammatory diseases and HIV. J Immunol 2001;166:2420–6.
2. Crabb BE. Pro and anti-inflammatory cytokines in human immunodeficiency virus infection and acquired immunodeficiency syndrome. Pharmacol Ther 2002;95:295–304.
3. Emmelkamp JM, Rockstroh JK. CCR5 antagonists: comparison of efficacy, side effects, pharmacokinetics and interactions—review of the literature. Eur J Med Res 2007;12(9):409–17.
4. Reinhardt RL, Kang SJ, Liang HE, et al. T helper cell effector fates—who, how, and where? Curr Opin Immunol 2006;18:271–7.
5. Keane NM, Price P, Lee S, et al. An evaluation of serum soluble CD30 levels and serum CD26 (DDPIV) enzyme activity as markers of type 2 and type 1 cytokines in HIV patients receiving highly active antiretroviral therapy. Clin Exp Immunol 2001;126:111–6.
6. Eggena MP, Barugahare B, Jones N, et al. Depletion of regulatory T cells in HIV infection is associated with immune activation. J Immunol 2005;174:4407–14.
7. Zandman-Goddard G, Shoenfield Y. HIV and autoimmunity. Autoimmun Rev 2002;1:329–37.
8. den Uyl D, Van der Horst-Bruinsma IE, Van Agtmael M. Progression of HIV to AIDS: a protective role of HLA-B27. AIDS Rev 2004;6:89–96.
9. Reveille JD. The changing spectrum of rheumatic disease in human immunodeficiency virus infection. Semin Arthritis Rheum 2000;30:147–66.
10. Zimmerman PA, Buckler-White A, Alkhasib G, et al. An inactivating mutation in the gene encoding CC chemokine receptor 5: impact on HIV-1 susceptibility and disease progression. Mol Med 1997;3:23–36.
11. Medina-Rodriguez F, Guzman C, Jara LJ, et al. Rheumatic manifestations in human immunodeficiency virus positive and negative individuals: a study of two populations with similar risk factors. J Rheumatol 1993;20:1880–4.
12. Berman A, Reboredo G, Spindler A, et al. Rheumatic manifestations in populations at risk for HIV infection. The added effect of HIV. J Rheumatol 1991;18:1564–7.
13. Massabki PS, Accetturi C, Nishie JA, et al. Clinical implications of autoantibodies in HIV infection. AIDS 1997;11:1845–50.
14. Asherson RA, Cervera R. Antiphospholipid antibodies and infections. Ann Rheum Dis 2003;62:388–93.
15. Cervera R, Asherson RA, Acevedo ML, et al. Antiphospholipid syndrome associated with infections: clinical and microbiological characteristics in 100 patients. Ann Rheum Dis 2004;63:1312–7.

16. Daar ES, Little S, Pitt J, et al. Diagnosis of primary HIV infection. Los Angeles County Primary HIV infection recruitment network. Ann Intern Med 2001;134: 25–9.

17. Berman A, Espinoza LR, Diaz JD, et al. Rheumatic manifestations of human immunodeficiency virus infection. Am J Med 1988;85:59–64.

18. Pouchot J, Simonpoli AM, Bortolotti V, et al. Painful articular syndrome and human immunodeficiency virus infection. Arch Intern Med 1992;152:646–9.

19. Mody GM, Parke FA, Reveille JD. Articular manifestations of human immunodeficiency virus infection. Best Pract Res Clin Rheumatol 2003;17:265–87.

20. Rowe IF, Forster SM, Sefert MH. Rheumatological lesions in individuals with human immunodeficiency virus infections. QJM 1989;73:1167–84.

21. Rynes RI, Goldberg DL, Digiacomo R, et al. Acquiredimmunodeficiency syndrome-associated arthritis. Am J Med 1998;84:810–6.

22. Espinoza LR, Aguilar JL, Espinoza CG, et al. HIV-associated arthropathy. HIV antigen demonstration in the synovial membrane. J Rheumatol 1990;17: 1195–201.

23. Njobvu P, McGill P, Kerr H, et al. Spondyloarthropathy and human immunodeficiency virus infection in Zambia. J Rheumatol 1998;25:1553–98.

24. Ornstein MH, Sperber K. The anti-inflammatory and antiviral effects of hydroxychloroquine in two patients with acquired immunodeficiency syndrome and active inflammatory arthritis. Arthritis Rheum 1996;39:157–61.

25. Adebajo AO, Mijiyawa M. The role of sulfasalazine in African patients with HIV-associated seronegative arthritis. Clin Exp Rheumatol 1998;16:629.

26. Kellner H, Fuessl HS, Herzer P. Seronegative spondyloarthropathies in HIV-infected patients: further evidence of uncommon features. Rheumatol Int 1994;13:211–3.

27. Weeratunge NC, Roldan J, Anstead GM. Jaccoud arthropathy: a rarity in the spectrum of HIV-associated arthropathy. Am J Med 2004;328:351–3.

28. Chinniah K, Mody GM, Bhimma R, et al. Arthritis in association with human immunodeficiency virus infection in black African children: causal or coincidental? Rheumatology 2005;44:915–20.

29. Calabrese LH, Kelley DM, Myers A, et al. Rheumatic manifestations and human immunodeficiency virus infection. The influence of clinical and laboratory variables in a longitudinal cohort study. Arthritis Rheum 1991;34:257–63.

30. Espinoza LR, Jara LJ, Espinoza CG, et al. There is an association between human immunodeficiency virus infection and spondyloarthropathies. Rheum Dis Clin North Am 1992;18:257–66 [abstract].

31. Reveille JD, Conant MA, Duvic M, et al. Human immunodeficiency virus associated psoriasis, psoriatic arthritis and Reiter's syndrome; a disease continuum? Arthritis Rheum 1990;33:1574–8.

32. Winchester R, Brancato L, Itescu S, et al. Implications from the occurrence of Reiter's syndrome and related disorders in association with advanced HIV infection. Scand J Rheumatol 1988;74:89–93.

33. Cuellar ML, Espinoza LR. Rheumatic manifestations of HIV-AIDS. Baillieres Best Pract Res Clin Rheumatol 2000;14:579–93.

34. Vessi Lopolous D, Challassani P, Jurado RL, et al. Musculoskeletal infections in patients with human immunodeficiency virus infection. Medicine 1997;76: 284–94.

35. Keat A. HIV and overlap with Reiter's syndrome. Baillieres Clin Rheumatol 1994; 8:363–77.

36. Duvic M, Johnson TM, Rapini RP, et al. Acquired immunodeficiency syndrome associated psoriasis and Reiter's syndrome. Arch Dermatol 1987;123: 1622–32.
37. Obuch ML, Maurer TA, Becker B, et al. Psoriasis and human immunodeficiency virus infection. J Am Acad Dermatol 1992;27:667–73.
38. Sugiyama H, Gyulai R, Toichi E, et al. Dysfunctional blood and target tissue CD4+CD25+ high regulatory T cells in psoriasis: mechanism underlying unrestrained pathogenetic effector T cell proliferation. J Immunol 2005;174:164–73.
39. Weiss L, Doukova-Petrini V, Caccavelli L, et al. Human immunodeficiency virus driven expansion of CD4+CD25+ regulatory T cells which suppress HIV specific CD4 T cells' responses in HIV-infected patients. Blood 2004;104: 3249–56.
40. Tourne L, Durez P, Van Vooren JP, et al. Alleviation of HIV-associated psoriasis and psoriatic arthritis with cyclosporine. J Am Acad Dermatol 1997;37:501–2.
41. Giuseppe VLDS, Stefano S, Giuliano S. Clinical improvement of psoriasis in an AIDS patient effectively treated with combination antiretroviral therapy. Scand J Infect Dis 2006;38(1):74–5.
42. Sellam J, Bouvard B, Masson C, et al. Use of infliximab to treat psoriatic arthritis in HIV-positive patients. Joint Bone Spine 2007;74:197–200.
43. Cepada EJ, William FM, Ishimori ML. The use of anti-tumor necrosis factor therapy in HIV-positive individuals with rheumatic diseases. Ann Rheum Dis 2008;67:710–2.
44. Linardaki G, Katsarau O, Ionnidou P, et al. Effective etanercept treatment for psoriatic arthritis complicating concomittant human immunodeficiency virus and hepatitis C virus infection. J Rheumatol 2007;34:1353–5.
45. Solomon G, Broncato L, Winchester R. An approach to the HIV-positive patient with a spondyloarthropathic disease. Rheum Dis Clin North Am 1991;17:43–59.
46. Belz J, Breneman DL, Nordlund JJ. Successful treatment of a patient with Reiter's syndrome and acquired immunodeficiency syndrome with etretinate. J Am Acad Dermatol 1989;20:898–903.
47. Williams HC, Vivier AW. Etretinate and AIDS-related Reiter's disease. Br J Dermatol 1991;124:389–92.
48. Spuber K, Kalb TH, Stecher V, et al. Inhibition of human immunodeficiency virus type 1 replication by hydrochloroquine in T cells and monocytes. AIDS Res Hum Retroviruses 1993;9:91–8.
49. Masson C, Chennebault JM, Leclech C. Is HIV infection a contraindication to the use of methotrexate in psoriatic arthritis? J Rheumatol 1995;22:2191.
50. Lopez-Lauea C, Njobvu PD, Gonzales S, et al. The HLA B*5703 allele confers susceptibility to the development of spondyloarthropathies in Zambian human immunodeficiency virus-infected patients with slow progression to acquired immunodeficiency syndrome. Arthritis Rheum 2005;52:275–9.
51. Ntsiba H, Lamini N. Is inflammatory disease in HIV-infected patients a form of spondyloarthropathy? Joint Bone Spine 2004;71:300–2.
52. Williams FM, Cohen PR, Jumshyd J, et al. Prevalence of the diffuse infiltrative lymphocytosis syndrome among human immunodeficiency virus type 1-positive outpatients. Arthritis Rheum 1998;41:863–8.
53. Rosenberg ZS, Jaffe DA, Itescu S. Spectrum of salivary gland disease in HIV-infected patients: characterization with GA-67 citrate imaging. Radiology 1992;184:761–4.

54. Schuval SJ, O'Reilly ME, Bonagura VR. Increased frequency of HLA Dr 11 in pediatric human immunodeficiency virus-associated parotid gland enlargement. Clin Diagn Lab Immunol 1997;4:258–60.

55. Olive A, Salavert A, Manriquez M, et al. Parotid lipomatosis in HIV-positive patients: a new clinical disorder associated with protease inhibitors. Ann Rheum Dis 1998;37:691–5.

56. Itescu S, Broncato LJ, Buxbaum J, et al. A diffuse infiltrative CD8 lymphocytosis syndrome in human immunodeficiency virus (HIV) infection. A host immune response associated with HLA-DR5. Ann Intern Med 1991;112:3–10.

57. Kazi S, Cohen PR, Williams F, et al. The diffuse infiltrative lymphocytosis syndrome. Clinical and immunological features in 35 patients. AIDS 1996;10:385–91.

58. Itescu S, Winchester R. Diffuse infiltrative lymphocytosis syndrome. A disorder occurring in human immunodeficiency virus 1 infection that may present as sicca syndrome. Rheum Dis Clin North Am 1972;18:683–97.

59. Itescu S, Rose S, Dwyer E, et al. Certain HLA DR 5 and DR6 major histocompatibility complex class 11 alleles are associated with a CD8 lymphocytotic host response to human immunodeficiency virus type 1 characterized by low lymphocyte viral strain heterogeneity and slow disease progression. Proc Natl Acad Sci U S A 1949;91:11472–6.

60. Itescu S, Dalton J, Zhang HZ, et al. Tissue infiltration in a Cd8 lymphocytosis syndrome associated with human immunodeficiency virus type 1 infection has the phenotypic appearance of an antigenically driven response. J Clin Invest 1993;91:2216–25.

61. Itescu S, Simonelli PF, Winchester RJ, et al. Human immunodeficiency virus type 1 strains in the lungs of infected individual evolve independently from those in peripheral blood and are highly conserved in C-terminal region of the envelope V3 loop. Proc Natl Acad Sci U S A 1994;91:11378–82.

62. Uccini S, Riva E, Antonelli G, et al. The benign cystic lymphoepithelial lesion of the parotid gland is a viral reservoir in HIV type 1-infected patients. AIDS Res Hum Retroviruses 1999;15:1339–44.

63. Kordossis T, Paikos S, Aroni K, et al. Prevalence of Sjogren's-like syndrome in a cohort of HIV-1 positive patients: descriptive pathology and immunopathology. Br J Rheumatol 1998;37:691–5.

64. McArthur CP, Africa CW, Castellani WJ, et al. Salivary gland disease in HIV/AIDS and primary Sjogren's syndrome; analysis of collagen 1 distribution and histopathology in America and African patients. J Oral Pathol Med 2003;32:544–51.

65. Munoz FS, Cardenal B, Balsa A, et al. Rheumatic manifestations in 556 patients with human immunodeficiency virus infection. Semin Arthritis Rheum 1991;21: 30–9.

66. Masanes F, Pedrol E, Grau JM, et al. Symptomatic myopathies in HIV-1 infected patients untreated with antiretroviral agents—a clinico-pathological study of 30 consecutive patients. Clin Neuropathol 1996;15:221–5.

67. Illa I, Nath A, Dalakas M. Immunocytochemical and virological characteristics of HIV-associated inflammatory myopathies. Similarities with seronegative polymyositis. Ann Neurol 1991;29:474–81.

68. Dalakas MC, Pezeshkpour GH, Gravell M, et al. Polymyositis associated with AIDS retroviruses. JAMA 1986;256:2381–3.

69. Leon-Monzon M, Lamperth L, Dalakais MC. Search for HIV proviral DNA and amplified sequences in the muscle biopsies of patients with HIV polymyositis. Muscle Nerve 1993;16:408–13.

70. Cuellar ML. HIV infection-associated inflammatory musculoskeletal disorders. Rheum Dis Clin North Am 1998;24:403–21.
71. Seidman R, Peress NS, Nuovo G. In situ detection of polymerase chain reaction-amplified HIV-1 nucleic acids in skeletal muscle in patients with myopathy. Mod Pathol 1994;7:369–75.
72. Chariot P, Dubreuil-Lemaire ML, Zhou JY, et al. Muscle involvement in human immunodeficiency virus infected patients is associated with marked selenium deficiency. Muscle Nerve 1997;20:386–9.
73. Johnson RW, Williams FM, Kasi S, et al. Human immunodeficiency virus-associated polymyositis; a longitudinal study of outcome. Arthritis Rheum 2003;49:172–8.
74. Attarian S, Mallecourt C, Donnet A, et al. Myositis in infiltrative lymphocytosis syndrome. Clinicopathological observations and treatment. Neuromuscul Disord 2004;14:740–3.
75. Gresh JP, Aguilar JL, Espinoza LR. Human immunodeficiency virus infection-associated dermatomyositis. J Rheumatol 1989;16:1397–8.
76. Cupler EJ, Leon-Monzon M, Miller J, et al. Inclusion body myositis in HIV-1 and HTLV-1 infected patients. Brain 1996;119:1887–93.
77. Dalakas MC, Pezeshkpour GH, Flaherty M. Progressive nemaline (rod) myopathy associated with HIV infection. N Engl J Med 1987;317:1602–3.
78. Feinberg DM, Spiro AJ, Weidenheim KM. Distinct light microscopic changes in human immunodeficiency virus associated nemaline myopathy. Neurology 1998;50:592–631.
79. Gonatas NK. The fine structure of the rod-like bodies in nemaline myopathy and their relation to the Z-discs. J Neuropathol Exp Neurol 1966;25:409–21.
80. Jocusch BM, Veidman H, Griffiths W, et al. Immuno-flourescence microscopy of a myopathy: alpha actinin is a major constituent of nemaline rods. Exp Cell Res 1980;127:409–20.
81. Dwyer BA, Mayer RF, Lee SC. Progressive nemaline rod myopathy as a presentation of human immunodeficiency virus. Arch Neurol 1992;49:440.
82. Chariot P, Ruet E, Authier FJ, et al. Acute rhabdomyolysis in patients infected by human immunodeficiency virus. Neurology 1994;44:1692–6.
83. Campa A, Yang Z, Lai S, et al. HIV-related wasting in HIV-infected drug users in the era of highly active antiretroviral therapy. Clin Infect Dis 2005;41:1179–85.
84. Abouzahir A, Bouchama R, Azennang M, et al. Tropical pyomyositis simulating septic arthritis in AIDS patients—two cases. Med Trop (Mars) 2004;34:672–4.
85. Espinoza LR, Berman A. Soft tissues and osteo-articular infections in HIV-infected patients and other immunodeficient states. Baillieres Best Pract Res Clin Rheumatol 1999;13:115–28.
86. Ansaloni L, Acaye GL, Re M. High HIV sero-prevalence among patients with pyomyositis in Northern Uganda. Trop Med Int Health 1996;1:210–6.
87. Marquez J, Restrepo CS, Candia L, et al. Human immunodeficiency virus associated rheumatic diseases in the HAART era. J Rheumatol 2004;31:741–6.
88. Simms RW, Zerbini CAF, Ferrate N, et al. Fibromyalgia syndrome in patients infected with human immunodeficiency virus. Am J Med 1992;92:368–74.
89. Gherardi R, Belec L, Mhiri C, et al. The spectrum of vasculitis in human immunodeficiency virus infected patients. A clinico-pathologic evaluation. Arthritis Rheum 1993;36:1164–74.
90. Font C, Miro O, Pedrol E, et al. Polyarteritis nodosa in human immunodeficiency virus infection: report of four cases and review of the literature. Br J Rheumatol 1996;35:796–9.

91. Bardin T, Gaudouen C, Kuntz D, et al. Necrotizing vasculitis in human immuno-deficiency virus (HIV) infection. Arthritis Rheum 1987;30:S105.

92. Cupps TR, Fauci AS. Systemic necrotizing vasculitis of the polyarteritis nodosa group. In: Smith LH, editor. Major problems in internal medicine, vol. 14. Phila-delphia: WB Saunders; 1981. p. 26–9

93. Nieuwhof CM, Damoiseaux J, Cohen Tervaert JW. Successful treatment of cere-bral vasculitis in an HIV-positive patient with anti-CD25 treatment. Ann Rheum Dis 2006;65:1677–8.

94. Javed MA, Sheppard MN, Pepper J. Aortic root dilation secondary to giant cell aortitis in a human immunodeficiency virus-positive patient. Eur J Cardiothorac Surg 2006;30:400–1.

95. Marks C, Kuskov S. Pattern of arterial aneurysms in acquired immunodeficiency disease. World J Surg 1995;19:127–37.

96. Chetty R, Batitang S, Nair R. Large artery vasculopathy in HIV-positive patients: another vasculitis enigma. Hum Pathol 2000;31:374–9.

97. Shingadia D, Das L, Klein-Gitelman M, et al. Takayasu's arteritis in a human immunodeficiency virus-infected adolescent. Clin Infect Dis 1999;29:458–9.

98. Bayrou O, Phlippoteau C, Antigou C, et al. Adult Kawasaki syndrome associated with HIV infection and anti cardiolipin antibodies. J Am Acad Dermatol 1993;29: 663–4.

99. Valez AP. Kawasaki-like syndrome possibly associated with immune reconstitu-tion syndrome in an HIV-positive patient. AIDS Read 2006;16:464–6.

100. Zhang S, Ma S. Epidemiology of HIV in China. Br Med J 2002;324:803–4.

101. Branagan TH III. Retroviral-associated vasculitis of the nervous system. Neurol Clin 1997;15:927–44.

102. Calabrese LH, Esyes M, Yen-Liebermann B, et al. Systemic vasculitis in associ-ation with human immunodeficiency virus infection. Arthritis Rheum 1989;32: 569–76.

103. Katsetos CD, Fincke JE, Legido A, et al. Angiocentric CD 3+ T cell infiltrates in human immunodeficiency virus type 1-associated central nervous system disease in children. Clin Diagn Lab Immunol 1996;6:105–14.

104. Garcia-Garcia JA, Marcias J, Castellanos V, et al. Necrotizing granulomatous vasculitis in advanced HIV infection. J Infect 2003;47:333–5.

105. Barbaro G, Barbarini G, Pellicelli AM. HIV-associated coronary arteritis in a patient with focal myocardial infarction. N Engl J Med 2001;23:1799–800.

106. Fabris P, Tositti G, Giordani MT, et al. Prevalence and clinical significance of circulating cryoglobulins in HIV-positive patients with and without co-infection with hepatitis c virus. J Med Virol 2003;69:339–43.

107. Kosmas N, Kantos A, Panayiota Kopoulos G, et al. Decreased prevalence of mixed cryoglobulinemia in the HAART era among HIV-positive, HCV-negative patients. J Med Virol 2006;78:1257–61.

108. Ventura G, Gasparani G, Lucia MB, et al. Osteo-articular bacterial infections are rare in HIV-infected patients. 14 cases found among 4023 HIV-infected patients. Acta Orthop Scand 1997;68:554–8.

109. Munoz-Fernandez S, Maciaus A, Pantoja L, et al. Osteoarticular infection in intravenous drug abusers: influence of HIV infection and differences with non-drug abusers. Ann Rheum Dis 1993;53:570–4.

110. Barzilai A, Varon D, Martinowitz U, et al. Characteristics of septic arthritis in human immunodeficiency virus-infected hemophiliacs versus other risk groups. Rheumatology 1999;38:139–42.

111. Ross JJ, Shamsuddin H. Sternoclavicular septic arthritis: review of 180 cases. Medicine 2004;83:139–48.

112. Saraux A, Taelman H, Blanche P, et al. HIV infection as a risk factor for septic arthritis. Br J Rheumatol 1997;36:333–7.

113. Saraux A, Blanche P, Taelman H, et al. Does septic arthritis occur in patients infected with the human immunodeficiency virus? Rev Rhum 1994;61:317–21.

114. Dubost JJ, Fis I, Deuis P, et al. Polyarticular septic arthritis. Medicine 1993;72: 296–310.

115. Louthrenoo W. Musculoskeletal manifestations of HIV infection in Thailand. An analysis of 100 cases. J Clin Rheumatol 1997;3:258–68.

116. Buskila D, Tenenbaum J. Septic bursitis in human immunodeficiency virus infection. J Rheumatol 1989;16:1374–6.

117. Hirsch R, Miller SM, Kazi S, et al. Human immunodeficiency virus-associated atypical mycobacterial skeletal infections. Semin Arthritis 1996;25:347–56.

118. Belzunegui J, Sauststeban M, Gorordo M, et al. Osteoarticular mycobacterial infections in patients with the human immunodeficiency virus. Clin Exp Rheumatol 2004;22:343–5.

119. Restrepo CS, Lemos DF, Gordillo H, et al. Imaging findings in musculoskeletal complications of AIDS. Radiographics 2004;24:1029–49.

120. Pouchot J, Vinceneux P, Barge J, et al. Tuberculous polymyositis in HIV infection. Am J Med 1990;89:250–1.

121. Louthrenoo W, Mahanuphab P, Scurguanmitra P, et al. Trichinosis mimicking polymyositis in a patient with human immunodeficiency virus infection. Br J Rheumatol 1993;32:1025–6.

122. Manfredi R, Mastroni A, Coronado OV, et al. Hyperuricemia and progression of HIV disease. J Acquir Immune Defic Syndr Hum Retroviral 1996;12:318–9.

123. Disla E, Stein S, Acevedo M, et al. Gouty arthritis in acquired immunodeficiency syndrome. An unusual but aggressive case. Arthritis Rheum 1995;38:570–2.

124. Manfredi R, Chiodo F. Longitudinal assessment of serum urate levels as a marker of HIV disease progression. Int J STD AIDS 1998;9:433–4.

125. Calabrese L, Kirchner E, Shrestha E. Rheumatic complications of human immunodeficiency virus (HIV) infection in the era of highly active antiretroviral therapy (HAART): emergence of a new syndrome of immune reconstitution and changing pattern of disease. Semin Arthritis Rheum 2005;35:166–74.

126. Basu D, Williams FM, Aln CW, et al. Changing spectrum of the diffuse infiltrative lymphocytosis syndrome. Arthritis Rheum 2006;55:466–72.

127. Mastroianni A. Emergence of Sjogren's syndrome in AIDS patients during highly active antiretroviral therapy. AIDS 2004;18:1349–52.

128. Chamberlain AJ, Hollowwood K, Turner RJ. Tumid lupus erythematosus occurring following highly active antiretroviral therapy for HIV infection: a manifestation of immune restoration. J Am Acad Dermatol 2004;51:161–5.

129. French MA, Price P. Immune restoration disease in HIV-infected patients after antiretroviral therapy. Clin Infect Dis 2001;32:325–6.

130. Foulon G, Wislez M, Maccache JM, et al. Sarcoidosis in HIV-infected patients in the era of highly active antiretroviral therapy. Clin Infect Dis 2004;38:418–25.

131. Gomez V, Smith PR, Burack J, et al. Sarcoidosis after antiretroviral therapy in a patient with acquired immunodeficiency syndrome. Clin Infect Dis 2000;31: 1278–80.

132. Lapadula G, Iannone F, Covelli M, et al. Interleukin-10 in rheumatoid arthritis. Clin Exp Rheumatol 1995;15:629–32.

133. Diri E, Lipsky PE, Bergreu RE. Emergence of systemic lupus erythematosus presenting with features suggestive of human immunodefficiency virus infection. J Rheumatol 2000;27:27111–4.

134. Muller S, Richalet P, Laurent-Crawford A, et al. Autoantibodies typical of nonorganspecific autoimmune diseases in HIV-seropositive patients. AIDS 1992;6:933–42.

135. Malin JK, Patel NJ. Arthropathy and HIV infection. A muddle of mimicry. Postgrad Med 1993;93(8):143–50.

136. Kopelman RH, Zolla-Pazner S. Association of human immunodeficiency virus infection and autoimmune phenomenon. Am J Med 1988;84:82–4.

137. Esteva MH, Blasini AM, Ogly D, et al. False positive results for antibody to HIV in two men with systemic lupus erythematosus. Ann Rheum Dis 1992;51:1071–3.

138. Bessen LJ, Greene JB, Louie E, et al. Severe polymyositis-like syndrome associated with zidovudine therapy of AIDS and ARC. N Engl J Med 1988;318:708.

139. Florence E, Shrooten W, Verdonck K, et al. Rheumatological complications associated with the use of indinavir and other protease inhibitors. Ann Rhum Dis 2002;61:82–4.

140. Leone J, Beguinot I, Dehlinger V, et al. Adhesive capsulitis of the shoulder induced by protease inhibitor therapy. Three new cases. Rev Rhum Engl Ed 1998;65:800–1.

141. Brooks JI, Gallicano K, Garber G, et al. Acute mono-arthritis complicating therapy with indinavir. AIDS 2000;14:2064–5.

142. Lebrecht D, Deveaud C, Beauvoit B, et al. Uridine supplementation antagonizes zidovudine induced mitochondrial myopathy and hyperlactatemia. Arthritis Rheum 2008;58:318–26.

143. Masanes F, Barriento A, Cebrian M, et al. Clinical, histological and molecular reversibility of zidovudine myopathy. J Neurol Sci 1998;159:226–8.

144. Fordet L, Cabame J, Kettaneh A, et al. Corticosteroid-induced lipodystrophy is associated with features of the metabolic syndrome. Rheumatology 2007;46:1102–6.

145. Carr A, Samaras K, Thorisdottin A, et al. Diagnosis, prediction and natural course of HIV-1 protease inhibitor associated lipodystrophy, hyperlipidemia and diabetes mellitus; a cohort study. Lancet 1999;353:2093–9.

146. Friis-Moller N, Sabin CA, Weber R, et al. Combination antiretroviral therapy and the risk of mycobacterial infarction. N Engl J Med 2003;349:1993–2003.

147. Walker UA, Hoffman C, Enters M, et al. High serum urate in HIV-infected persons: the choice of the antiretroviral drug matters. AIDS 2006;20:1556–8.

148. Mineo I, Tarui S. Myogenic hyperuricemia. What can we learn from metabolic myopathies? Muscle Nerve 1993;3:575–81.

149. Enomoto A, Kimura H, Chiroungdue A, et al. Molecular identification of a renal urate anion exchange that regulates blood urate levels. Nature 2002;417:447–52.

150. Glesby MJ. Bone disorders in human immunodeficiency virus infection. Clin Infect Dis 2003;37(Suppl 2):91–5.

151. Tebas P, Powderly WG, Claxton S, et al. Accelerated bone loss in HIV-infected patients receiving potent antiretroviral therapy. AIDS 2000;14:63–7.

152. Carr A. Osteopenia in HIV infection. AIDS Clin Care 2001;13(8):281–91.

153. Fairfield WP, Finkelstein JS, Klibanski A, et al. Osteopenia in eugonadal men with acquired immune deficiency syndrome: wasting syndrome. J Clin Endocrinol Metab 2001;86:2020–6.

154. Negredo E, Martinez-Lopez E, Paredes R, et al. Reversal of HIV 1-associated osteoporosis with once weekly alendronate. AIDS 2005;19:343–5.

155. Guaraldi G, Orlando G, Madeddu G, et al. Alendronate reduces bone resorption in HIV-associated osteopenia/osteoporosis. HIV Clin Trials 2004;5:269–77.
156. Verheist D, Mange M, Meyland J, et al. Fanconi syndrome and renal failure induced by tenofovir: a first case report. Am J Kidney Dis 2002;40:1331–3.
157. Glesby MJ, Hoover DR, Vaamonde CM. Osteonecrosis in patients infected with human immunodeficiency virus: a case control study. J Infect Dis 2001;184: 519–23.
158. Brown A. Anti-CCR5 monoclonal antibody has strong anti-HIV activity. J Infect Dis 2008;198:1345–52.
159. Buskila D, Gladman DD, Langevitz P, et al. Rheumatologic manifestations of infection with the human immunodeficiency virus (HIV). Clin Exp Rheumatol 1990;8:563–73.
160. Berman A, Cahn P, Perez H, et al. Human immunodeficiency virus infection-associated arthritis: clinical characteristics. J Rheumatol 1999;26:1158–62.
161. Chen F, Day SL, Metcalfe RA, et al. Characteristics of autoimmune thyroid disease occurring as a late complication of immune reconstitution in patients with advanced human immunodeficiency virus (HIV) disease. Medicine 2005; 84:98–106.
162. Patzakis MJ. Septic arthritis in patients with human immunodeficiency virus. Clin Orthop Relat Res 2006;451:46–9.
163. Njobvu P, McGill P. Human immunodeficiency virus-related reactive arthritis in Zambia. J Rheumatol 2005;32:1299–304.
164. Njobvu P, McGill P. Soft tissue rheumatic lesions and HIV infection in Zambians. J Rheumatol 2006;33:2493–7.
165. Zhang X, Li H, Li T, et al. Distinctive rheumatic manifestations in 98 patients with human immunodeficiency virus infection in China. J Rheumatol 2007;34:1760–4.
166. Medina F, Perez Saleme L, Fuentes J, et al. Impact of highly active antiretroviral therapy on rheumatic manifestations in human immunodeficiency virus-infected patients. Arthritis Rheum 2004;48:S185.
167. Kulthanan K, Jiamton S, Omcharoen V, et al. Autoimmune and rheumatic manifestations and antinuclear antibody study in HIV-infected Thai patients. Int J Dermatol 2002;41:417–22.

Latent Infection and Tuberculosis Disease in Rheumatoid Arthritis Patients

Eduardo Acevedo-Vásquez, MD, DR[a,b,*], Darío Ponce de León, MD[c],
Rocío Gamboa-Cárdenas, MD[b]

KEYWORDS

- Tuberculosis • Latent tuberculosis infection
- Rheumatoid arthritis • Biologic therapy • Inmmunosenescence

Even though it is likely that tuberculosis emerged in the American continent approximately 10,000 years ago coinciding with the presence of its first inhabitants, archeologic evidence of tuberculosis dates back only to the past 2000 years.[1] These findings have been confirmed by DNA, bacteriologic, and anatomopathologic studies of suspicious tissues that have been adequately preserved in mummy tissues from the southern desertic area in Peru.[2] As it is today, the disease likely was a public health problem, its onset and dissemination occurring in the presence of malnutrition and crowded conditions resulting from multiple socioeconomic problems not uncommon in the face of natural disasters and wars.[1,2]

EPIDEMIOLOGY OF LATENT TUBERCULOSIS INFECTION AND TUBERCULOSIS DISEASE

The World Health Organization (WHO) estimates that approximately one third of the world's population, or approximately 2 billion people, are latently infected with *Mycobacterium tuberculosis,* the causative agent of tuberculosis. In 2006 the WHO reported a global incidence of 139 per 100,000 population, indicating that more than 1 million people develop active tuberculosis disease every year and approximately 2 million die as a result. Approximately every 20 minutes, 64 people die of tuberculosis, 320 fall ill with it, and an astounding 3200 become infected with *M tuberculosis*. The rates

[a] School of Medicine, Universidad Nacional Mayor de San Marcos, Lima, Perú
[b] Department of Rheumatology, Guillermo Almenara Hospital, 111 Buen Retiro Street, Lima 41, Perú
[c] Division of Internal Medicine, Guillermo Almenara Hospital, EsSALUD, 800 Grau Avenue, Lima 13, Perú
* Corresponding author. Department of Rheumatology, Guillermo Almenara Hospital, 111 Buen Retiro Street, Lima 41, Perú.
E-mail address: edacvas@terra.com.pe (E. Acevedo-Vásquez).

Rheum Dis Clin N Am 35 (2009) 163–181
doi:10.1016/j.rdc.2009.03.008
0889-857X/09/$ – see front matter © 2009 Elsevier Inc. All rights reserved.

of incidence around the world vary from a low of 4.4 per 100,000 in the United States to a high of 363 per 100,000 inhabitants in Africa. In Latin America the majority of countries exhibit intermediate or lower rates than the global prevalence.[3–5]

IMMUNE RESPONSE IN TUBERCULOSIS INFECTION
The Life Cycle of Mycobacterium tuberculosis in Infected Individuals

The immune response mounted to the infection generally is successful in containing, although not eliminating, the pathogen; thus, the infection becomes latent. M tuberculosis becomes dormant, residing in granulomas; as a result, infected individuals are asymptomatic and noninfectious.[6] This latency often extends throughout a lifetime. Reactivation of latent tuberculosis infections (LTBIs), however, can occur in response to perturbations of the immune response, with active tuberculosis ensuing. Thus, a constant battle between the host (which tries to contain the infection) and the mycobacterium (which tries to reactivate and replicate) is waged.[7]

Role of Cytokines in Granuloma Formation and Containment of Mycobacterium tuberculosis

An effective host response against M tuberculosis involves the coordinated action of the innate and adaptive immunologic responses. As the mycobacteria arrive in the lung, macrophages and dendritic cells readily engulf them. An important first step is the recruitment of intravascular immune cells to the proximity of the infective focus. This process is controlled by adhesion molecules and chemokines. Chemokines, such as chemokine (C-C motif) receptor 2 (CCR2), CCR3, CCR4, and CCR5, contribute to the formation and maintenance of granuloma in tuberculosis infection,[8] recruiting macrophages, dendritic cells, and others to the infected lungs.[9] The influx of macrophages and formation of the granuloma occurs at sites of infection, and some investigators believe that an identical type of reaction (delayed-type hypersensitivity reaction) occurs in the skin after the injection of purified protein derivative (PPD).[10] In most individuals, however, this initial innate immune response is insufficient to control mycobacterial replication. As a result, the infection spreads to regional lymph nodes and transient hematogenous dissemination commonly occurs before the infection ultimately is contained by an adaptive immune response, composed of $\gamma\delta$T-cells and CD4+ and CD8+ T-cells.[11] Tumor necrosis factor α (TNF-α) contributes to granuloma formation and maintenance by regulation of chemokines or chemokine receptors. M tuberculosis, alternatively, induces an increase in mRNA for many proinflammatory genes, such as interferon-γ (IFN-γ), TNF-α, lymphotoxin, interleukin (IL) 2, and IL-1.

The Current Role of Tumor Necrosis Factor α and Other Cytokines in the Defense Against Mycobacterium tuberculosis

Different cytokines participate in the containment of M tuberculosis, which in LTBI is surrounded by macrophages and dendritic cells within the granuloma formed for this purpose. In mice that lack the TNFRp55 receptor, granuloma formation is delayed and inefficient[12]; alternatively, knockout mice for TNF-α have shown a diminished survival when affected with M tuberculosis and, in autopsies, disseminated forms of tuberculosis with abscesses throughout the lungs, liver, spleen, and kidneys were found. Using histopathology, many necrotic areas with acid-alcohol resistant bacilli were found; mature granulomas were not found in the areas of necrosis.[13] In the late phases of the disease, when the granuloma has been established, its maintenance also is a TNF-α–dependent action.[14] IFN-γ is an extracellular pro-inflammatory cytokine that activates the innate and adaptive arms of the immune system. Its effects include stimulating the production of other pro-inflammatory cytokines, such as TNF-α and IL-12; inhibiting the production of anti-inflammatory cytokines, such as IL-4; upregulating major histocompatibility complex class II expression on the surface of macrophages and other antigen-presenting cells; stimulating immunoglobulin production by B lymphocytes; promoting differentiation of T-helper lymphocytes into the Th1 phenotype; and promoting apoptosis of anti-inflammatory Th2 lymphocytes.[15]

IFN-γ leads to the modulation of nuclear gene expression via the Janus kinase–signal transducer and activator of transcription signaling pathway. The functions of these genes include promotion of major histocompatibility complex class I and II expression, modulation of leukocyte-epithelial cell interactions, and promotion of inflammatory cytokine synthesis and free radical formation.[16] These functions are key aspects of the innate and acquired immune responses to most microbial pathogens and are pertinent as systemic defenses against mycobacterial disease.[17]

Recent evidence suggests that IL-17–producing T-helper lymphocyte cells (so-called Th17 cells) participate in protection against tuberculosis, although their role is less clear.[18] Probably they provide a first line of defense against *M tuberculosis* and participate in the early steps of granuloma formation.[19] IL-6 and IL-23 are secreted to induce differentiation of precursor cells to Th17 cells and to elicit an acute phase response. The role of IL-6 in the protection against mycobacterial infections has not been elucidated. Studies in mice have shown that a decreased production of IL-6 results in the exacerbation of infection by *M avium*[20] while at the same time conditioning a reduced production of IFN-γ[21]; therefore, it is reasonable to hypothesize that IL-6 plays a protective role in infections by mycobacteria. Despite the absence IL-6, however, it has been shown that it is possible to contain and control bacterial growth and mount a satisfactory immune response; thus, some investigators consider IL-6 a nonessential cytokine in the protection against *M tuberculosis* infection.[22]

Although the regulation of mycobacterial infections typically is attributed to the CD4+Th1 cells of the cellular immune response, and little is known about the contribution of the humoral response, several recent studies suggest that peripheral B cells are important in host defense against mycobacteria. In a murine tuberculosis model, B cells were an important constituent of formed granulomas and B-cell knockout mice failed to contain tuberculosis infection and died.[23]

The protective and pathologic response to *M tuberculosis* is complex and multifaceted, involving many components of the immune system. Current biologic agents and innovative agents that are in the development phase for the treatment of rheumatoid arthritis (RA) have as a target the main host mechanisms of protection against tuberculosis, therefore are likely to increase patients' susceptibility to mycobacterial disease or to the reactivation of LTBI.

TUBERCULOSIS AND RHEUMATOID ARTHRITIS

New drug classes have been developed over the past 10 years based on human or chimeric antibodies against cytokines or receptors with pivotal roles in the inflammatory pathways of immune-mediated inflammatory disease. These agents are collectively referred to as *biologics*. Anti–TNF-α agents carry the largest infection risk of all the biologics, predisposing patients to mycobacterial infections. This is not surprising, as TNF has an important role in granuloma formation and maintenance, which is essential for host defense against mycobacteria. Among the anti-TNF agents, infliximab and adalimumab are associated with a greater risk for infection than etanercept.[24]

Risk for Tuberculosis Infection Before the Availability of Biologic Therapy

The incidence of tuberculosis among patients who have RA and are not on biologic therapy is controversial and studies performed to this end are few and difficult to compare. In Spain, Carmona and colleagues found a risk for RA of 4.13 in patients who had RA as compared with that in the general population (adjusted for age and gender). The source of information used for each of the groups examined, however, was different: EMECAR, which oversees all forms of tuberculosis, was used for the patients who had RA and the National Network of Epidemiological Surveillance of Spain was used to estimate the incidence in the global population; however, this system only oversees the pulmonary and meningeal forms of the infection. The under-estimation of the incidence of tuberculosis in the general population could be a factor that makes comparison between these populations difficult.[25] In Asia, tuberculosis was reported to occur three times more frequently in patients who had RA than in the general population; this was a nonstandardized rate.[26] Alternatively, Yamada and colleagues[27] found a risk three times higher for the occurrence of tuberculosis in patients who had RA compared with the general population (relative risk [RR] 3.21; 95% CI, 1.21–8.55).

In Peru, the authors examined the risk for tuberculosis in patients who had RA and in gender- and age-matched controls free of autoimmune disease and of the same socioeconomic stratum. The authors found 15 cases of tuberculosis in the cohort of patients who had RA, which represented 216 per 100,000 person-years. Even though a higher rate of tuberculosis was present in the patients who had RA, significant differ-ence in the incidence density between them and the control group was not found (the adjusted hazard ratio was 1.69; 95% CI, 0.26–10.93).[28]

In the United States, Wolfe and colleagues examined the incidence density of tuber-culosis in approximately 11,000 patients who had RA and found it no more than expected in the general population (6.2 per 100,000 versus 5.8 per 100,000). The inci-dence rates were not adjusted, however, and the CIs were wide. Furthermore, the ethnic composition of the cohort was not representative of the general population and the identification of the infection was based on a survey in which persons were asked about the positivity of the tuberculin skin test (TST) or the presence of tubercu-losis at any point during their lifetime, which could provide biased information.[29]

Risk for Tuberculosis Infection During Biologic Therapy

The arrival of biologic therapy for the management of RA has marked a milestone comparable to the discovery of cortisone approximately half a century ago. Currently, there are three TNF-α inhibitors approved by the Food and Drug Administration (FDA) in clinical use: infliximab, a chimeric mouse-human monoclonal antibody against anti-TNF-α; etanercept, a fusion protein Fcγ1 receptor of TNF-p75 soluble of TNF-α; and adalimumab, a human monoclonal antibody against anti–TNF-α.

Tuberculosis and Inhibitors of Tumor Necrosis Factor α

With the introduction of TNF-α inhibitors as therapy for RA, the most serious adverse event of concern with their use has been tuberculosis infection. In an analysis per-formed with the BIOBADASER, a database for biologic products from the Spanish Society for Rheumatology, which included 1548 patients receiving biologic agents (86% with infliximab and 14% with etanercept), 17 patients developed tuberculosis (65% of cases with extrapulmonary involvement), with an incidence of tuberculosis of 1893 per 100,000 patients exposed in the year 2000 and 1113 in 2001 in compar-ison with the calculated rate for patients who had RA not exposed to infliximab of 95 per 100,000 patient years for RR of 90.1 and 53.0, respectively; in this study the incidence rates were standardized adequately for age and gender and the tuberculosis infection was identified by mycobacterium isolation.[24]

In a study performed in Asia using the obligatory reports database, the Tuberculosis Surveillance System (KTBS), a RR of 30.1 (95% CI, 7.4–122.3) in patients who had anti–TNF-α therapy versus a RR of 8.9 (95% CI, 4.6–17.2) in subjects who did not have biologic therapy was found.[30] Likewise, in a study performed in the United States, the incidence of tuberculosis in 15,940 patients who had RA (2327 received etanercept, 6460 received infliximab, and 558 received both infliximab and etanercept) was 52.5 (14.3–134.4) per 100,000 patient-years of exposure whereas the incidence rate for tuberculosis in the United States population was 6.4 per 100,000 persons according to the Centers for Disease Control and Prevention (CDC).[29]

In a postmarketing study, Askling and colleagues[31] in Sweden reported that the risk for hospitalization related to tuberculosis was fourfold higher in subjects who had RA and who received anti–TNFα therapy during the period 1999 to 2004 compared with a similar patient group who did not receive anti–TNF-α therapy (RR 4.0; 95% CI, 1.3–12). The relationship between the use of anti–TNF-α and onset of granulomatous infection was examined by Wallis and coworkers using data collected through the Adverse Event Reporting System (AERS) of the FDA. Tuberculosis was the disease reported most frequently (approximately 144 and 35 per 100,000 infliximab-treated and etanercept-treated patients, respectively).[32]

The increased susceptibility to tuberculosis and its atypical presentation are not limited to infliximab and are common to all anti–TNF-α therapies. The association between tuberculosis and etanercept seem less evident compared with infliximab[31] and 4.1 times greater among infliximab than etanercept users.[32] In a cohort of 112,300 patients who had RA, the risk for tuberculosis for each disease-modifying antirheumatic drug (DMARD) was examined independently: only anti-TNF compounds showed an increased risk for tuberculosis as compared with other DMARDs (RR for infliximab 1.8; 95% CI, 1.0–2.6; RR for etanercept 1.2; 95% CI, 0.9–1.8).[33]

For adalimumab, given that the data available are only from clinical studies and that surveillance programs occurred later, a head-to-head comparison with other biologic agents of the risk for tuberculosis cannot be established; however, adalimumab probably carries a similar increased risk for tuberculosis reactivation than infliximab, with most cases occurring in the first 8 months after adalimumab therapy. Burmester and colleagues[34] found a high incidence of tuberculosis among patients who had RA and who used adalimumab (50 per 100 000 person-years of follow up).

Tuberculosis and Non–Antitumor Necrosis Factor α Biologic Therapy

In addition to the anti–TNF-α agents, three new classes of drugs have become available for the treatment of RA: human IL-1 receptor antagonist, anti-CD20 antibodies, and CD4+T-cell costimulatory modulators.

Anakinra was the first IL-1 receptor antagonist approved by the FDA. Fleishmann studied the long-term safety of anakinra in a cohort of 1346 patients who had RA, of whom 510 had received 36 consecutive months of treatment. Even though the cumulative rate of serious infections was more than triple with anakinra than with placebo, only a single case of nonspecified, nontuberculosis mycobacterial (NTM) infection was diagnosed in a patient receiving anakinra and concomitant prednisone and methotrexate. An important demographic datum to consider is that 90% of the patients were white, who in general are at lower risk for tuberculosis.[35] Likewise, in a meta-analysis of three randomized clinical trials, which included approximately 2800 patients treated with anakinra with a follow-up of 24 weeks, no cases of tuberculosis were demonstrated. In these analyses, patients who had certain comorbidities that increase the risk for tuberculosis were excluded, introducing a bias.[36] For active tuberculosis, Brassard and colleagues[33] found 19 cases among 1414 patients treated with anakinra in their cohort of 112,300 patients; however, the risk for tuberculosis was increased significantly only in past users of corticosteroids who received anakinra (adjusted rate ratio 1.7; 95% CI, 1.1–2.8). In this study, however, the investigators identified the cases of tuberculosis based on the code number present in an administrative document, which could produce an overdiagnosis of tuberculosis; this could explain the relative high rate of tuberculosis reported with anakinra. Additionally, reactivation of previous tuberculosis infection in a 77-year-old patient who had RA after 23 months of anakinra monotherapy has been reported.[37]

Rituximab is the only available anti-CD20 antibody. A meta-analysis of three randomized controlled trials failed to demonstrate a significant increase in the rituximab-associated risk for serious infection (pooled OR 1.45; 95% CI, 0.56–3.73) and no cases of tuberculosis were found.[36] An important role of peripheral B cells in the immune response against *M tuberculosis* has been suggested in some studies; furthermore, B cells are important components of the established granuloma. Even though a clear association between rituximab and LTBI reactivation, like the one occurring with anti–TNF-α inhibitors, has not been demonstrated, the first case of mycobacterial disease related to rituximab use was reported recently.[38] Likewise, two cases of nontuberculous mycobacteria were reported in patients who had inflammatory myopathies and were treated with rituximab.[39]

Abatacept is the only approved CD4+ T-cell costimulatory modulator. A meta-analysis of five randomized controlled trials found no increase in the risk for serious infection associated with abatacept therapy (pooled OR 1.35; 95% CI, 0.78–2.32).[36] The drug has been shown, however, to increase the infection risk in patients already using a biologic agent but not to impair the capacity to control *M tuberculosis* infection in a murine model.[40]

Tuberculosis and the New Biologic Agents

Improved understanding of the pathophysiology of RA has revealed that although TNF-α is central to autoimmune inflammation, it is not the cornerstone of RA pathogenesis; rather, TNF-α is part of a network of cytokines that not only interact closely but also have important effects of their own. This may be one of the reasons why anti–TNF-α compounds have not turned out to be a universal tool that fits all and fixes all. The success of anti–TNF-α agents along with their shortcomings (including lack of efficacy in a significant proportion of patients, loss of efficacy over time, associated risk for LTBI reactivation, and high cost) have triggered an enormous research effort to identify novel potential targets. These new targets include costimulatory molecule inhibitors, adhesion molecule inhibitors, cytokine inhibitors, kinase modulators, B-cell targeting therapies, complement inhibitors, chemokine inhibitors, and RANK/RANKL modulators. Some of them already are approved for its use in RA whereas others are being considered for approval. Just as with anti–TNF-α therapies, the targets of these new biologics agents are indispensable for the formation and maintenance of the tuberculosis granuloma; therefore, special care is in order for patients at high risk for tuberculosis.

As future targets for new biologic therapies are under development, with the potential for adverse immunologic functions against mycobacteria, the need to implement mycobacterial infection screening strategies for patients who are candidates for biologic agents should be stressed. Golimumab is a human monoclonal antibody that neutralizes TNF-α with high affinity. In a phase III study, the rate of serious infections in 137 patients treated with golimumab for up to 52 weeks was not greater than the risk observed by the placebo group; furthermore, no cases of tuberculosis were observed. Before the study, however, a rigorous screening took place and patients who had a history or clinical evidence of LTBI were excluded; therefore, the association between golimumab and an increased risk for tuberculosis, comparable to what occurs with the currently available anti-TNF compounds, cannot be ruled out.[41]

IL-6 is a pleiotropic cytokine that affects the function of B cells and is found overexpressed in the synovial tissue and peripheral blood of patients who have RA,[42] making this cytokine a potential therapeutic target. In a 2008 phase III trial, treatment with tocilizumab, a humanized monoclonal antibody that binds to the IL-6 receptor, no mycobacterial infections were noted.[43] Although IL-6 has proved important in the initial containment of M tuberculosis infection in a mouse model, late containment occurs independently of IL-6,[22] suggesting that IL-6 is not essential for the host defense against tuberculosis and that inhibition of IL-6 would not be anticipated to increase the risk for reactivation of LTBI. The issue, however, of whether or not tocilizumab confers an increased risk for mycobacterial disease remains controversial and demands careful investigation before approval of the drug.

IL-17 and IL-23 also represent promising novel targets. IL-17 has the capacity to induce chronic destructive arthritis independent of IL-1 and TNF-α. Anti–IL-17A cytokine therapy has been successful in mouse models of arthritis but awaits clinical trials in humans.[44] IL-17 and IL-23 have important roles in all stages of the immune response against mycobacterial infection, from neutrophil recruitment in the early phase to granuloma formation and maintenance in later stages.[45] Therapeutic agents that influence these cytokines, therefore, are likely to alter a patient's susceptibility to mycobacterial disease or could reactivate LTBI.

AGING, RHEUMATOID ARTHRITIS, AND THE RESPONSE OF THE IMMUNE SYSTEM TO *MYCOBACTERIUM TUBERCULOSIS* INFECTION

Aging is a physiologic process that occurs over time in every living being and that is characterized by structural and functional changes at the cellular, organ, and system levels. The aging of the immune system, a process known as immunosenescence, usually parallels chronologic age; however, in autoimmune diseases, such as RA, this process can accelerate, resulting in further dysregulation of the immune system.[46] This dysregulation in turn contributes to an increase susceptibility to infections and possibly to cancer and other autoimmune diseases. Aging is associated not only with a decline in the number of responsive T cells but also with a decline on their performance when compared with T cells from younger individuals. There is clinical and experimental evidence that abnormalities in several aspects of the adaptive immune response do occur with aging. With thymic involution, there is a reduction in the activation of regulatory T cells, which may result in diminished antiself responses.[47] During thymic involution, the epithelial layer of the gland, which is responsible for the selection and maturation of T cells, is replaced by fatty cells, resulting in a reduction of the output of recent thymic emigrants. A space-filling autoproliferative mechanism, known as homeostatic proliferation, keeps peripheral T cells at constant levels throughout the lifespan and becomes important as age progresses. Homeostatic proliferation, however, can induce replicative stress on peripheral T cells resulting in a shift of the phenotype of circulating T cells, specifically a decrease in the number of naïve T cells (CD45RA) and an increase in the number of memory T cells (CD45RO). This shift, which occurs in normal and in accelerated aging (as in RA), may result in inappropriate adaptive immune response.[48] Shortening of the lymphocytic telomeric length may lead to an excessive turnover of cells in these patients. CD4 telomeres are shortened several times over the course of the disease; these findings suggest that CD4 T cells have cycled excessively, causing telomeres to erode prematurely, leading to immunosenescence. As a result of this process, the production of T cells by the thymus is insufficient, forcing T cells to hyperproliferate. This compensatory self-replication of T cells leads to contraction of the T-cell receptors repertoire and down-regulation of the CD28 costimulatory molecule with an increased percentage of $CD4^+CD28^{null}$ and $CD8^+CD28^{null}$ T cells, limiting the ability of the immune system to secret them properly.[49] Other important changes in these senescent cells include an altered pattern of cytokine expression (from T helper on TH1 to TH2), resulting on the increased production of some autoantibodies, a resistance to apoptosis, and the expression of many genes that generally are found on natural killer cells.

M tuberculosis infection usually does not lead to active disease, given that the immune response generally is successful in containing, albeit not eliminating, the pathogen. Acute tuberculosis can result in a small percentage of infections probably because of an inadequate immune response. In most cases, however, individuals have asymptomatic and noninfectious latency, which usually extends over the lifespan. In response to perturbation of the immune system, however, reactivation of a latent infection can occur, resulting in an active infection process. A good control of infection by *M tuberculosis* requires of a robust antigen-specific CD4 T-cell response and the production of Th1 cells–associated cytokines, IFN-γ, IL-12, and TNF-α.[7] As discussed previously, however, during aging or accelerated aging, the immune system may not be able to mount an adequate response favoring the occurrence of active tuberculosis or LTBI reactivation. The infections in these patients can be subtle rather than overt and oftentimes are accompanied by false-negative TST for LTBI.[50]

LATENT TUBERCULOSIS INFECTION IN PATIENTS WHO HAVE RHEUMATOID ARTHRITIS

The cases of tuberculosis that occur in patients who have RA and are receiving anti–TNF-α therapy are, for the most part, the result of the reactivation of LTBI,[51] which makes its diagnostic and treatment compulsory. The diagnosis begins with an adequate clinical history to detect the presence of risk factors predisposing to the development of tuberculosis. Even though the radiologic findings of granulomatous diseases are not specific, and abnormalities in LTBI are detected in only 10% to 20% of patients, it is necessary to obtain a chest radiograph to detect changes suggestive of previous tuberculosis infectionand to detect active tuberculosis.

The diagnostic tests to detect LTBIs traditionally have been based on the TST. The TST is a recall response to soluble antigens previously encountered during tuberculosis infection. After intradermal tuberculin challenge in a sensitized individual, antigen-specific T cells are activated to secrete cytokines that mediate a hypersensitivity reaction. This infiltrate is constituted predominantly by CD4+ T cells.[52] The TST has a low sensitivity, however, being particularly poor at detecting LTBIs in high-risk immunocompromised patients. For example, in countries with high rates of LTBI, LTBIs may not be detected using the TST in more than half the subjects who have RA (**Fig. 1**).[16] This decreased reactivity to TST in patients who have RA can be attributed to the dysfunction of T cells associated with RA. The TST has low specificity and the positive results may reflect previous exposure to atypical mycobacteria or to vaccination with the Calmette-Guérin bacillus. Patients who have RA, however, and who have an altered immune response are more likely to have false-negative TST

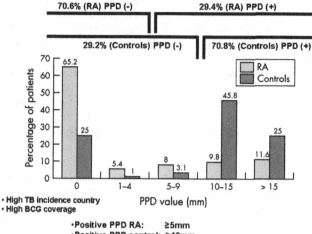

**Induration sizes to PPD in patients with RA and healthy Controls
Bars depicts positivity for PPD by risk group**

Fig.1. Induration sizes to PPD in patients who had RA and healthy controls from a population highly endemic for tuberculosis. PPD positive results occurred significantly less frequently in patients who had RA than in the healthy controls (29.4% versus 70.8% respectively; P<.001). (*Data from* Ponce de León D, Acevedo-Vásquez E, Sánchez-Torres A, et al. Attenuated response to purified protein derivative in patients with rheumatoid arthritis: study in a population with a high prevalence of tuberculosis. Ann Rheum Dis 2005;64:1360–1.)

results; for this reason, it is recommended to use a cutoff point of greater than or equal to 5 mm for the test to be considered positive. This lower threshold point increases the sensitivity albeit at the expense of a lower specificity. In this context, LTBI could be diagnosed erroneously in some patients due to the false-positive results. In patients who have autoimmune disorders, however, such as RA, a false-negative TST result is more dangerous given that the risk for tuberculosis is greater for them. Therefore, it is better to increase the sensitivity even though the specificity diminishes, given that preventive therapy can be offered to a larger number of patients.

Advances in mycobacterial genomics have led to the development of two new blood IFN-γ release assays (IGRAs) in response to two unique antigens, ESAT-6 and CFP-10, that are highly specific for *M tuberculosis* and which are absent from *M bovis*, *M avium*, and most other nontuberculous mycobacteria. One assay, the enzyme-linked immunospot (ELISPOT) (T-SPOT.*TB*, Oxford Immunotec, Oxford, UK) enumerates IFN-γ–secreting T cells; the other measures IFN-γ concentration in the supernatant using ELISA (QuantiFERON-TB Gold [QFT-G], Cellestis, Carnegie, Australia). The latest improvement to this technology is the Quantiferon-TB Gold In-Tube (QFT-IT) test, which incorporates another specific tuberculosis antigen (TB 7.7), and in which whole blood is drawn directly into a vacutainer tube precoated with antigens ready for incubation.[53]

Given that there is no gold standard for the diagnosis of LTBI, the exact sensitivity of these tests cannot be determined. An indirect method of determining this sensitivity is to assess the correlation between risk factors for tuberculosis in persons who have low incidence of tuberculosis, whereas patients who live in endemic tuberculosis areas are assessed by comparing them with a control group who have the same risk factors but who do not have an autoimmune disorder. One study has correlated IGRA and TST results with risk factors for LTBI. QFT-IT was associated significantly more closely with the presence of risk factors for LTBI (odds ratio [OR] 23.8; 95% CI, 5.14 to 110) than TST (OR 2.77; 95% CI; 1.22 to 6.27) ($P = .009$) in 142 patients who had inflammatory diseases and lived in areas of low endemicity for tuberculosis.[54] The authors' group studied the positivity of the TST and QFT-IT and compared their positivities with their respective control groups. A much higher approximation was found between QFT-IT and its controls (75%) compared with those for TST (41%).[55] Recent recommendations from the CDC, however, indicate that the IGRAs have not been assessed in immunocompromised patients, because the information available regarding these in vitro tests for the diagnosis of tuberculosis in the elderly is scarce.[56] T-SPOT-*TB* also has shown promise in immunocompromised patients, as it has been found more sensitive than TST in HIV patients, immunosuppressed hematologic patients, and young children who have HIV infection and malnutrition.

How can We Adequately Detect Latent Tuberculosis Infections in the most Vulnerable Patients who have Rheumatoid Arthritis? The Elderly Rheumatoid Arthritis Group

As discussed previously, patients who have RA and who develop tuberculosis are, for the most part, older than 60; therefore, it is necessary to evaluate the performance of these tests in this age group. One of the few studies conducted to this end is from Kobashi and colleagues, who studied 130 nonimmunosuppressed patients who had active tuberculosis, 30 of whom were older individuals. A difference in the reactivity to TST was found between the older (27%) and the younger patients (70%) ($P = .012$); however, no differences were found with the QFT-IT (77% versus 87%; $P = .185$).[57]

Comparison of Tuberculin Skin Test and Quantiferon-TB Gold in Tube Test in Patients who had Rheumatoid Arthritis Versus Control Patients

To determine the performance of TST and QFT-IT in the diagnosis of LTBI in older individuals (≥ 60 years), the authors performed a subanalysis of recently studied patients (**Fig. 2**); we found a much lower proportion of TST reactivity in the older patients who had RA (8/45; 17%) than in control individuals from the same age group (29/41; 71%) ($P<.001$); this difference persisted for patients aged 40 to 60 ($P<.001$) but not in the younger patients (age 20–40) (45% versus 36%; $P = .622$).[55] When the performance of QFT-IT was examined, the author found, as with the TST, a much lower reactivity in patients older than 60 (40%) than in controls from the same age group (71%) ($P = .004$); in contrast, there was no difference between patients and controls in the younger age group. These data are depicted in **Fig. 3**.

These findings demonstrate that the sensitivity of the currently available diagnostic tests for the detection of LTBI is influenced by two factors: the test used and age. A decreased reactivity to QFT-IT in older adults (≥ 60 years) is noted but this decreased reactivity is discovered even earlier with TST. These findings could be related to the dysregulation, which is characteristic of the process of immunosenescence and which is evident at earlier age with TST.[46] This suggests that IGRAs have a better sensitivity for LTBI compared with TST in patients who have RA; however, the performance of both diagnostic tools are impaired in those patients older than 60 years. These data may have important clinical implications, given that LTBI screening before anti–TNF-α therapy in the elderly may not be sufficiently trustworthy to adequately prevent the development of tuberculosis using the tests currently available.

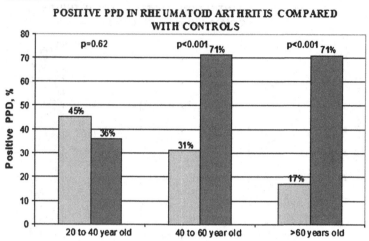

Fig. 2. Induration sizes to PPD in patients who had RA and healthy control subjects according to patient age in a population highly endemic for tuberculosis. (*Data from* Ponce de Leon D, Acevedo-Vasquez E, Alvizuri S, et al. Comparison of an interferon-γ assay with tuberculin skin testing for detection of tuberculosis infection in patients with rheumatoid arthritis in a TB-endemic population. J Rheumatol 2008;35:776–81.)

SCREENING TEST FOR TUBERCULOSIS BEFORE THE INITIATION OF BIOLOGIC THERAPY IN PATIENTS WHO HAVE RHEUMATOID ARTHRITIS: CURRENT RECOMMENDATIONS

Several countries have generated national guidelines that address LTBI before TNF-α blocker therapy is initiated, and these should be consulted.[58] There are some notable differences between countries, which probably reflect local prevalence and other conditions of care.

Similar to any other diagnostic test, the predictive value of the IGRAs results depends on the prevalence of *M tuberculosis* infection in the population being tested. Results should be interpreted in conjunction with other epidemiologic, medical history, physical examination, and diagnostic findings.

As with a negative TST result, negative IGRA results should not be used alone to exclude LTBI, especially in the elderly. With any of the testing methods, persons who have a negative test result still can have LTBI. Those who have a negative result but who have higher clinical suspicion for risk factors for tuberculosis might need treatment or closer monitoring for disease.

It is recommended that all patients who have RA be screened for the presence of active tuberculosis or LTBI before the use of biologic agents. Screening should include a detailed history aimed at the ascertainment of risk factors for tuberculosis, including past history of tuberculosis, trips to endemic areas, country of origin, exposure to cases of active tuberculosis, overcrowded living conditions (prisons, nursing homes, or areas of low socioeconomic status), health care workers, or history of a positive

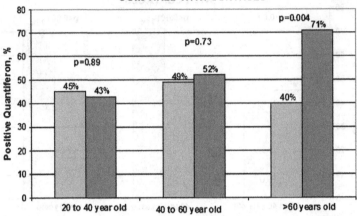

Fig. 3. Induration sizes to QFT-IT in patients who had RA and healthy control subjects in a population highly endemic for tuberculosis. (*Data from* Ponce de Leon D, Acevedo-Vasquez E, Alvizuri S, et al. Comparison of an interferon-γ assay with tuberculin skin testing for detection of tuberculosis infection in patients with rheumatoid arthritis in a TB-endemic population. J Rheumatol 2008;35:776–81.)

TST; a chest radiograph also should be obtained and may demonstrate evidence of tuberculosis sequelae.

Some authorities advocate not using the TST for screening purposes in view of the several disadvantages of this test. Its sensitivity is lower in immunosuppressed patients than in healthy subjects, and some patients, therefore, may have a false-negative TST result. Furthermore, TST is poorly reproducible, requires two visits for its performance, and is subject to observer error. These limitations have led Swiss authorities to replace the use of TST for an IGRA test for screening purposes.[59]

The CDC[60] states that patients should undergo the TST test. Indurations of 5 mm or greater should be interpreted as a positive result; however, a TST induration of less than 5 mm does not exclude *M tuberculosis* infection. Anergy panel testing (eg, Candida) is not recommended; the same is true for the two-step or booster tuberculin test. In July 2005, the CDC convened a meeting of consultants and researchers who had expertise in the field to review scientific evidence and clinical experience with QFT-G. On the basis of this review and discussion, the CDC recommended that QFT-G may be used in all circumstances in which the TST currently is used.Because of the lack of screening data in immunosuppressed populations, however, it is unknown whether or not these IGRAs behave similarly to the TST in these individuals. Given that IGRAs have higher specificity than the TST, it is tempting to use one of these tests to confirm a positive TST result. Given the lack of information on the relative sensitivities of these tests in immunosuppressed populations, the rationale for use IGRAs in these patients currently is unsupported.[56]

The British Thoracic Society does not recommend routine use of the TST in this setting, because most patients considered for anti-TNF therapy are immunosuppressed and likely to have false-negative TST results.[61] Recently, the Public Health

Agency of Canada released a national statement about recommendations on the use of IGRAs for specific subgroups. According to these recommendations, the TST should be the initial test used to detect LTBI in immunocompromised individuals. In light of the known problems with false-negative TST results in immunocompromised populations, however, these guidelines advise that an IGRA test may be performed in immunocompromised patients who have a negative initial TST result.[62]

The prevalence of LTBI varies throughout the world and, therefore, it is not surprising that the screening guidelines for LTBI vary between regions. The usefulness of the TST is dependent on the background prevalence of tuberculosis, in that a positive TST has a high positive predictive value in regions where tuberculosis is highly prevalent.

Efficacy of Screening Protocols

There is a strong evidence of the efficacy for screening and treatment of LTBI before the initiation of anti-TNF therapy. Wolfe and colleagues found four cases of tuberculosis in a cohort of more than 6000 patients who had RA and who received infliximab in the United States between January 2000 and June 2002. All cases were in patients who had not been screened for LTBI before initiation of anti-TNF therapy, whereas no cases of tuberculosis were seen in patients who complied with the formal screening protocol.[29] In clinical trials of adalimumab, once tuberculosis screening was incorporated, Perez and colleagues[63] reported an 85% reduction in the occurrence of cases of tuberculosis. Similarly, in Spain, Carmona and colleagues[64] described a decreased of 83% in the incidence of tuberculosis after screening and treatment recommendations were instituted.

As discussed previously, studies conducted in North America, Europe, and Spain have shown that the follow-up of patients receiving TNF-α antagonists with screening programs is necessary and that the treatment of LTBI decreases the risk for developing tuberculosis by nearly 80%. Infection may occur, however, even with negative tuberculosis screening in patients before biologic therapy is started. Data are limited in those countries with high tuberculosis and LTBI prevalence; however, the impact of screening surveillance in highly endemic areas is predicted to be higher than that reported in low endemic areas.

The following recommendations are suggested:

- A TST test should be done before biologic therapy is initiated. An induration of less than 5 mm does not exclude *M tuberculosis* infection.
- Patients who have risk factors for tuberculosis and a negative TST should be considered for treatment of LTBI after active tuberculosis is ruled out. Those patients who have a negative TST should have an in vitro test (eg, QFT-IT) according to local recommendations, given its better sensitivity.
- Patients who have positive TST result (≥ 5 mm) or positive IGRA test must receive prophylactic therapy after active tuberculosis has been ruled out.
- The drug of choice for the treatment of LTBI is isoniazid (at a dosage of 10 mg/kg/day), with a maximum daily dose of 300 mg for 9 consecutive months.
- In patients who have LTBI, it is recommended that biologic therapy be initiated at least 4 weeks after starting tuberculosis prophylaxis.
- Tuberculosis prophylaxis for patients who are candidates for biologic therapy and exposed to contacts with active tuberculosis, regardless of TST results, should be administered.
- The persistence of fever and respiratory symptoms must be considered serious in patients receiving biologic therapy and the suspicion of tuberculosis must be high.

- Cases of tuberculosis must be reported to public health authorities to facilitate their treatment and the identification of all exposed individuals.

NONTUBERCULOSIS MYCOBACTERIAL DISEASE IN PATIENTS UNDERGOING ANTI-TUMOR NECROSIS FACTOR α THERAPY

NTM infections are caused a group of more than 100 species of bacteria that are ubiquitous in soil and water and which exhibit varied pathogenicity. NTM infections are opportunistic, requiring defects in local or systemic host immunity to cause disease in humans. Unlike tuberculosis, disease from NTM infection is due to exposure to environmental organisms; cases of human-to-human transmission have never been documented.[65] Patients who have pre-existing structural lung disease are known to be at risk for NTM infection as there are defects of cell-mediated immunity, including abnormalities of the IL-12/IFN-γ axis. NTM infections are classified based on the rate of growth in culture; M avium complex (MAC) and M kansasii are slow growers whereas M abscessus and M fortuitum are rapidly growing mycobacteria. Unlike tuberculosis, NTM infections does not cause reactivation disease, and skin testing using NTM antigens analogous to the PPD used to test for tuberculosis infection has not been useful for diagnosis of NTM disease.

Few data on the emergence of NTM disease in patients undergoing anti-TNF therapy have been published. Wallis and colleagues[32] examined the relationship between the use of etanercept and infliximab and onset of granulomatous infection, including NTM, using data collected through the AERS of the FDA from January 1998 to September 2002. In this database, 639 reported cases of granulomatous infectious diseases, including 374 cases of tuberculosis and 37 of unspecified NTM infections, were identified in approximately 346,000 United States patients treated over a 4.75-year period. Despite sharing a common therapeutic target, the risk for unspecified NTM infections was 2.08-fold greater among patients who received infliximab (12.9 per 100,000 patients) than among those who received etanercept (6.2 per 100,000 patients).

An FDA advisory committee reviewed the safety of TNF inhibitors in 2001 and noted that in more than 170,000 patients worldwide treated with infliximab, 84 developed tuberculosis and none developed atypical mycobacterial infection. For etanercept, out of approximately 104,000 patients, 11 developed tuberculosis and eight developed atypical mybobacteria, including six cases of MAC and one case each of M kansasii and M marinaruum.[66] Several cases of NTM disease in patients who have RA associated with anti-TNF-α have been reported.

Etanercept therapy has been reported in association with the development of fatal and nonfatal NTM infections. Fatal cases included complicated psoas abscess 12 months after initiation of etanercept in a 79-year-old patient who had RA in whom MAC cultures grew[67]; MAC lung disease with multiple positive MAC sputum cultures in a patient who had RA[68]; pulmonary M xenopi infection in a 71-year-old man who had RA fewer than 12 months after initiation of etanercept[69]; and pulmonary M abscessus infection in a 56-year-old patient who had RA.[70] Nonfatal cases reported included M chelonae endophthalmitis in a patient receiving etanercept for psoriatic arthritis, M xenopi spinal osteomyelitis in a patient who had RA,[71] and M marinum tenosynovitis and pulmonary M szulgai infection in patients who had RA.[72]

Infliximab therapy also has been associated with fatal and nonfatal cases of NTM infection. Fatal M peregrinum pneumonia has been reported in a 68-year-old patient who had refractory polymyositis shortly after institution of infliximab.[73] Nonfatal cases reported included M abscessus soft tissue infection with rapid growing in a

67-year-old patient 13 months after initiation of infliximab therapy.[74] Okubo and coworkers reported pulmonary MAC without dissemination in a 67-year-old patient who had RA 6 weeks after introduction of infliximab.[75] Finally, the case of a patient who developed *M fortuitum* granulomatous hepatitis has been reported.[76]

The authors recommend that physicians maintain a high level of vigilance for late-onset NTM infection in persons using anti–TNF-α therapy, especially in communities in which mycobacterial organisms are highly prevalent.

The range of NTM species involved in anti–TNF-α–associated mycobacterial disease is intriguing, as it includes pulmonary, extrapulmonary, and disseminated disease and species of high (eg, *M marinum*, *M xenopi*, and *M szulgai*) and low (eg, *M fortuitum* and *M peregrinum*) pathogenicity. This might reflect not only geographic distribution of cases but also the importance of host factors in these infections.

According to the WHO, one third of the world's population is believed to have a LTBI. There is no evidence of a latent phase for NTM infections, however, which, in part, explains the low frequency of NTM disease compared with tuberculosis reactivation in patients undergoing anti-TNF treatment. Furthermore, NTM infections usually present after at least 12 months of anti-TNF treatment and, therefore, are considered new infections. The generally lower pathogenicity of NTM species as opposed to *M tuberculosis* could further explain the lower frequency of anti-TNF–associated NTM disease. Moreover, underdiagnosis of NTM disease as a result of insufficient awareness of the pathogenic potential of NTM species is a recognized problem. The prominent role of TNF in the pathogenesis of NTM infection is proved in mouse models in which anti-TNF treatment increased the mycobacterial burden.[77]

SUMMARY

Patients receiving biologic therapies are at higher risk for developing tuberculosis than patients who have similar diseases and are not receiving these treatments or the general population; a definite risk exists particularly with anti-TNF agents. All patients who are candidates for the use of biologic agents should be screened for latent and active tuberculosis before its initiation. Despite a considerable reduction in the incidence of tuberculosis after initiation of anti-TNF therapy achieved with screening procedures, new cases of tuberculosis or reactivation of LTBI may occur during the course of treatment, so a high level of vigilance is highly recommended. QFT-IT seems more sensitive than TST for detecting LTBI in patients who have RA but seems less sensitive in elderly patients who have RA than in immunocompetent patients. The diagnostic tests to detect LTBI in elderly patients who have RA do not have adequate sensitivity (TST and QFT-IT); therefore, the onset of biologic therapy in this group of patients, particularly in areas highly endemic for tuberculosis, must be done carefully. Immunosenescence usually parallels an individual's chronologic age; however, in autoimmune diseases, such as RA, this process can accelerate, resulting in further dysregulation of the immune system, which in turn contributes to an increased susceptibility to infections and, as documented in this article, possibly contributes to the poor performance of LTBI diagnostic tests in elderly patients who have RA. Serious infectious with MNT may ensue in patients receiving biologic therapy, especially anti–TNF-α compounds.

ACKNOWLEDGMENTS

The authors are grateful to Graciela S. Alarcón, MD, MPH, for her comments and suggestions in an earlier version of this article and for her help editing the English version.

REFERENCES

1. Gomez J, Mendonça de Souza S. Prehistoric tuberculosis in America: adding comments to literature review. Mem Inst Oswaldo Cruz 2002;98:S151–9.
2. Acevedo-Vasquez E, Ponce De León D, Gamboa R. [Tuberculosis as emergent diseases associated to medical treamtment of rheumatoid arthritis.] In: Caballero C, editor. [Challenges for diagnosis and treatment for rheumatoid arthritis in Latin America.] 1st edition. Barranquilla (Columbia): Uninorte; 2006. p. 349–71.
3. World Health Organization. Global tuberculosis control. WHO/HTM/TB/2008.393. Geneva, Switzerland: World Health Organization; 2008.
4. Lonnroth K, Raviglione M. Global epidemiology of tuberculosis: prospects for control. Semin Respir Crit Care Med 2008;29:481–91.
5. Dye C, Watt C, Bleed D, et al. Evolution of tuberculosis control and prospects for reducing tuberculosis incidence, prevalence, and deaths globally. JAMA 2005; 293:2767–75.
6. Manabe YC, Bishai WR. Latent Mycobacterium tuberculosis persistence, patience, and winning by waiting. Nat Med 2000;6:1327–9.
7. Flynn J, Chan J. Immunology of tuberculosis. Annu Rev Immunol 2001;19:93–129.
8. Algood H, Chan J, Flynn J. Chemokines and tuberculosis. Cytokine Growth Factor Rev 2003;14:467–77.
9. Salgame P. Host innate and Th1 responses and the bacterial factors that control Mycobacterium tuberculosis infection. Curr Opin Immunol 2005;17:374–80.
10. Orme I, Cooper A. Cytokine/chemokine cascades in immunity to tuberculosis. Immunol Today 1999;20:307–12.
11. Cassidy J, Bryson D, Gutierrez M, et al. Lymphocyte subtype in experimentally induced early-stage bovine tuberculous lesions. J Comp Pathol 2001;124:46–51.
12. Ehlers S, Benini J, Kutsch S. Fatal granuloma necrosis without exacerbated mycobacterial growth in tumor necrosis factor receptor p55 gene-deficient mice intravenously infected with Mycobacterium avium. Infect Immun 1999;67: 3571–9.
13. Kaneko H, Yamada H, Mizuno S, et al. Role of tumor necrosis factor-alpha in Mycobacterium- induced granuloma formation in tumor necrosis factor alpha-deficient mice. Lab Invest 1999;79:379–86.
14. Mohan V, Scanga C, Yu K, et al. Effects of tumor necrosis factor alpha on host immune response in chronic persistent tuberculosis: possible role for limiting pathology. Infect Immun 2001;69:1847–55.
15. Schroder K, Hertzog P, Ravasi T, et al. Interferon-γ: an overview of signals, mechanisms and functions. J Leukoc Biol 2004;75:163–89.
16. Boehm U, Klamp T, Groot M, et al. Cellular responses to interferon-γ. Annu Rev Immunol 1997;15:749–95.
17. Sexton P, Harrison A. Susceptibility to nontuberculous mycobacterial lung disease. Eur Respir J 2008;31:1322–33.
18. Khader S, Bell G, Pearl J, et al. IL-23 and IL-17 in the establishment of protective pulmonary CD4 (+) T cell responses after vaccination and during Mycobacterium tuberculosis challenge. Nat Immunol 2007;8:369–77.
19. Ouyang W, Kolls JK, Zheng Y. The biological functions of T helper 17 cell effectors cytokines in inflammation. Immunity 2008;28:454–67.
20. Appelberg R, Castro A, Pedrosa J, et al. Role of interleukin-6 in the induction of protective T cells during mycobacterial infections in mice. Immunology 1994;82: 361–4.

21. Leal I, Smedegard B, Andersen P, et al. Interleukin-6 and interleukin-12 partici-
    pate in induction of a type 1 protective T-cell response during vaccination with
    a tuberculosis subunit vaccine. Infect Immun 1999;67:5747–54.
22. Saunders B, Frank A, Orme I, et al. Interleukin-6 induces early gamma interferon
    production in the infected lung but is not required for generation of specific immu-
    nity to Mycobacterium tuberculosis infection. Infect Immun 2000;68:3322–6.
23. Maglione P, Xu J, Chan J. B cells moderate inflammatory progression and
    enhance bacterial containment upon pulmonary challenge with Mycobacterium
    tuberculosis. J Immunol 2007;178:7222–34.
24. Gomez-Reino J, Carmona L, Rodriguez V, et al. Treatment of rheumatoid arthritis
    with tumor necrosis factor inhibitors may predispose to significant increase in
    tuberculosis risk. A multicenter active-surveillance report. Arthritis Rheum 2003;
    48:2122–7.
25. Carmona L, Hernández-García C, Vadillo C, et al. Increased risk of tuberculosis
    in patients with rheumatoid arthritis. J Rheumatol 2003;30:1436–9.
26. Yoshinaga Y, Tatsuya K, Tomoko M, et al. Clinical characteristics of Mycobacte-
    rium in rheumatoid arthritis patients. Mod Rheumatol 2004;14:143–8.
27. Yamada T, Nakajima A, Inoue E, et al. Elevated risk of tuberculosis in patients with
    rheumatoid arthritis in Japan. Ann Rheum Dis 2006;65:1661–3.
28. Gamboa R, Acevedo-Vásquez E, Gutiérrez C, et al. [Risk of tuberculosis disease
    in rheumatoid arthritis patients.] Anales de la Facultad de Medicina de Montevi-
    deo 2006;67:310–7.
29. Wolfe F, Michaud K, Anderson J, et al. Tuberculosis infection in patients with rheu-
    matoid arthritis and the effect of infliximab therapy. Arthritis Rheum 2004;50:
    372–9.
30. Seong S, Choi C, Woo J, et al. Incidence of tuberculosis in Korean patients with
    rheumatoid arthritis (RA): effects of RA itself and of tumor necrosis factor
    blockers. J Rheumatol 2007;34:706–11.
31. Askling J, Fored CM, Brandt L, et al. Risk and case characteristics of tuberculosis
    in rheumatoid arthritis associated with tumor necrosis factor antagonists in
    Sweden. Arthritis Rheum 2005;52:1986–92.
32. Wallis R, Broder M, Wong J, et al. Granulomatous infectious diseases associated
    with tumor necrosis factor antagonists. Clin Infect Dis 2004;38:1261–5.
33. Brassard P, Kezouh A, Suissa S. Antirheumatic drugs and the risk of tuberculosis.
    Clin Infect Dis 2006;43:717–22.
34. Burmester G, Mariette X, Montecucco C, et al. Adalimumab alone and in combi-
    nation with disease-modifying antirheumatic drugs for the treatment of rheuma-
    toid arthritis in clinical practice: the Research in Active Rheumatoid Arthritis
    (ReAct) trial. Ann Rheum Dis 2007;66:732–9.
35. Fleischmann R. Safety of extended treatment with anakinra in patients with rheu-
    matoid arthritis. Ann Rheum Dis 2006;65:1006–12.
36. Salliot C. Risk of serious infections during rituximab, abatacept and anakinra ther-
    apies for rheumatoid arthritis: meta-analyses of randomized placebo-controlled
    trials. Ann Rheum Dis 2008;68:25–32.
37. Settas L, Tsimirikas G, Vosvotekas G, et al. Reactivation of pulmonary tubercu-
    losis in a patient with rheumatoid arthritis during treatment with IL-1 receptor
    antagonists. J Clin Rheumatol 2007;13:219–20.
38. Winthrop K. Mycobacterial and other serious infections in patients receiving anti-
    tumor necrosis factor and other newly approved biologic therapies: case finding
    through the Emerging Infections Network. Clin Infect Dis 2008;46:1738–40.

39. Lutt J, Pisculli M, Weinblatt M, et al. Severe nontuberculous mycobacterial infection in 2 patients receiving rituximab for refractory myositis. J Rheumatol 2008;35:1683–6.

40. Bigbee C, Gonchoroff D, Vratsanos G, et al. Abatacept treatment does not exacerbate chronic *Mycobacterium tuberculosis* infection in mice. Arthritis Rheum 2007;56:2557–65.

41. Kay J. Golimumab in patients with active rheumatoid arthritis despite treatment with methotrexate: a randomized, double-blind, placebo-controlled, dose-ranging study. Arthritis Rheum 2008;58:964–75.

42. Ponce de León D, Pastor C, Beraun Y, et al. Patrón de citocinas séricas en pacientes con artritis reumatoide de acuerdo a su reactividad al PPD. Reum Clin 2006;2:289–93.

43. Smolen JS. Effect of interleukin-6 receptor inhibition with tocilizumab in patients with rheumatoid arthritis (OPTION study): a double-blind, placebo-controlled, randomized trial. Lancet 2008;371:987–97.

44. Lubberts E. IL-17/Th17 targeting: on the road to prevent chronic destructive arthritis? Cytokines 2008;41:84–91.

45. Khader S, Cooper A. IL-23 and IL-17 in tuberculosis. Cytokines 2008;41:79–83.

46. Weyand C, Fulbright J, Goronzy J. Immunosenescence, autoimmunity, and rheumatoid arthritis. Exp Gerontol 2003;38:833–41.

47. Linton P, Dorshkind K. Age-related changes in lymphocyte development and function. Nat Immunol 2004;5:133–9.

48. Thewissen M, Somers V, Venken K, et al. Analysis of immunosenescence markers in patients with autoimmnune disease. Clin Immunol 2007;123:209–18.

49. Weyand C, Goronzy J. Premature immunosenescence in rheumatoid arthritis. J Rheumatol 2002;29:1141–6.

50. Ponce de León D, Acevedo-Vásquez E, Sánchez-Torres A, et al. Attenuated response to purified protein derivative in patients with rheumatoid arthritis: study in a population with a high prevalence of tuberculosis. Ann Rheum Dis 2005;64:1360–1.

51. Gardam M, Keystone E, Menzies R. Anti-tumour necrosis factor agents and tuberculosis risk: mechanisms of action and clinical management. Lancet Infect Dis 2003;3:1–14.

52. Roitt I, Brostoff J, Male D. Hypersensitivity type IV. In: Cook L, editor. Immunology. 4th edition. Barcelona: Mosby; 1998. p. 255.5.

53. Menzies D, Pai M, Comstock G. Meta-analysis: new tests for the diagnosis of latent tuberculosis infection: areas of uncertainty and recommendations for research. Ann Intern Med 2007;146:340–54.

54. Matulis G, Juni P, Villiger P, et al. Detection of latent tuberculosis in immunosuppressed patients with autoimmune diseases: performance of a *Mycobacterium tuberculosis* antigen-specific interferon γ assay. Ann Rheum Dis 2008;67:84–90.

55. Ponce de Leon D, Acevedo-Vasquez E, Alvizuri S, et al. Comparison of an interferon-γ assay with tuberculin skin testing for detection of tuberculosis (TB) infection in patients with rheumatoid arthritis in a TB-endemic population. J Rheumatol 2008;35:776–81.

56. Mazurek GH, Jereb J, Lobue P, et al. Guidelines for using the QuantiFERON-TB-Gold test for detecting *Mycobacterium tuberculosis* infection, United States. MMWR Recomm Rep 2005;54(RR-15):49–55.

57. Kobashi Y, Mouri K, Yagui S, et al. Clinical utility of the QuantiFERON TB-2G test for elderly patients with active tuberculosis. Chest 2008;133:1196–202.

58. Keane J, Bresnihan B. Tuberculosis reactivation during immunosuppressive therapy in rheumatic diseases:diagnostic and therapeutic strategies. Curr Opin Rheumatol 2008;20:443–9.

59. Beglinger C, Dudler J, Mottet C, et al. Screening for tuberculosis infection before the initiation of an anti-TNF-alpha therapy. Swiss Med Wkly 2007;137:620–2.
60. Centers for Disease Control and Prevention. Tuberculosis associated with blocking agents against tumor necrosis factor-alpha-California-2002–2003. MMWR Morb Mortal Wkly Rep 2004;53:683–6.
61. British Thoracic Society, Standards of Care Committee. BTS recommendations for assessing risk and for managing *Mycobacterium tuberculosis* infection and disease in patients due to start anti-TNF-alpha treatment. Thorax 2005;60:800–5.
62. Canadian Tuberculosis Committee. Updated recommendations on interferon gamma release assays for latent tuberculosis infection Can Commun Dis Rep 2008;34:1–13
63. Perez JL, Kupper H, Spencer-Green GT. Impact of screening for latent TB before initiating anti-TNF therapy in North America and Europe. Ann Rheum Dis 2005; 64(Suppl 3):265.
64. Carmona L, Gomez-Reino J, Rodriguez-Valverde V, et al. Effectiveness of recommendations to prevent reactivation of latent tuberculosis infection in patients treated with tumor necrosis factor antagonists. Arthritis Rheum 2005;52:1766–72.
65. Johnson M, Waller E, Leventhal J. Nontuberculous mycobacterial pulmonary disease. Curr Opin Pulm Med 2008;14:203–10.
66. American College of Rheumatology Hotline. FDA advisory committee reviews safety of TNF inhibitors. Available at: http://www.rheumatology.org/publications/hotline/0901tnf.asp?aud=mem. Accessed April 2009.
67. Phillips K, Husni M, Karlson E, et al. Experience with etanercept in an academic medical center; are infection rates increased? Arthritis Rheum 2002;47:17–21.
68. Jaffery SH, Carrillo M, Betensley AD. Fatal pulmonary nontuberculous mycobacterial infection in a patient receiving etanercept for rheumatoid arthritis. Chest 2004;126:944S.
69. Maimon N, Bruton J, Chan A, et al. Fatal pulmonary *Mycobacterium xenopi* in a patient with rheumatoid arthritis receiving etanercept. Thorax 2007;62:739–40.
70. Thomas JE. Fatal pulmonary *Mycobacterium abscessus* infection in a patient using etanercept. Hawaii Med J 2006;65:12–5.
71. Yim K. Recurrent *Mycobacterium xenopi* infection in a patient with rheumatoid arthritis receiving etanercept. Scand J Infect Dis 2004;36:150–4.
72. Van Ingen J. Pulmonary *Mycobacterium szulgai* infection and treatment in a patient receiving anti-tumor necrosis factor therapy. Nat Clin Pract Rheumatol 2007;3:414–9.
73. Marie I, Heliot P, Roussel F, et al. Fatal *Mycobacterium peregrinum* pneumonia in refractory polymyositis treated with infliximab. Rheumatology 2005;44:1201–2.
74. Mufti A, Toye B, McKendry R, et al. *Mycobacterium abscessus* infection after use of tumor necrosis factor alpha inhibitor therapy: case report and review of infectious complications associated with tumor necrosis factor alpha inhibitor use. Diagn Microbiol Infect Dis 2005;53:233–8.
75. Okubo H, Iwamoto M, Yoshio T, et al. Rapidly aggravated *Mycobacterium avium* infection in a patient with rheumatoid arthritis treated with infliximab. Mod Rheumatol 2005;15:62–4.
76. Boulman N, Rozenbaum M, Slobodin G, et al. *Mycobacterium fortuitum* infection complicating infliximab therapy in rheumatoid arthritis. Clin Exp Rheumatol 2006; 24:723.
77. Bala S, Kenneth, Kazempour K, et al. Inhibition of tumour necrosis factor alpha alters resistance to mycobacterium complex avium in mice. Antimicrobial Agents Chemother 1998;42:2336–41.

Infectious Complications of Biologic Agents

Emilio Martin-Mola, MD, PhD*, Alejandro Balsa, MD, PhD

KEYWORDS

- Infections • Tuberculosis • Rheumatoid arthritis
- Biologic agents • TNF-antagonists • Rituximab
- Abatacept • Tocilizumab

Rheumatoid arthritis (RA) is a chronic and debilitating condition that requires the continuous use of treatment that may include nonsteroidal anti-inflammatory drugs; classic disease-modifying antirheumatic drugs (DMARDs); glucocorticoids; and the new biologic DMARDS, such as tumor necrosis factor (TNF) antagonists, rituximab (RTX), abatacept (ABA), and tocilizumab (TCZ). Along the course of the disease, severe infections may develop that could be life threatening if not treated rapidly and adequately.

RA itself may increase patients' risk for infections. In 2002, Doran and colleagues[1] showed an increased risk for infection in patients who had RA compared with controls from the general population. Similarly, Smitten and colleagues[2] demonstrated that patients who had RA (n = 24,530) had an increased risk for hospitalization-related infections compared with patients who did not have RA (n = 500,000), with an adjusted hazard ratio (HR) of 2.03 (95% CI, 1.93–2.13). A study performed in Spain demonstrated an increased incidence of tuberculosis (TB), a common infection in immunocompromised patients, in patients who had RA.[3]

Medications probably are contributing to this risk. Patients who have RA and are receiving chronic treatment with glucocorticoids have an increased rate of hospitalization due to pneumonia (HR 1.7; 95% CI, 1.5–2.0).[4] Even more, it seems that a dose-response relationship exists between prednisone and pneumonia risk. Recently, a retrospective study in patients who had RA who were older than 65 revealed an increased rate of serious bacterial infections requiring hospitalization in patients starting glucocorticoids or cytotoxic DMARDs compared with patients

EM-M and AB have received honoraria, less than 10,000 Euros, for educational programs and as advisors for Wyeth, Abbott, Roche, and Schering-Plough.

Department of Rheumatology, Hospital Universitario La Paz, Paseo de la Castellana 261, 28046 Madrid, Spain

* Corresponding author.

E-mail address: emartinmola.hulp@salud.madrid.org (E. Martin-Mola).

doi:10.1016/j.rdc.2009.03.009
0889-857X/09/$ – see front matter © 2009 Elsevier Inc. All rights reserved.
rheumatic.theclinics.com

receiving methotrexate (MTX).[5] The increased infection rate was more pronounced within the first 90 days of treatment, and glucocorticoids showed a clear dose-response relationship with infections, with a relative risk (RR) of 2.97 and 5.48 for a starting dose of 10 to 19 mg per day and greater than 20 mg per day, respectively.[5] Glucocorticoids also are associated with a dose-related effect on the risk for infections in the study by Smitten and colleagues[2]; patients on more than 10 mg of prednisone had an almost threefold increased risk for being hospitalized due to infections compared with patients who had RA and were treated with less than 5 mg daily.

Since biologics were launched, many safety reports of patients treated with these drugs have been published, including randomized controlled trials (RCTs) and meta-analyses, prospective cohorts and registries, and retrospective series and case reports. In most of these studies, biologics have been associated with an increased incidence of severe and nonsevere infections. Nonetheless, these findings have not been consistent, and the reported risks for developing infection differ among studies. This article provides an overview of which studies the authors consider the most relevant.

INFECTIONS ASSOCIATED WITH TUMOR NECROSIS FACTOR ANTAGONISTS

Most of the pivotal RCTs did not report an increase rate of infections.[6–8] Short-term follow-up, selection bias, and low statistical power for detecting infrequent adverse events may explain the results. Nonetheless, this finding has not been consistent, with some investigators describing an increased rate of infections. Keystone and colleagues,[9] in a 52-week trial of adalimumab, found that the proportion of patients who had a serious infection was 3.8% versus 0.5% in the placebo group (P<.02). In another report, St. Clair and colleagues[10] described a significant increase in serious infections, especially pneumonia, among patients receiving infliximab. Other studies have demonstrated that a combination of ABA and anti-TNF biologics results in increased risk for serious infections, leading to the recommendation against the combined use of biologics.[11,12]

The safety of etanercept was tested in open-label extension trials of 3-years' duration in RA,[13] 192 weeks in ankylosing spondylitis,[14] and 8-years' duration in juvenile RA.[15] Overall, no unexpected complications appeared, and efficacy was consistently maintained. The most frequent infections were localized to the upper respiratory tract. In the RA study, however, ten patients died during or after discontinuing participation in the study; of those ten, seven presented with infection as a major contributory factor to their death.[13] A placebo-controlled randomized trial was performed to ascertain the safety of etanercept in patients who had at least one comorbidity. The incidence of medically important infections was the primary endpoint of the trial. The study ended early because of low enrollment and lower than predicted rates of infections. Although no firm conclusions could be drawn due to the small number of events and broad CIs, the data suggested that the rate of severe infections was not increased in patients who had comorbidities.[16]

A meta-analysis from nine RCTs of infliximab and adalimumab in RA concluded that there was an increased risk for severe infections: the odds ratio was 2.0 (95% CI, 1.3–3.1), with a number needed to harm of 59 (95% CI, 39–125) within a treatment period of 3 to 12 months.[17] A posterior meta-analysis that included etanercept and that corrected the toxicity effect for the duration of exposure did not confirm the increased risk of TNF antagonist for serious infection when used at the recommended doses (OR 1.21; 95% CI, 0.89–1.63).[18]

Evidence from biologics registries shows the complexity of the association with infections. In 2005, Listing and colleagues[19] published the results of the German register, RABBIT (Rheumatoid Arthritis–oBservation of BIologic Therapy). The rate of infections in patients who had RA treated with biologics was compared with that of patients treated with classic DMARDs (control population). The total number of infections per 100 patient-years was 22.6 (95% CI, 18.7–27.2), 28.3 (95% CI, 23.1–34–7), and 6.8 (95% CI, 5.0–9.4) for the etanercept, infliximab, and control groups, respectively. When only severe infections were analyzed, the percentages dropped to 6.4, 6.2, and 2.3, respectively. To provide a more accurate result, propensity scores were applied (ie, patients who had an estimated likelihood of less than 40% for receiving biologics were excluded from the analysis—9.2% etanercept/infliximab and 59.2% controls). The adjusted RR for the total number of infections compared with the control group was 2.31 (95% CI, 1.4–3.9) for etanercept and 3.01 (95% CI, 1.8–5.1) for infliximab. The adjusted RR for severe infections remained elevated, with odds ratios of 2.16 (0.9–5.4) for etanercept and 2.13 (0.8–5.5) for infliximab. When different sites of infections were analyzed, both severe and nonsevere infections in the respiratory tract, skin, and subcutaneous tissue were found more frequent with both etanercept and infliximab when compared with controls.

Data from the British register were published in 2006.[20] In this prospective study, 1354 DMARD-treated patients were compared with 7664 anti–TNF-treated patients. During a period of approximately 4 years, 525 serious infections versus 56 in the control group were detected. In spite of this difference, the incidence rate ratio (IRR) adjusted for baseline risk did not show differences between patients and the control group: IRR 1.03 (95% CI, 0.68–1.57). The frequency of severe skin and soft tissue infections, however, in the anti–TNF-treated patients increased: adjusted IRR 4.28 (95% CI, 1.06–17.17).

Askling and colleagues[21] analyzed three databases: (1) ARTIS, which included 4167 patients who had RA starting anti-TNF; (2) the Swedish Inpatient Cohort, which included 44,946 patients who had RA who had been hospitalized for any reason; and (3) patients from the Inpatient Cohort who had been hospitalized because of an infection. By cross-referencing these datasets, they found that within the Inpatient Register data, the adjusted RR for hospitalization with infection associated with TNF blockers was 1.43 (95% CI, 1.18–1.73) during the first year of treatment and 1.15 and 0.82 in the second and third years of treatment, respectively.

The data obtained from the Spanish registry for patients taking biologics, BIOBADASER, showed an incidence rate of infections of any severity with TNF antagonists of 53 cases per 1000 patient-years among patients treated with these agents for any rheumatic condition. The median time to emergence of infection was 8 months (data provided from BIOBADASER by L. Carmona, personal communication, 2009).

Observational studies are subject to methodologic variables that may explain the apparently different results. One of them is the definition of serious infection and another is the definition of the exposure. Exposure may be confined to the period during which patients receive treatment, may be increased to the period from treatment start to a lag period without treatment, or even may be increased to the period from treatment start until the end of follow-up period, irrespective of the time point when the patients discontinued treatment. Using this strategy, the data from the British register were reanalyzed,[22] and the results showed that the adjusted IRR for serious infections while patients were receiving treatment was 1.22 (95% CI, 0.88–1.69). Also, when the at-risk period was limited to the first 90 days after the start of anti-TNF therapy, the adjusted IRR rose to 4.6 (95% CI, 1.8–11.9). It was concluded that the risk for infections increases during early phases of treatment, although some confounding factors, such as an unexpectedly low rate of infections in the early stages of treatment with classic DMARDs, may have contributed to these results (**Table 1**).[22] The increased risk during the first months of treatment is confirmed by data from the Spanish registry, which show that the risk for infection during the first months of treatment may be up to four times greater than the risk in later stages of treatment (data provided from BIOBADASER by Loreto Carmona, personal communication, January 2009).

The increased risk in the first months can be interpreted in several ways. A lower threshold for hospitalization of patients on anti-TNF could be one of the main reasons,[23] although greater dropout of patients who had severe infections also might have played a role. Whatever the cause of the increase in infections during early

Table 1
Rates of severe infections applying different at-risk periods

Severe infections (receiving treatment)	Disease-modifying antirheumatic drugs (n = 2170)	All anti–tumor necrosis factors (n = 8659)
Person-years	2908	13,277
No. infections	114	737
Rate per 1000 person-years	39.2 (32.3–47.1)	55.5 (51.7–59.5)
Adjusted incidence ratio	Referent	1.22 (0.88–1.69)
Severe infections (receiving treatment, first 90 days of exposure)	**Disease-modifying antirheumatic drugs (N = 2170)**	**All anti–tumor necrosis factors (n = 8659)**
Person-years	532	2091
No. infections	13	151
Rate per 1000 person-years	24.4 (13.1–41.4)	72.2 (61.5–84.2)
Adjusted IRR	Referent	4.6 (1.8–11.9)[a]
Severe infections (receiving treatment, plus 90 days lag window)	**Disease-modifying antirheumatic drugs (n = 2170)**	**All anti–tumor necrosis factors (n = 8659)**
Person-years	2908	13,823
No. infections	114	842
Rate per 1000 person-years	39.2 (32.3-47.1)	60.9 (57.0–65.0)
Adjusted IRR	Referent	1.3 (0.93–1.78)
Severe infections (ever received treatment)	**Disease-modifying antirheumatic drugs (n = 2170)**	**All anti–tumor necrosis factors (n = 8659)**
Person-years	2908	15,420
No. infections[b]	114	975
Rate per 1000 person-years	39.2 (32.3–47.1)	63.2 (59.4–67.2)
Adjusted IRR	Referent	1.35 (0.99–1.85)

[a] 95% CI.
[b] Adjusted for age, sex, disease duration and severity, extra-articular RA, baseline steroid use, diabetes, chronic obstructive pulmonary disease, and smoking history.
Modified from Dixon WG, Symmons DP, Lunt M, et al. Serious infection following anti-tumor necrosis factor alpha therapy in patients with rheumatoid arthritis: lessons from interpreting data from observational studies. Arthritis Rheum 2007;56:2896–04.

phases of treatment, however, clinicians must be aware that severe infections may occur at any time in RA; therefore, close monitoring for safety is mandatory.

Other differences may explain the different results among registries. The Japanese registry included 5000 patients who had RA treated with infliximab and were monitored for 6 months, as required by the health authorities in Japan.[24] Bacterial pneumonia developed in 2.2% and TB developed in 0.4% (n = 14). These findings are comparable to the safety results from a RCT of infliximab conducted in Japan.[25] When both populations of Japanese origin, the one in the RCT and the one in the registry, were compared with that of the ATTRACT trial,[26] some differences appeared. Japanese patients take lower doses of MTX (8 mg/wk is the maximum dose approved in Japan) and higher doses of glucocorticoids than the others, and more patients are in late Steinbrocker stages. Therefore, the results from Japanese studies cannot be extrapolated easily to a Western setting.

A retrospective study conducted in a tertiary referral center reviewed the records of 709 patients who had RA and other rheumatic conditions and who received at least one TNF-α blocker. The incidence of infection during the first anti-TNF course was compared with the rate during the period immediately before receiving such therapy. Forty-seven infections in 44 patients fulfilled the definition for severe infection. The incidence rate of serious infection was 3.4 ± 38.7 per 100 patient-years and 10.5 ± 86.9 per 100 patient-years before and after anti-TNF treatment, respectively (P = .03). The most frequent sites of infection were the upper respiratory tract, lung, and skin. Although no differences in the type of infections were observed between the three TNF blockers, a trend toward more infections was observed with infliximab.[27]

A recent retrospective cohort study of patients who had RA and were treated with anti-TNF or MTX identified serious infections (ie, patients admitted in the hospital because of bacterial infections). The investigators required that infections be identified within 6 months of the most recent exposure to anti-TNF or MTX and that the diagnosis of infection be preceded by a rigorous procedure, including a review of the medical records by two infectious disease specialists blinded to the treatment received, to ensure an agreed-on definite diagnosis of infection. The multivariate-adjusted hazard ratio for hospitalization due to infection was 1.9 (1.3–2.8) for definite infection in patients receiving biologics compared with those exclusively on MTX.[28] In another recent study,[2] current treatment with anti-TNF agents was associated with a slightly increased risk for hospitalized infection, with an adjusted rate ratio of 1.21 (95% CI, 1.03–1.43), whereas treatment with MTX or hydroxychloroquine was associated with decreased risk. Nevertheless, two studies addressing a similar topic did not support that finding.[4,5] Again, several factors, including differences in the methodology used to identify infections, might have caused these discrepancies.

Is the risk for infection a class effect? In a brief report,[29] infliximab and not etanercept was associated with the highest incidence of serious infections during the first 6 months of therapy compared with MTX (the adjusted IRR for infliximab was 2.4 [95% CI, 1.23–4.68] and for etanercept was 1.61 [95% CI, 0.75–3.47]). Similar to other studies, a time-dependent risk also was observed. Thus, the IRR of severe infection was not significant when the data from 6 months beyond the initiation of treatment were analyzed. Adalimumab was excluded from the study because of the low number of patients receiving this agent. Data from the Spanish registry of patients who were exposed to their first anti-TNF agent showed a trend toward more infections in patients treated with TNF antibodies compared with etanercept (ie, infliximab, 75 [95% CI, 70–81]; etanercept, 47 [95% CI, 41–53]; and adalimumab, 68 [95% CI, 58–81]) (data provided from BIOBADASER by Loreto Carmona, personal communication, January 2009). In contrast, when data from the German and the British registers were analyzed, no differences were found among any of the anti-TNF[19,20] treatments. British data, however, using an at-risk period limited to the first 90 days after the start of anti-TNF therapy, showed a trend toward more infections with infliximab compared with etanercept or adalimumab (the rate per 1000 person-years was 95.4 [75.0–119.2] for infliximab, 59.9 [39.8–85.9] for adalimumab, and 60.0 [45.5–77.4] for etanercept).[22] The large induction dose of infliximab during initial months, lower half-life of etanercept, and different mechanistic properties of anti-TNF antibodies and etanercept might account for these differences.[29,30] Confounding variables between the different populations, however, such as the use of concomitant drugs, comorbidities, and different thresholds of disease severity for access to biologics, also might have played a role in the different results obtained.

Few studies have addressed the risk for perioperative infections in patients receiving anti-TNF.[31,32] In one such study, the infection frequency after orthopedic procedures was 6.5%, although therapy interruptions before surgery did not significantly reduce the rate of complications. In another study, perioperative continuation of anti-TNF did not increase the risk for infection at the surgical site. A recent abstract suggested that in patients who had a history of anti-TNF exposure, the risk for serious postoperative infections was twofold lower in patients not receiving the drug for 28 days presurgery compared with those receiving the biologic during that same period.[33] As recommended by other investigators,[34,35] it seems logical that biologic therapy should be discontinued before elective surgery.

INFECTIONS ASSOCIATED WITH NON–TUMOR NECROSIS FACTOR ANTAGONISTS

Besides the three TNF antagonists, other biologic DMARDs targeting different molecules or sites, such as ABA and RTX, have been developed and approved to treat RA.

TCZ is a humanized monoclonal antibody targeting the interleukin 6 receptor that was licensed in Japan to treat RA and juvenile idiopathic arthritis; it also has been approved in the European Union and in other countries for treatment of RA. Most of the safety data obtained for these agents come from RCTs. Overall, an increased risk for infection has been found when compared with placebo, although no new severe complications have been identified. An analysis of 601 patients included in the six major Japanese TCZ trials and five long-term, open-label extension studies showed that serious infection was the most frequent severe adverse event, with an incidence rate of 6.34 per 100 patient-years. When the incidence of infections was analyzed in the pooled data of three RCTs, however, the total infection rate in the TCZ-treated group was not elevated when compared with that in the control population (40.1% versus 43.1%).[36] Alternatively, an analysis of data comparing the incidence of infection in the patients who had RA included in the RCTs from 1999 to 2007 in Japan with the incidence of infection in an observational cohort of Japanese patients who had RA revealed different results. When adjusted for male gender and older age, the standardized incidence ratio (SIR) of respiratory and urinary infections in patients treated with TCZ was increased (SIR 5.08 [95% CI 3.52–7.09] and 3.31 [95% CI 1.33–6.81], respectively).[37] The main limitations of these data were due to the comparison of two different populations (ie, an RCT group and an observational cohort, for which infection rates or other side-effects might have been underreported).

RTX, a chimeric monoclonal antibody targeting CD20 B cells that was approved years ago for non-Hodgkin's lymphoma, induces a sustained B-lymphocyte depletion that may last for several months. Results from major RCTs did not show a relevant increase in infections.[38–41] Recently, data from 119 patients treated with RTX and followed for up to 6 months (and who were included in the RABBIT register) were presented. Eleven nonserious infections developed, most of which were respiratory infections. Furthermore, 10 events that could be considered serious adverse events were observed; of these, two were infections, cystitis and herpes zoster.[42]

One subject of concern has been the risk for infection in patients who have B-cell depletion who need to be treated with another biologic if RTX is not effective or produces severe intolerance. Data from a long-term follow-up (median 11 months) of patients included in the RTX trials who were treated with TNF antagonists or ABA after receipt of RTX recently have been published. The median time from the last dose of RTX until a different biologic was administered was 7 months and, at this time point, most of the patients were B-cell depleted. The results did not reveal an increase in severe infections when compared with the post-RTX treatment period before administration of another biologic (6.99 serious infections per 100 patient-years post-RTX versus 5.49 serious infections per 100 patient-years after another biologic). An analysis also was performed to assess patients treated exclusively with a TNF antagonist and, again, no increase in severe infection was observed.[43]

ABA is a fully human fusion protein that binds to CD80/CD86 and prevents full T-cell activation. Data regarding serious infections due to the RA ABA clinical program have been presented. When the safety data from published articles were analyzed, an increase in serious infection was found in ABA-treated patients compared with patients on placebo (n = 61, 2.8% versus n = 21, 1.9%). When the results were analyzed in detail, however, it became apparent that the increase was concentrated in a subgroup of patients who were treated concomitantly with another biologic.[44] In another analysis, the incidence of hospitalized infections over time was compared with the expected number of infections in four RA cohorts not treated with biologics, two of which were made up of patients who had early arthritis. A total of 4150 ABA-trial patients (10,365 patient-years) with a median exposure time of 26.2 months had, in the cumulative ABA experience, an incidence rate of hospitalized infections of 2.73 per 100 patient-years. The SIR varied depending on the RA cohort compared, and it was increased slightly when compared with the two early arthritis cohorts: SIR 1.88 (95% CI 1.7–2.1) for the NOAR (British early cohort) and SIR 1.44 (95% CI 1.3–1.6) for the ERA (Swedish early cohort).[45]

A recent meta-analysis that examined data from 12 RCTs performed with RTX, ABA, and anakinra did not show an increase of serious infections with RTX or ABA. Anakinra increased the risk, however, especially when comorbidity factors were associated.[46]

OPPORTUNISTIC AND RARE INFECTIONS

In recent years, various unusual infections that usually occur in immunocompromised patients have been reported to be associated with the use of TNF blockers. Case reports published include infections by toxoplasma,[47] listeria,[48,49] histoplasma,[50] leishmania,[51] coccidioidomycosis,[52] and legionella infections,[53,54] among others. In France, a registry of patients who had opportunistic or severe infections registered over a 1-year reported 10 consecutive cases of pneumonia due to legionella. Of these, six patients received adalimumab, two infliximab, and two etanercept. When compared with the general population, the RR for acquiring a legionella infection in patients receiving anti-TNF was between 16.5 and 21.0.[54]

A fatal and rare demyelinating disease caused by JC or BK polyomavirus (progressive multifocal leukoencephalopathy) has been described in patients treated with RTX. Most of the cases occurred in patients receiving RTX in combination with chemotherapy or as part of a hematopoietic stem cell transplant.[55] A few cases of systemic lupus erythematosus and two cases of RA, however, also have been reported.[56]

TUBERCULOSIS AND OTHER MYCOBACTERIAL INFECTIONS WITH TUMOR NECROSIS FACTOR ANTAGONISTS

TB is a major cause of illness and death worldwide, especially in Asia and Africa. An estimated 1.5 million people died from TB in 2006. In addition, another 200,000 people who had HIV died from HIV-associated TB.[57]

As discussed previously, a study conducted in Spain demonstrated a fourfold increase (RR 3.68; 95% CI, 2.36–5.92) in TB among patients who had RA in the prebiologics era when compared with the general population, with a mean annual incidence of 124 per 100,000 patients. In Spain, the mean incidence of TB has been estimated as 23 per 100,000 persons, which can be considered in the upper range of countries with low rates of TB. The number of cases in that cohort was so small, however, with only seven cases, that it was impossible to evaluate factors that could have increased or influenced the development of TB.[3] An increase in TB also was confirmed in a recent Swedish study based on an analysis of data from the general population and data from four different patients cohorts, demonstrating that patients not treated with anti-TNF had a twofold increased risk for TB compared with the general population (2.0; 95% CI, 1.2–3.4).[58] In 2007, a report from South Korea, a country with a higher incidence rate of TB in the general population (ie, 67.2 per 100,000 persons), showed that patients who had RA who were not treated with TNF antagonists had an adjusted risk ratio of TB of 8.9 (95% CI, 4.6–17.2) compared with the general population.[59] Another study performed in the United States, however, did not demonstrate such an increase. That study surveyed 10,782 patients who had RA in 1998–1999, before the use of anti-TNF, and detected a TB rate of 6.2 cases (95% CI, 1.6–34.4) per 100,000 patients. The recent incidence rates of TB in the United States population were 6.4 (for year 1999) and 5.8 (for year 2000) per 100,000 persons.[60]

The use of different disease-modifying antirheumatic drug therapies for RA and the association with the risk for developing TB has been investigated. Recently, a Canadian cohort study of 112,300 patients who had RA identified 386 cases of TB, and anti-TNF and traditional DMARDs were independently associated with TB (RR for DMARDs, 1.2; 95% CI, 1.0–1.5).[61]

TNF is essential for granuloma formation, which is necessary for containment of intracellular infections.[30,62] Therefore, treatment with these agents had been associated with an increase in infections not only with *Mycobacterium tuberculosis* but also with *Listeria monocytogenes* and *Histoplasma capsulatum*.[30] TB may develop after the administration of any of the three TNF inhibitors.

In 2001, Keane and colleagues[63] published the results of the Food and Drug Administration (FDA) Adverse Event Reporting System, which receives spontaneous reports of suspected adverse events. They described 70 cases of TB after treatment with infliximab since this drug was launched in 1998 through May 29, 2001. A similar number of people were exposed to etanercept, and nine cases of TB were reported to the FDA at that time. Infliximab-associated cases had unusual characteristics that caused the TB infection to be especially severe; 40 out of 70 cases presented extrapulmonary disease (17 of which were disseminated) and 64 of these were from countries with a low incidence of TB. The TB characteristics observed differed from those that occur in immunocompetent patients, who exhibit pulmonary infections as a prominent feature. The median interval between starting infliximab therapy and the development of infection was only 12 weeks, supporting the hypothesis that most infections were reactivations of latent TB.[63]

In 2003, the Spanish Society of Rheumatology published what was considered, at that time, the largest observational study on the safety of TNF inhibitors based on data obtained from a national registry, BIOBADASER, in which safety data were actively collected.[64] In that report, 17 patients who had TB were reported, all of which were receiving infliximab. As in the study described previously,[63] many extrapulmonary cases were detected (65% of the patients). The estimated incidence of TB associated with infliximab was 1893 cases per 100,000 patients in 2000 and 1113 cases per 100,000 patients in 2001. Considering that the incidence background of TB in Spain in 2000 was 21 cases per 100,000 persons, a risk ratio can be estimated of 90.1 (95% CI, 58.8–146.0) for patients treated with infliximab. The risk ratio of TB in patients who had RA treated with infliximab compared with patients who had RA and who received non–anti-TNF therapy was 19.9 (95% CI, 16.2–24.8) in 2000.[3,64]

Other studies also have demonstrated an increase in TB in patients receiving TNF blockers. For example, Wolfe and colleagues[60] found an incidence rate of 52.5 (95% CI, 14.3–134.4) per 100,000 patient-years in patients who had RA and were treated with infliximab versus an incidence rate of 6.4 per 100,000 persons in the general United States population. In Sweden, a fourfold increase (95% CI, 1.3–12) in the risk for TB was reported for patients who had RA treated with anti-TNF compared with patients who had RA not receiving anti-TNF therapy.[58] Finally, a Korean report found an adjusted risk ratio for TB of 30.1 (95% CI, 7.4–122.3) compared with the general population.[59] Nineteen bacterial intracellular infections have been reported in the British register, among which 10 were due to TB. A predominance of the extrapulmonary pattern again was confirmed, and a median time of only 3 months between treatment initiation and TB development was observed for the seven infliximab-treated patients.[20] Only one case of TB was detected in the German register.[19] The fact that the TB problem was already known by the time this register was launched could have influenced this result if it is assumed that all patients had been screened and treated for latent TB.

Whether or not anti-TNF antibodies might increase the incidence of TB compared with etanercept is a matter of debate. As discussed previously, the dose of infliximab at the beginning of treatment or the lower half-life of etanercept may have influenced the results. Furthermore, different modes of action that hypothetically might play a role have been reviewed.[30] These differences may stem from the apoptosis-inducing activity observed with infliximab but not with etanercept, the different avidities of the agents for soluble versus transmembrane TNF, and, finally, the irreversible high association with TNF and the fast rate of TNF binding exhibited by infliximab compared with etanercept.[30]

Wallis and colleagues,[65,66] using data collected from the adverse event reporting system of the FDA, found an increase in TB and other granulomatous infections (ie, histoplasma and listeria) associated with infliximab compared with etanercept (54 versus 32 TB cases per 100,000 patients treated; $P<.001$). The data analyzed were obtained from the time that etanercept and infliximab were approved until the third quarter of 2002. There also were differences in the time point at which TB developed. For infliximab, 44% of the cases appeared within the first 90 days of treatment versus 10% among patients receiving etanercept. These differences might suggest that infliximab-related TB cases were particularly related to the reactivation of latent TB, whereas the linearity of the TB infection curve until late phases of treatment with etanercept could be related not only to reactivation but also to new TB infections.[66] Adalimumab was not included in the study because it had not been licensed by that time. Alternatively, the Swedish register of patients using anti-TNF found an increased incidence of TB with infliximab (145 per 100 patient-years; 95% CI, 58–129) compared with etanercept (80 per 100 patient-years; 95% CI, 16–232). Nonetheless, the difference observed between the drugs was not as high as that observed previously.[58] Data from the British registry also found an increase in TB cases due to infliximab compared with etanercept.[20] The Spanish database, BIOBADASER, showed that TB could be associated with any of the TNF antagonists, with a trend toward more cases associated with infliximab. The low power of the sample to detect significant differences made it impossible to derive a firm conclusion.[67] Furthermore, as stated by Winhtrop,[62] several circumstances also might explain the different rates of TB. For example, the MedWatch database is a voluntary database and, therefore, early cases of TB at the beginning of infliximab therapy might have prompted physicians to report them, whereas the TB cases that occur randomly with etanercept treatment might be unrecognized or underreported. Regardless of the cause, no head-to-head studies have been conducted to resolve the issue.

After TB was identified as a major problem, many countries implemented their own screening procedures to diagnose and treat latent TB before initiating treatment with TNF antagonists. In 2005, the authors published the first report demonstrating the effectiveness of using such measures. Before the official recommendations were implemented, there were 32 cases of TB in 6126 patient-years of observation, and all these patients were receiving infliximab. The risk was 20.9-fold higher than the background risk in the Spanish population. After the official recommendations were applied, the risks were similar for patients who had RA who were treated and who were not treated with biologics (RR 3.8; 95% CI, 0.1–23.3).[68] In a later report performed after the official recommendations were launched, 15 cases were registered in the authors' database. Of these, only two originated after fully implementing the screening recommendations. As a consequence, the lack of adherence to the official recommendations increased the probability of developing TB sevenfold (95% CI, 1.60–64.69) (**Table 2**).[67] A Greek retrospective study[69] showed that anti-TB chemoprophylaxis had only partial preventive success. In contrast to the Spanish recommendations, only patients who had a 10-mm positive cutoff point (versus 5 mm in Spain) were considered positive for latent TB, and chemoprophylaxis with isoniazid lasted only 6 months (versus 9 in Spain). Although the difference in rates was not significant, a lower frequency of active TB was observed in patients taking their chemoprophylaxis treatment properly compared with those who did not.[69]

TUBERCULOSIS WITH NON–TUMOR NECROSIS FACTOR ANTAGONISTS

As discussed previously, TNF is a relevant cytokine that promotes granuloma formation, which prevents active TB development. Therefore, it is not surprising that blocking other cytokines or sites has not been associated with similar increases in TB infections. Another circumstance that might have contributed to this situation is the increased awareness of the need to prevent this infection. Nonetheless, a few cases of TB associated with the administration of ABA and TCZ[36,70] have been described. Screening for TB now is recommended before initiating treatment with ABA and TCZ but not with RTX.

Furthermore, the inclusion criteria for latent TB infection in the major RCTs differed for ABA, TCZ, and RTX. In the ABA trials, patients who had latent TB infection were excluded from the study[70]; in the Japanese TCZ studies, no screening for TB was performed[36]; and in Western countries, patients who had latent TB infection could be recruited with the implementation of the national recommendations for treating

Table 2
Active tuberculosis before and after implementing Spanish recommendations

Treatment Starts	Patient-Years of Exposure to Tumor Necrosis Factor Antagonists	Cases	Tuberculosis Rate per 100,000 Patient-Years	Incidence Rate Ratio Versus General Population (95% CI)	Incidence Rate Ratio Versus EMECAR[a] (95% CI)
Before March 2002 (before TB recommendations)	8671	41	472 (384–642)	19 (11–32)	5.8 (2.5–15, 4)
After March 2002 (before TB recommendations)	8717	15	172 (103–285)	7 (3–13)	2.4 (0.8–7.2)
100% compliance	4576	2	43 (11–175)	1.8 (0.28–7.1)	Unlimited
<100% compliance	4170	13	311 (181–636)	13 (6–25)	4.8 (1.04–44.3)

[a] EMECAR, historical RA prospective cohort of non–biologic-treated patients.
Modified from Gomez-Reino JJ, Carmona L, Angel DM. Risk of tuberculosis in patients treated with tumor necrosis factor antagonists due to incomplete prevention of reactivation of latent infection. Arthritis Rheum 2007;56:2896–904.

this condition.[71,72] Finally, in the RTX study,[39] no PPD testing was performed, and patients were excluded only if they demonstrated a history of significant recurrent infection. How these different recruitment criteria might have had an impact on the development of active TB infection remains unknown.

In a recent study performed in the United States and Canada, three cases of TB were associated with RTX. No details were provided about TB development in relation to the timing of RTX administration, levels of B lymphocytes, or number of RTX infusions in these patients. RTX administration is provided with high doses of gluco-corticoids and patients on this therapy usually receive concomitant therapy with MTX or other DMARDs in addition to chronic treatment with glucocorticoids. Whether or not RTX is directly associated with TB, physicians need to be aware that opportunistic infections, such as TB, may develop in any immunosuppressed population. Although there is no evidence for the need to perform a systematic screening for latent TB,[73] it seems prudent to implement any measure that may reduce infections. Furthermore, RTX is licensed only in the United States and in Europe for patients who have failed to respond to TNF blockers; therefore, in most patients receiving RTX, a routine procedure to exclude latent TB already should have been performed.

NONTUBERCULOUS MYCOBACTERIAL INFECTIONS

Nontuberculous mycobacterial (NTM) infections usually are acquired from environmental sources. Most species are less aggressive than *M tuberculosis*; therefore, symptomatic infections usually are associated with immunocompromised patients. The most frequent clinical locations of NTM infections are the skin and lungs; however, patients who have HIV infection, patients who are immunosuppressed due to transplants, and patients receiving anti-TNF therapy are susceptible to developing disseminated disease.[74] In a recent study, Winthrop and colleagues[75] reported 49 cases of mycobacterial infection in patients receiving anti-TNF or other approved biologic agents. Of these, 32 were NTM infections and 17 were TB infections. Compared with the most recent FDA data, this report revealed increased numbers of NTM versus TB infections (**Table 3**). Eight patients died while receiving treatment for the infection, and five of these patients had NTM infection. Anti-TNF agents and RTX, but not ABA, were associated with TB and NTM infection. Effective measures to prevent TB may have inverted the TB/NTM ratio in favor of TB; however, rheumatologists need to be aware that other mycobacterial agents may underlie severe infections with fatal consequences.

Table 3
Mycobacterial tuberculosis and nontuberculous mycobacterial infections in two reports

Infections due to	Wallis et al[66]	Winthrop et al[75]
M tuberculosis (%)	43 (n = 323)	34.7 (n = 17)
NTM (total in %)	8.7 (n = 29)	65.3 (n = 32)
NTM infections by agent	—	Winthrop et al[75]
M avium (%)	ND	33 (n = 16)
M chelonae (%)	ND	10 (n = 5)
M abscessus (%)	ND	6 (n = 3)
M marinum (%)	ND	6 (n = 3)
Other NTM infections (%)	ND	10 (n = 5)

Abbreviation: ND, not determined.

SUMMARY

Infection is a frequent complication in RA and other autoimmune diseases. Since 2000 the spectrum of therapeutic possibilities (ie, biologic agents) for treating RA has expanded rapidly. Most of the reports have described an increase of infections with the use of TNF antagonists that also may apply to severe infections, especially when TNF blockers are administered at higher doses than recommended. TB is associated with the use of TNF blockers. In most cases, TB is the result of latent TB reactivation, although new infection cannot be excluded, especially in those cases that appear several months after the start of the treatment. The increased awareness of this complication and the implementation of screening measures to detect and treat latent TB has dropped TB infection to figures close to those of the general population.

ACKNOWLEDGMENTS

We are indebted to the Spanish Society of Rheumatology, especially to Loreto Carmona, for providing unpublished data for the BIOBADASER database. We also thank her for reviewing and providing invaluable suggestions for improving the quality of this manuscript.

REFERENCES

1. Doran MF, Crowson CS, Pond GR, et al. Frequency of infection in patients with rheumatoid arthritis compared with controls: a population-based study. Arthritis Rheum 2002;46:2287–93.
2. Smitten AL, Choi HK, Hochberg MC, et al. The risk of hospitalized infection in patients with rheumatoid arthritis. J Rheumatol 2008;35:387–93.
3. Carmona L, Hernandez-Garcia C, Vadillo C, et al. Increased risk of tuberculosis in patients with rheumatoid arthritis. J Rheumatol 2003;30:1436–9.
4. Wolfe F, Caplan L, Michaud K. Treatment for rheumatoid arthritis and the risk of hospitalization for pneumonia: associations with prednisone, disease-modifying antirheumatic drugs, and anti-tumor necrosis factor therapy. Arthritis Rheum 2006;54:628–34.
5. Schneeweiss S, Setoguchi S, Weinblatt ME, et al. Anti-tumor necrosis factor alpha therapy and the risk of serious bacterial infections in elderly patients with rheumatoid arthritis. Arthritis Rheum 2007;56:1754–64.
6. Furst DE, Schiff MH, Fleischmann RM, et al. Adalimumab, a fully human anti tumor necrosis factor-alpha monoclonal antibody, and concomitant standard antirheumatic therapy for the treatment of rheumatoid arthritis: results of STAR (Safety Trial of Adalimumab in Rheumatoid Arthritis). J Rheumatol 2003;30:2563–71.
7. Klareskog L, van der Heijde D, de Jager JP, et al. Therapeutic effect of the combination of etanercept and methotrexate compared with each treatment alone in patients with rheumatoid arthritis: double-blind randomised controlled trial. Lancet 2004;363:675–81.
8. Genovese MC, Bathon JM, Fleischmann RM, et al. Longterm safety, efficacy, and radiographic outcome with etanercept treatment in patients with early rheumatoid arthritis. J Rheumatol 2005;32:1232–42.
9. Keystone EC, Kavanaugh AF, Sharp JT, et al. Radiographic, clinical, and functional outcomes of treatment with adalimumab (a human anti-tumor necrosis factor monoclonal antibody) in patients with active rheumatoid arthritis receiving concomitant methotrexate therapy: a randomized, placebo-controlled, 52-week trial. Arthritis Rheum 2004;50:1400–11.

10. St. Clair EW, van der Heijde DM, Smolen JS, et al. Combination of infliximab and methotrexate therapy for early rheumatoid arthritis: a randomized, controlled trial. Arthritis Rheum 2004;50:3432–43.

11. Weinblatt M, Schiff M, Goldman A, et al. Selective costimulation modulation using abatacept in patients with active rheumatoid arthritis while receiving etanercept: a randomised clinical trial. Ann Rheum Dis 2007;66:228–34.

12. Weinblatt M, Combe B, Covucci A, et al. Safety of the selective costimulation modulator abatacept in rheumatoid arthritis patients receiving background biologic and nonbiologic disease-modifying antirheumatic drugs: a one-year randomized, placebo-controlled study. Arthritis Rheum 2006;54:2807–16.

13. Klareskog L, Gaubitz M, Rodriguez-Valverde V, et al. A long-term, open-label trial of the safety and efficacy of etanercept (Enbrel) in patients with rheumatoid arthritis not treated with other disease-modifying antirheumatic drugs. Ann Rheum Dis 2006;65:1578–84.

14. Davis JC Jr, van der Heijde DM, Braun J, et al. Efficacy and safety of up to 192 weeks of etanercept therapy in patients with ankylosing spondylitis. Ann Rheum Dis 2008;67:346–52.

15. Lovell DJ, Reiff A, Ilowite NT, et al. Safety and efficacy of up to eight years of continuous etanercept therapy in patients with juvenile rheumatoid arthritis. Arthritis Rheum 2008;58:1496–504.

16. Weisman MH, Paulus HE, Burch FX, et al. A placebo-controlled, randomized, double-blinded study evaluating the safety of etanercept in patients with rheumatoid arthritis and concomitant comorbid diseases. Rheumatology (Oxford) 2007;46:1122–5.

17. Bongartz T, Sutton AJ, Sweeting MJ, et al. Anti-TNF antibody therapy in rheumatoid arthritis and the risk of serious infections and malignancies: systematic review and meta-analysis of rare harmful effects in randomized controlled trials. JAMA 2006;295:2275–85.

18. Leombruno JP, Einarson TR, Keystone EC. The safety of anti-Tumor Necrosis Factor treatments in rheumatoid arthritis: meta and exposure adjusted pooled analyses of serious adverse events. Ann Rheum Dis 2008; [epub ahead of print].

19. Listing J, Strangfeld A, Kary S, et al. Infections in patients with rheumatoid arthritis treated with biologic agents. Arthritis Rheum 2005;52:3403–12.

20. Dixon WG, Watson K, Lunt M, et al. Rates of serious infection, including site-specific and bacterial intracellular infection, in rheumatoid arthritis patients receiving anti-tumor necrosis factor therapy: results from the British Society for Rheumatology Biologics Register. Arthritis Rheum 2006;54:2368–76.

21. Askling J, Fored CM, Brandt L, et al. Time-dependent increase in risk of hospitalisation with infection among Swedish RA patients treated with TNF antagonists. Ann Rheum Dis 2007;66:1339–44.

22. Dixon WG, Symmons DP, Lunt M, et al. Serious infection following anti-tumor necrosis factor alpha therapy in patients with rheumatoid arthritis: lessons from interpreting data from observational studies. Arthritis Rheum 2007;56:2896–904.

23. Patkar NM, Teng GG, Curtis JR, et al. Association of infections and tuberculosis with antitumor necrosis factor alpha therapy. Curr Opin Rheumatol 2008;20:320–6.

24. Takeuchi T, Tatsuki Y, Nogami Y, et al. Postmarketing surveillance of the safety profile of infliximab in 5000 Japanese patients with rheumatoid arthritis. Ann Rheum Dis 2008;67:189–94.

25. Abe T, Takeuchi T, Miyasaka N, et al. A multicenter, double-blind, randomized, placebo controlled trial of infliximab combined with low dose methotrexate in Japanese patients with rheumatoid arthritis. J Rheumatol 2006;33:37–44.

26. Maini R, St Clair EW, Breedveld F, et al. Infliximab (chimeric anti-tumour necrosis factor alpha monoclonal antibody) versus placebo in rheumatoid arthritis patients receiving concomitant methotrexate: a randomised phase III trial. ATTRACT Study Group. Lancet 1999;354:1932–9.

27. Salliot C, Gossec L, Ruyssen-Witrand A, et al. Infections during tumour necrosis factor-alpha blocker therapy for rheumatic diseases in daily practice: a systematic retrospective study of 709 patients. Rheumatology (Oxford) 2007;46:327–34.

28. Curtis JR, Patkar N, Xie A, et al. Risk of serious bacterial infections among rheumatoid arthritis patients exposed to tumor necrosis factor alpha antagonists. Arthritis Rheum 2007;56:1125–33.

29. Curtis JR, Xi J, Patkar N, et al. Drug-specific and time-dependent risks of bacterial infection among patients with rheumatoid arthritis who were exposed to tumor necrosis factor alpha antagonists. Arthritis Rheum 2007;56:4226–7.

30. Ehlers S. Tumor necrosis factor and its blockade in granulomatous infections: differential modes of action of infliximab and etanercept? Clin Infect Dis 2005; 41(Suppl 3):S199–203.

31. den Broeder AA, Creemers MC, Fransen J, et al. Risk factors for surgical site infections and other complications in elective surgery in patients with rheumatoid arthritis with special attention for anti-tumor necrosis factor: a large retrospective study. J Rheumatol 2007;34:689–95.

32. Ruyssen-Witrand A, Gossec L, Salliot C, et al. Complication rates of 127 surgical procedures performed in rheumatic patients receiving tumor necrosis factor alpha blockers. Clin Exp Rheumatol 2007;25:430–6.

33. Dixon WG, Lunt M, Watson K, et al. Anti-TNF therapy and the risk of serious postoperative infection: results from the BSR biologics register (BSRBR) [abstract]. Ann Rheum Dis 2007;66(Suppl II):118.

34. Askling J, Dixon W. The safety of anti-tumour necrosis factor therapy in rheumatoid arthritis. Curr Opin Rheumatol 2008;20:138–44.

35. Bongartz T. Elective orthopedic surgery and perioperative DMARD management: many questions, fewer answers, and some opinions. J Rheumatol 2007;34:653–5.

36. Nishimoto N, Miyasaka N, Yamamoto K, et al. Safety profile of tocilizumab in Japanese patients with rheumatoid arthritis. Incidences of infections in Japanese long-term clinical studies [abstract]. Ann Rheum Dis 2008;67(Suppl II):335.

37. Hoshi D, Nishimoto N, Inoue E, et al. Incidence of infections in Japanese rheumatoid arthritis patients treated with tocilizumab (TCZ) in clinical studies in comparison to those in an observational cohort of Japanese patients, IORRA. Ann Rheum Dis 2008;67(Suppl II):200.

38. Edwards JC, Szczepanski L, Szechinski J, et al. Efficacy of B-cell-targeted therapy with rituximab in patients with rheumatoid arthritis. N Engl J Med 2004; 350:2572–81.

39. Emery P, Fleischmann R, Filipowicz-Sosnowska A, et al. The efficacy and safety of rituximab in patients with active rheumatoid arthritis despite methotrexate treatment: results of a phase IIB randomized, double-blind, placebo-controlled, dose-ranging trial. Arthritis Rheum 2006;54:1390–400.

40. Cohen SB, Emery P, Greenwald MW, et al. Rituximab for rheumatoid arthritis refractory to anti-tumor necrosis factor therapy: Results of a multicenter, randomized, double-blind, placebo-controlled, phase III trial evaluating primary efficacy and safety at twenty-four weeks. Arthritis Rheum 2006;54:2793–806.

41. Keystone E, Fleischmann R, Emery P, et al. Safety and efficacy of additional courses of rituximab in patients with active rheumatoid arthritis: an open-label extension analysis. Arthritis Rheum 2007;56:3896–908.

42. Strangfeld A, Hierse F, Listing J, et al. RA patients treated with Rituximab. Routine care data of the German Biologics Register RABBIT [abstract]. Arthritis Rheum 2008;58(Suppl):S305.

43. Genovese MC, Breedveld FC, Emery P, et al. Safety of biologic therapies following rituximab treatment in rheumatoid arthritis patients. Ann Rheum Dis 2009; [epub ahead of print].

44. Hochberg MC, Simon TA. Safety of abatacept in patients with rheumatoid arthritis [abstract]. Ann Rheum Dis 2008;67(Suppl II):36.

45. Smitten AL, Simon TA, Qi K, et al. Hospitalized infections in the abatacept RA clinical development program: an epidemiological assessment with >10,000 person-years of exposure [abstract]. Arthritis Rheum 2008;58(Suppl):S786–7.

46. Salliot C, Dougados M, Gossec L. Risk of serious infections during rituximab, abatacept and anakinra treatments for rheumatoid arthritis: meta-analyses of randomised placebo-controlled trials. Ann Rheum Dis 2009;68:25–32.

47. Lassoued S, Zabraniecki L, Marin F, et al. Toxoplasmic chorioretinitis and anti-tumor necrosis factor treatment in rheumatoid arthritis. Semin Arthritis Rheum 2007;36:262–3.

48. Gluck T, Linde HJ, Scholmerich J, et al. Anti-tumor necrosis factor therapy and Listeria monocytogenes infection: report of two cases. Arthritis Rheum 2002;46:2255–7.

49. Aparicio AG, Munoz-Fernandez S, Bonilla G, et al. Report of an additional case of anti-tumor necrosis factor therapy and Listeria monocytogenes infection: comment on the letter by Gluck et al. Arthritis Rheum 2003;48:1764–5.

50. Jain VV, Evans T, Peterson MW. Reactivation histoplasmosis after treatment with anti-tumor necrosis factor alpha in a patient from a nonendemic area. Respir Med 2006;100:1291–3.

51. Tektonidou MG, Skopouli FN. Visceral leishmaniasis in a patient with psoriatic arthritis treated with infliximab: reactivation of a latent infection? Clin Rheumatol 2008;27:541–2.

52. Bergstrom L, Yocum DE, Ampel NM, et al. Increased risk of coccidioidomycosis in patients treated with tumor necrosis factor alpha antagonists. Arthritis Rheum 2004;50:1959–66.

53. Li GF, Benucci M, Del RA. Pneumonitis caused by Legionella pneumoniae in a patient with rheumatoid arthritis treated with anti-TNF-alpha therapy (infliximab). J Clin Rheumatol 2005;11:119–20.

54. Tubach F, Ravaud P, Salmon-Ceron D, et al. Emergence of Legionella pneumophila pneumonia in patients receiving tumor necrosis factor-alpha antagonists. Clin Infect Dis 2006;43:e95–100.

55. FDA. Available at: www.fda.gov/cder/foi/label/2006/103705s5230-s5231lbl.pdf. Accessed Feb 2009.

56. FDA. Available at: www.fda.gov/medwatch/safety/2008/rituxan_DHCP_Final% 209411700.pdf. Accessed Feb 2009.

57. WHO. Tuberculosis. Available at: http://www.who.int/tb/en/. Accessed Feb 2009.

58. Askling J, Fored CM, Brandt L, et al. Risk and case characteristics of tuberculosis in rheumatoid arthritis associated with tumor necrosis factor antagonists in Sweden. Arthritis Rheum 2005;52:1986–92.

59. Seong SS, Choi CB, Woo JH, et al. Incidence of tuberculosis in Korean patients with rheumatoid arthritis (RA): effects of RA itself and of tumor necrosis factor blockers. J Rheumatol 2007;34:706–11.

60. Wolfe F, Michaud K, Anderson J, et al. Tuberculosis infection in patients with rheumatoid arthritis and the effect of infliximab therapy. Arthritis Rheum 2004;50:372–9.

61. Brassard P, Kezouh A, Suissa S. Antirheumatic drugs and the risk of tuberculosis. Clin Infect Dis 2006;43:717–22.
62. Winthrop KL. Risk and prevention of tuberculosis and other serious opportunistic infections associated with the inhibition of tumor necrosis factor. Nat Clin Pract Rheumatol 2006;2:602–10.
63. Keane J, Gershon S, Wise RP, et al. Tuberculosis associated with infliximab, a tumor necrosis factor alpha-neutralizing agent. N Engl J Med 2001;345: 1098–104.
64. Gomez-Reino JJ, Carmona L, Valverde VR, et al. Treatment of rheumatoid arthritis with tumor necrosis factor inhibitors may predispose to significant increase in tuberculosis risk: a multicenter active-surveillance report. Arthritis Rheum 2003; 48:2122–7.
65. Wallis RS, Broder MS, Wong JY, et al. Granulomatous infectious diseases associated with tumor necrosis factor antagonists. Clin Infect Dis 2004;38: 1261–5.
66. Wallis RS, Broder M, Wong J, et al. Granulomatous infections due to tumor necrosis factor blockade: correction. Clin Infect Dis 2004;39:1254–5.
67. Gomez-Reino JJ, Carmona L, Angel DM. Risk of tuberculosis in patients treated with tumor necrosis factor antagonists due to incomplete prevention of reactivation of latent infection. Arthritis Rheum 2007;57:756–61.
68. Carmona L, Gomez-Reino JJ, Rodriguez-Valverde V, et al. Effectiveness of recommendations to prevent reactivation of latent tuberculosis infection in patients treated with tumor necrosis factor antagonists. Arthritis Rheum 2005; 52:1766–72.
69. Sichletidis L, Settas L, Spyratos D, et al. Tuberculosis in patients receiving anti-TNF agents despite chemoprophylaxis. Int J Tuberc Lung Dis 2006;10:1127–32.
70. Sibilia J, Westhovens R. Safety of T-cell co-stimulation modulation with abatacept in patients with rheumatoid arthritis. Clin Exp Rheumatol 2007;25:S46–56.
71. Genovese MC, McKay JD, Nasonov EL, et al. Interleukin-6 receptor inhibition with tocilizumab reduces disease activity in rheumatoid arthritis with inadequate response to disease-modifying antirheumatic drugs: the tocilizumab in combination with traditional disease-modifying antirheumatic drug therapy study. Arthritis Rheum 2008;58:2968–80.
72. Emery P, Keystone E, Tony HP, et al. IL-6 receptor inhibition with tocilizumab improves treatment outcomes in patients with rheumatoid arthritis refractory to anti-tumour necrosis factor biologicals: results from a 24-week multicentre randomised placebo-controlled trial. Ann Rheum Dis 2008;67:1516–23.
73. Smolen JS, Keystone EC, Emery P, et al. Consensus statement on the use of rituximab in patients with rheumatoid arthritis. Ann Rheum Dis 2007;66:143–50.
74. von Reyn CF, et al. Nontuberculous mycobacteria. In: Fauci AS, Braunwald E, editors. Harrison's principles of internal medicine. 17th edition. New York: McGraw-Hill Companies, Inc.; 2008. p. 1027–32.
75. Winthrop KL, Yamashita S, Beekmann SE, et al. Mycobacterial and other serious infections in patients receiving anti-tumor necrosis factor and other newly approved biologic therapies: case finding through the Emerging Infections Network. Clin Infect Dis 2008;46:1738–40.

Index

Note: Page numbers of article titles are in **boldface** type.

A

Abatacept, infections due to, 168, 188–189, 192

Abscess, epidemic (pyomyositis), 47–48, 146

Acinetobacter infections, in systemic lupus erythematosus, 79

Acquired immunodeficiency syndrome. *See* Human immunodeficiency virus infection.

Acrodermatitis, papular, in hepatitis B, 132

Acute intermittent painful articular syndrome, in HIV infection, 142

Adalimumab, infections due to, 165, 184, 187–189

Aging, rheumatoid arthritis in, tuberculosis response in, 169–170, 172

AIDS. *See* Human immunodeficiency virus infection.

Anaerobic infections, bacterial arthritis in, 69

Anakinra, tuberculosis risk with, 167–168

Antibiotics
    for bacterial arthritis, 69–70
    for pyomyositis, 48
    for reactive arthritis, 35

Antibody(ies)
    in parvovirus B19 infections, 103
    in rheumatic disease, in HIV infection, 141–142
    in Sjögren's syndrome, 114

Anticardiolipin antibodies, in hepatitis C, 115–116

Anti–liver-kidney microsome antibodies, in hepatitis C, 115–116

Antimitochondrial antibodies, in hepatitis C, 116–117

Antinuclear antibodies
    in hepatitis C, 115–116
    in Sjögren's syndrome, 114

Antiphospholipid syndrome, in hepatitis C, 116–117

Antisynthetase syndrome, necrotizing fasciitis in, 46

Aplastic crisis, in parvovirus B19 infections, 99

Arteritis, in HIV infection, 147

Arthralgia, in HIV infection, 142

Arthritis
    biologic agents for, infectious complications of, 166–167,
        183–199
    in hepatitis B, 131–132
    in hepatitis C, 112–113
    in HIV infection, 142–143
    in parvovirus B19 infections, 99–103
    infections and. *See* Infections; *specific infections and organisms.*
    reactive. *See* Reactive arthritis.
    rheumatoid. *See* Rheumatoid arthritis.
    septic, **63–73,** 147

Rheum Dis Clin N Am 35 (2009) 201–213
doi:10.1016/S0889-857X(09)00032-5
0889-857X/09/$ – see front matter © 2009 Elsevier Inc. All rights reserved.

rheumatic.theclinics.com

S

Sacroiliitis, in reactive arthritis, 26, 33
Salmonella infections
   in systemic lupus erythematosus, 78
   pyomyositis in, 47–48
   reactive arthritis in, 27–28
      epidemiology of, 2, 23
      pathophysiology of, 31–32
   septic arthritis in, 147
Sarcoidosis, in HIV infection, 148
Septic arthritis. *See* Bacterial arthritis.
Septic bursitis, 50–54
Septic tenosynovitis, 48–50
Serologic testing, in parvovirus B19 infections, 104
Serratia marcescens infections, bursitis in, 51
Shigella infections, reactive arthritis in, 2, 23, 28
Shoulder, bursitis of, 52
Sialadenitis, in hepatitis C, 113–114
Sicca symptoms, in hepatitis C, 113–114
Signal transducer and activator of transcription (STAT) proteins, in parvovirus B19 infections, 97
Sjögren's syndrome, in hepatitis C, 113–114, 116–117
Skin manifestations
   of hepatitis B, 132
   of reactive arthritis, 25–26
SOCS (suppressor of cytokine signaling) proteins, in parvovirus B19 infections, 97
Soft tissue infections, **45–62**
   evaluation of, 54
   necrotizing fasciitis, 45–46
   pyomyositis, 47–48, 146
   septic bursitis, 50–54
   septic tenosynovitis, 48–50
   treatment of, 54
Spondyloarthropathies, in HIV infection, 143
Sporotrichosis
   bursitis in, 52
   septic arthritis in, 147
   tenosynovitis in, 50
Staphylococcal infections, osteomyelitis in, 147–148
Staphylococcus aureus infections
   bursitis in, 51–52
   in systemic lupus erythematosus, 78–79
   necrotizing fasciitis in, 45–46
   pyomyositis in, 47–48
   septic arthritis in, 66, 68–70, 147
   tenosynovitis in, 49
Staphylococcus epidermidis infections, tenosynovitis in, 49
STAT (signal transducer and activator of transcription) protein, in parvovirus B19 infections, 97
Still disease, necrotizing fasciitis in, 46

Moving?

Make sure your subscription moves with you!

To notify us of your new address, find your **Clinics Account Number** (located on your mailing label above your name), and contact customer service at:

E-mail: elspcs@elsevier.com

800-654-2452 (subscribers in the U.S. & Canada)
314-453-7041 (subscribers outside of the U.S. & Canada)

Fax number: 314-523-5170

Elsevier Periodicals Customer Service
11830 Westline Industrial Drive
St. Louis, MO 63146

*To ensure uninterrupted delivery of your subscription, please notify us at least 4 weeks in advance of move.

Printed in the United States
By Bookmasters